Concepts in
Pediatrics
CARDIOLOGY

Concepts in
Pediatrics
CARDIOLOGY

Atul Choube MD

Professor and Head
Department of Pediatrics
KD Medical College
Mathura, UP

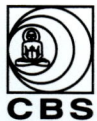

CBS

CBS Publishers & Distributors Pvt Ltd

New Delhi • Bengaluru • Chennai • Kochi • Kolkata • Mumbai
Hyderabad • Nagpur • Patna • Pune • Vijayawada

Concepts in
Pediatrics
CARDIOLOGY

ISBN: 978-93-86310-62-0

Copyright © Author and Publisher

First Edition: 2017

Published by Satish Kumar Jain and produced by Varun Jain for

CBS Publishers & Distributors Pvt Ltd
4819/XI Prahlad Street, 24 Ansari Road, Daryaganj, New Delhi 110 002, India.
Ph: 23289259, 23266861, 23266867   Website: www.cbspd.com
Fax: 011-23243014   e-mail: delhi@cbspd.com; cbspubs@airtelmail.in.
Corporate Office: 204 FIE, Industrial Area, Patparganj, Delhi 110 092
Ph: 4934 4934   Fax: 4934 4935   e-mail: publishing@cbspd.com; publicity@cbspd.com

Branches

- **Bengaluru:** Seema House 2975, 17th Cross, K.R. Road,
  Banasankari 2nd Stage, Bengaluru 560 070, Karnataka
  Ph: +91-80-26771678/79   Fax: +91-80-26771680   e-mail: bangalore@cbspd.com
- **Chennai:** 7, Subbaraya Street, Shenoy Nagar, Chennai 600 030, Tamil Nadu
  Ph: +91-44-26680620, 26681266   Fax: +91-44-42032115   e-mail: chennai@cbspd.com
- **Kochi:** Ashana House, No. 39/1904, AM Thomas Road, Valanjambalam,
  Ernakulam 682 016, Kochi, Kerala
  Ph: +91-484-4059061-65   Fax: +91-484-4059065   e-mail: kochi@cbspd.com
- **Kolkata:** 6/B, Ground Floor, Rameswar Shaw Road, Kolkata-700 014, West Bengal
  Ph: +91-33-22891126, 22891127, 22891128   e-mail: kolkata@cbspd.com
- **Mumbai:** 83-C, Dr E Moses Road, Worli, Mumbai-400018, Maharashtra
  Ph: +91-22-24902340/41   Fax: +91-22-24902342   e-mail: mumbai@cbspd.com

Representatives

- **Hyderabad** 0-9885175004 • **Nagpur**   0-9021734563 • **Patna** 0-9334159340
- **Pune**   0-9623451994 • **Vijayawada** 0-9000660880

Printed at: Paras Offset Pvt. Ltd, New Delhi, India

to
_____

loving memories of my parents

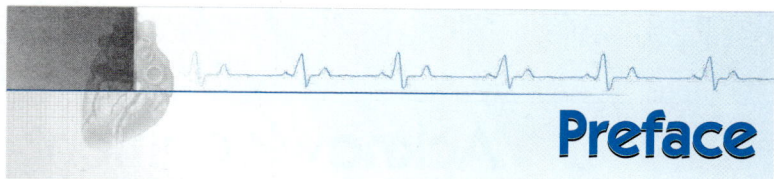

Preface

O Lord lead us from darkness of ignorance to the light of knowledge

With the grace of God this book has seen the light of the day and is in your hands now.

Throughout my teaching career, I have emphasized to my students that the child is not a compressed adult and the complicated aspects should be presented in as simple a manner as a child. I sincerely hope that this book will fulfill this doctrine.

The book's strong points are its no frills text in concise and compact format and hence affordable to students of pediatrics in India and other developing nations.

The book's reach includes the postgraduate and doctoral students of pediatrics as well as practitioners of medicine who are interested in attaining knowledge of childhood diseases.

God bless.

Atul Choube

Acknowledgment

I gratefully acknowledge the inspiration and help given by Anugrih Choube in the preparation of the manuscript.

Atul Choube

Contents

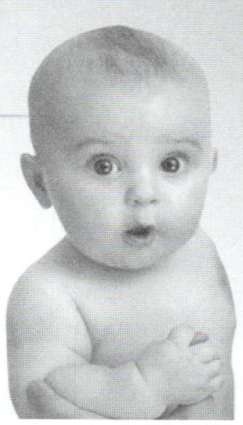

1

Heart Disease and Chromosomal Abnormalities

CYTOGENETICS

The 23 pair of chromosomes in man have been classified into seven groups from A to G according to similarity in size and shape and numbered in descending order of size. The shape is determined by position of centromere seen as a constricted region at or near the centre (metacentric), closer to one end (submetacentric) or at one end (acrocentric).

Any variation from the normal diploid number of chromosomes is termed aneuploidy. Trisomy refers to the presence of three homologous chromosomes and in monosomy only one is present.

Aneuploidy results from abnormal segregation or nondysjunction during formation of the gamete.

Among the autosomal abnormalities the most familial is trisomy 21 or Down syndrome.

Best known sex chromosome aneuploidy are Turner's syndrome and Klinefelter's syndrome.

Mosaicism: The presence of two or more different cell lines in a subject is found for all chromosome aberrations but most frequently involves the sex chromosome.

Although trisomies are usually not inherited a familial tendency to nondysjunction is sometimes apparent. This may be caused by a gene or chromosomal variant.

In most instances chromosome segregation is best influenced by environmental factors, among which the late maternal age

1

is best documented. Evidence of radiation and viruses is also mounting.

The most common structural aberration is translocation. A reciprocal translocation is formed when two nonhomologous chromosomes break and exchange segments. Since no chromatin material is lost, carriers of the reciprocal translocation are phenotypically normal. Three viable combinations—normal, carriers, abnormal should be found in equal frequencies among the offspring but the actual proportion of abnormal children varies with the chromosome involved and is usually less than expected frequency.

Most unbalanced translocations are not inherited and arise *de novo* in gamete. They are caused by chromosome breaking agents, such as ionizing radiation, viruses, drugs and chemicals.

Deletions are another form of common aberration. When both ends of a chromosome are deleted, the broken ends may fuse to form a ring. Deletions are lethal in absence of mosaicism.

Y-chromosome may vary in length and shape. This variation being caused by loss or duplication of the distal portion of long arm. This region appears to be genetically inert since the Y variant affect neither the phenotype or reproductive capacity.

A special type of deficiency and duplication is isochromosome formed by misdivision of centromere, it may divide across the transverse rather than the longitudinal plane. The result will be one chromosome carrying two long arms carrying identical genes with no short arm and the other chromosome with two short arms. Isochromosomes for long arm are most frequent in patients with atypical Turner syndrome.

Inversions arise when two breaks occur in a single chromosome and the segment between is inverted. The order of the genes is disarranged but since none are lost or duplicated the carrier of an inversion is usually phenotypically normal. The change in order may cause difficulty when chromosomes synapse during meiosis and induce abnormal segregation and nondysjunction. Inversions are frequently seen in chromosome 9.

The simplest cell to study for cytogenetic analysis is peripheral blood small lymphocytes. Bone marrow cell is examined in blood dyscrasia and fibroblasts are cultured from abortuses. Techniques have been developed to culture amniotic fluid for prenatal diagnosis. The chromosomes of male and female meiotic cells can be examined to look for the cause of reduced fertility or sterility.

Additional aids for chromosome diagnosis are sex chromatin and dermatoglyphic analysis. A simple technique to screen for X-chromosome aberration is examination of interphase nuclei for the presence of sex chromatin or Barr body. The principle underlying formation of sex chromatin body is the inactivation of all X-chromosomes in excess of one, i.e. Lyon hypothesis. The number of Barr bodies in a cell is thus one less than the total number of X-chromosomes present. Complete karyotyping is essential for X abnormalities.

The correlation between dermatoglyphics and abnormal karyotype is clear. The diagnostic criteria are type and size of patterns on the distal phalanges of fingers. The position of axial triradius on palm. The type of pattern on hallucal area of sole and type and number of flexion creases on palm and little finger. This technique is of most value in diagnosis of autosomal trisomies and less value in deficiency disorders and sex chromosome aberrations. Dermatoglyphics is useful in places where there is no cytogenetics service.

Patients with chromosome aberrations have an array of physical and mental disorders of unknown origin. They have unusual facies, abnormal ears, malformations of heart and kidney, abnormalities of hands and feet and disturbances in dermal configuration and flexion creases.

HEART DEFECTS AND CHROMOSOME

About 3.5% of all pregnancies contain a recognizable chromosomal abnormality. After abortions number reduce to 0.5% of live birth. In survivors heart is involved in varying proportion ranging from a few to 100% in specific syndromes, the most striking are trisomy 13 and trisomy 18, with 90–100%. Intermediate in frequency are trisomy 21, partial short arm deletion of chromosome 4 and partial long arm deletion of chromosome 18 (40–50%). Less common frequencies are reported in partial short arm deletion of chromosome 5 and Turner syndrome (20%). The frequency in chromosomally abnormal births is about 1 in 700. In most studies minor structural chromosomal changes were encountered in fewer than 10% of the population sampled. Transmission of the variations in phenotypically normal individuals constitute a chromosomal structural load that might produce maldevelopment of heart. The evidence suggests a polygenic cause for heart malformation.

HEART IN DOWN SYNDROME

TRISOMY 21 (MONGOLISM)

Characterized by gross mental retardation, muscle hypotonia, multiple congenital malformations and characteristic facies, typical dermatoglyphics, reduced acetabular angle, disturbance of tryptophane metabolism and failure of polymorphonuclear leucocytes to mature fully. More variable traits include brachycephaly, third fontanel, deformed middle phalanx of little finger, Brushfield spots and congenital malformations of heart, alimentary tract and lungs.

Genetics

The disorder is associated with an extra chromosome identified as the smallest in human karyotype.

Regular trisomies form 95% of patients with Down syndrome. 4% are translocations involving mostly 14 and 21 or two chromosomes 21.1% exhibit mosaicism.

Nondysjunction is responsible for most cases of trisomy. The majority are born to older mothers. Translocation mongolism is not associated with parental age. The relation between age and nondysjunction is uncertain. Suggestions to causations include:

- X-radiation
- Hormonal imbalances
- Infection.

It is estimated that one in ten children of translocation carrier mothers will be affected rather than expected one-third, while half the offsprings of a trisomic female will be also trisomic. In twins monozygous pairs are concordant except for the rare event when nondysjunction occurs after zygote formation to give rise to monozygous twins with different chromosome patterns. Double nondysjunction with trisomy 21 and XXY Klinefelter syndrome has been observed.

Frequency

One in 600 to 700 births in Europe. Incidence of heart malformations is 19% in mongolism.

In newborns using stringent diagnostic criteria for diagnosis of mongolism 40% have heart defects.

About 5% of all CHD deaths are associated with mongolism.

Nature of Cardiac Defect

Persistent atrioventricular canal is the common cardiac anomaly in mongoloids.

Defects of cardiac septa account for over three quarters of the heart malformations in mongoloids.

AND, VSD and AV canal defects are commonest.

Isolated PDA, aberrant right subclavian artery have high incidence in mongolism.

Frankly cyanotic lesions are less common, e.g. TOF, PS, TGV. Coarctation of aorta, AS, truncus arteriosus, mitral atresia, endocardial fibroelastosis and single ventricle are rare in Down syndrome but not unknown.

The VSD is in membranous septum and AV canal position in equal proportions. Spontaneous closure of VSD by tricuspid valve adhesion can occur in mongolism.

TOF may be associated with complete AV canal defect or not in a possibly equal division.

A third of complete AV canal defect have added disturbance, e.g. parachute deformity, plastered valve, double orifice, free floating leaflet, etc.

The proportion of membranous ventricular septum is increased from normal 2 to 9% in individuals with Down syndrome. In summary septal defects account for most heart malfornations in mongolism, AV canal defects form a higher proportion of heart disease in mongoloids than nonmongoloids and the relatively uncommon purely cyanotic lesion in a mongoloid will often prove to be TOF than complete TGV.

CLINICAL FEATURES

General

The diagnosis of mongolism by inspection at birth is possible in all but about 1% of cases by the characteristic facies.

Confirmation is by dermatoglyphics and cytogenetic analysis. It is especially important to analyze the chromosomes of affected offspring of a young mother and the young mother herself in case a translocation is present. If an inherited translocation is found a search for carriers in all close relatives is indicated.

Cardiovascular

Mongoloid infants exhibit more cyanosis and coldness of extremities than normal infants and it is believed that their peripheral vasculature has some differences from the normal. Postnatal transitional circulation may be delayed in these subjects in the sense that high PAP and functional left to right shunt through the ductus may occur for a longer than usual period afterbirth. Pulmonary vascular obstructive disease may develop in patients having large interventricular communications or aorticopulmonary defects and Down syndrome earlier than would be found in phenotypically normal patients with defects of similar size. A possible explanation for these differences could lie in low grade mildly hypoxic state present most of the time in many patients with trisomy as a result of airway obstruction, weak thoracic musculature or a combination. Frank cyanosis is rare. The presenting feature is a heart murmur in second week of life. Correct diagnosis of heart defect is possible after one month of life. Majority of mongoloids with VSD have a QRS ranging from +50° to +150°.

Systemic Examination

1. *Head*: Brachycephaly, short neck and straight fine hair.
2. *Face*: Tongue protrudes, delayed dentition, epicanthic folds and Brushfield spots.
3. *Heart*: Malformations in 45% of cases. AV canal and VSD in 75% ASD, PDA, TOF.
4. *Abdomen*: Prominent, increased frequency of duodenal atresia and cryptorchidism.
5. *Extremities*: Short broad hands, clinodactyly 5th finger, gap between 1st and 2nd toe and simian crease.
6. *Dermatoglyphics*: Distal axial triradius, radial loop on 4th and 5th fingers, ulnar loop on 1st, 2nd and 3rd fingers simian crease.
7. *Miscellaneous*: Decreased acetabular angle; psychomotor retardation and high incidence of leukemia.

Prognosis

Those infants with CHD or other serious associated malformations die in infancy. After infancy premature deaths occur due to infections particularly respiratory which are poorly tolerated in mongoloid children. Those with a normal heart die of gastrointestinal anomalies (tracheoesophageal fistula, imperforate anus and duodenal atresia) and infections. Trisomy 21 being frail members of the species do not tolerate insults like angiocardiography.

Leukemia is 20 times more frequent in Down syndrome. This observation led to the assumption that Philadelphia chromosome found in CML probably represented a deletion of part of long arm of chromosome 21 and was accepted as the connecting link between mongolism and leukemia. This argument broke down when chromosome banding identified the Philadelphia chromosome 22 and rather being deleted the broken end was translocated to chromosome 9.

Treatment

There is no cure for Down syndrome. For many in addition to providing a favorable climate for the best intellectual development possible the only acceptable program is one that includes all therapeutic measures available to any child for any illness including cardiac surgery.

Preventive Measures

The incidence could be reduced about 30% by avoiding pregnancy after the 4th decade. Recurrence risks for pregnancies subsequent to an affected birth does not increase with increasing maternal age (1/90 for all age groups). The chance that a subsequent sib will be mongoloid is 1:90 from less than 25 years to 44 years age for trisomies.

Translocation carriers are at particular risk (1:10). In the rare case where the mother is 21q 21q carrier 100% of her offsprings will be affected.

Amniocentesis for prenatal diagnosis is indicated for mothers who have balanced translocations, a previous trisomic infant or who are over age of 40 years. Since cumulative X-ray exposure can influence nondysjunction efforts should be directed at reducing such exposures in females.

HEART IN EDWARDS' SYNDROME

Described by Smith and Edwards separately in 1960. This is a syndrome of multiple congenital anomalies caused by an extra chromosome in the E group. The small delicate facial features distinguish the patients from other trisomies. The chief signs are small for date, scaphocephaly, low set malformed ears, micrognathia, a nonfixed flexion deformity of fingers, deformed feet, spasticity and mental retardation. Renal, gastrointestinal and skeletal anomalies occur less uniformly. Failure to thrive and heart malformations are almost invariable.

Genetics

The incidence of this disorder is 1:4000 births. Late maternal age is etiologically important. Females are more affected. Sex ratio 4:1. Chromosome 18 is involved. Identification at 16.5 weeks gestation by amniotic fluid cell culture and subsequently confirmed at 20 weeks by induced abortion has been reported.

Mosaics and double trisomies have been recorded. Translocations are rare and give rise to partial trisomy syndromes, i.e. only part of the chromosome 18 is in triplicate.

Clinical Features

General: Hydramnios and small placenta.

• Mean birth weight 2200 gm.
• More females affected.
• Most die by 1 year.
• Hypertonia.
• Failure to thrive.
• Mental retardation.

Head: Scaphocephaly with prominent occiput.

Face: Low set malformed ears.

Heart: CHD is present in almost all cases. VSD 96%, ASD 22%, PDA 69%, DORV, aneurysmal transformation around a VSD has been observed in partial trisomies. Bicuspid aortic valve, AS, PS.

Occasionally VSD occurs as part of a complex situation, e.g. coarctation of aorta, ASD, TGV, AV canal defect or mitral atresia. Myocardial fibrosis or endocardial fibroelastosis is the subject of many reports.

Abdomen: Single umbilical artery, renal anomalies, e.g. horse-shoe kidney, cystic kidney, double ureter.

Diaphragmatic eventeration and Meckel's diverticulum.

Extremities: Clinodactyly, Rocker bottom feet, short dorsiflexed hallux.

Single crease on fifth finger, high frequency of arches on fingers and toes is the characteristic dermatoglyphic pattern. Less than 6 arches or more than 2 whorls strongly argues against diagnosis. Death during early infancy is common. Most trisomy 18 cases are sporadic and second recurrence is rare. Parental mosaicism in trisomy 18 has been reported. Parents of children with trisomy 18 should be investigated for their chromosome constitution.

HEART IN PATAU SYNDROME

A syndrome of multiple congenital anomalies associated with an extra chromosome of D group first reported by Patau in 1960.

Genetics

Incidence is 1:7000 to 1:14500 live births. Increased maternal age is noted in patients with nondysjunction and not with translocation. Mosaics occur in 5–10% cases.

Clinical Features

General: The average birth weight is lower limit of normal. Mental retardation, seizures, deafness and failure to thrive are usual. 75% die by 6 months of age.

Head: Arhinecephaly, microcephaly and scalp defects.

Face: Microphthalmia or anophthalmia, colobomata, cataract, ear deformity, capillary hemangioma over forehead, cleft lip and palate.

Heart: CHD in 88% cases, VSD 60%, ASD 44%, PDA 48%, dextrocardia 65%, TGV 11%,. Truncus arteriosus, hypoplastic left heart, atrioventricularis communis and Ebstein disease are associated rarely.

Abdomen: Midline wall defect, malrotation of gut, polycystic kidneys, hydronephrosis, renal agenesis, absent renal artery, inguinal or abdominal cryptorchidism with anomalous scrotal development. Bicornuate uterus is common in females.

Extremities: Polydactyly, hyperconvex nails and flexion deformities of hands.

Miscellaneous: Abnormal elevation of fetal hemoglobin. Polymorphonuclear leukocytes have nuclear projections about 12 times more frequently than normal. Abnormal external genitalia, hemangioma.

Dermatoglyphics: Simian crease, distal axial triradius, arch fibular pattern hallucal area.

Prognosis

Average life is 100 days. Cardiac lesion is usually responsible for death. Apnea and aspiration from cerebral abnormalities, renal agenesis and hypoplastic kidneys are additional factors in early demise. Parents of children with trisomy D should be studied for their chromosome constitution. Amniocentesis should be available for mothers with a previously affected infant.

HEART IN TURNER'S SYNDROME

Originally described by Turner in 1938 in a group of 6 women with short stature, absence of breast development, small amount of pubic and axillary hair, webbing of neck and cubitus valgus. In addition these phenotype females have raised urinary gonadotropin excretion and replacement of ovaries by streaks of connective tissue. Short stature is a uniform finding even at birth while broad chest, congenital lymphedema or its sequelae, low posterior hair line, prominent ears, narrow high arch palate, abnormal nails and a small mandible are found in 80% of cases. Lymphedema of feet may be confused with edema of CHF in newborn with CHD.

Genetics

About 94% of Turner syndrome have 45XO constitution. Six percent have mosaic 45X/46XX. A second group of patients with Turner phenotype but without webbing of neck have been labelled 'ovarian dysgenesis'. 50% of these have 45XO. 25% are mosaic. 25% have structural chromosomal abnormalities, such as deletions or isochromosomes. Phenotypic variation in Turner syndrome thus appears to be related to sex chromosome mosaicism, deletion or a combination of both. Other patients with short or normal stature, with or without neck webbing or other somatic abnormalities but with normal ovarian function and 46XX constitution without mosaicism have been labelled Bonnevie-Ullrich syndrome. A group of males with similar phenotype are termed Turner syndrome in male if the patient has abnormal sexual development, such as undescended testis or Bonnevie-Ullrich syndrome in male if there is no sexual abnormalities.

MacKusic in 1972 by karyotype approach combined Bonnevie-Ullrich syndrome and male Turner syndrome and named it Noonan syndrome. While the total digital ridge count is higher than normal in classic and mosaic Turner syndrome, it is normal in Noonan syndrome.

Clinical Features

General: Low birth weight, short stature, sexual infantilism, webbed neck, normal intelligence.

Extremities: Short 4th metacarpal, hypolastic nails.

Dermatoglyphics: Large whorls and loops.

Miscellaneous: Cubitus valgus, shield chest, multiple pigmented naevi, lymphedema.

Heart: CHD incidence 20%. Commonest are coarctation of aorta, aortic stenosis and VSD. Dextrocardia, aortic atresia and PS in mosaics. There are two main groups of CVS lesions. Coarctation of aorta is present in 70% of patients with heart disease and 45X constitution but not in mosaics or Noonan syndrome. PS with or without ASD is present in 90% of patients with Noonan syndrome or mosaic Turner syndrome but never in true 45X Turner syndrome with heart disorder.

The clinical consequence is that if a patient with apparent Turner phenotype is found to have PS, the chromosome constitution is not 45X. If the patient has coarctation of aorta, she cannot have pure 46XX but will have 45X.

Hypertension is noted in 25% of cases. It is mild and unrelated to renal or vascular disease.

There is high frequency of renal anomalies. By 40 years age the incidence of hypertension is 80%.

The high incidence of hypertension, diabetes and old for age appearance in these subjects suggests that precocious aging may be part of Turner syndrome.

2

Heart in Infective Myocarditis

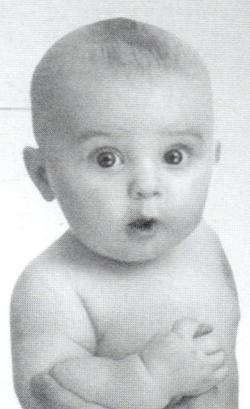

PREVALENCE

- 6.8% of autopsies in pediatric age group.
- Rheumatic carditis 32%
- Abscess in myocardium 16%
- Bronchopneumonia or lobar pneumonia 15%
- Poliomyelitis 7%
- Infective endocarditis 7%
- Bacterial endocarditis 5%
- Meningitis 4%
- Tuberculosis 4%
- Nephritis 3%
- Nonspecific myocarditis 3%

Other causes—measles, mumps, chickenpox, diphtheria, scarlet fever, whooping cough, influenza, anemia, croup, erythema multiform bullosum, coxsackievirus, infectious mononucleosis, encephalomyocarditis, silicosis, viral hepatitis, Chagas', disease, scrub typhus, Rocky Mountain spotted fever, epidemic typhus and echovirus.

There is a slight tendency for cases of myocarditis of unrecognized etiology to occur in summer or winter months. Maximum incidence in July and August.

The most commonly identified organism in pediatric age group today is coxsackievirus. This is specially true of newborn period and then 1 to 3 years age group. During epidemics rubella myocarditis may be recognized.

PATHOLOGY

The heart is flabby, pale and hypertrophied with enlarged ventricular chambers and a wall that appears thin but by weight is hypertrophied.

Histologically myocarditis is characterized by an interstitial infiltration of lymphocytes, polymorphs and plasma cells. The muscle fibers may show focal necrotic lesions at times and a diffuse degeneration at others. When septicemia has preceded death leukocytes clumped in abscess formation may appear throughout myocardium. Interstitial edema is common. In chronic cases fibrosis may appear.

A virus infection, such as poliomyelitis, virus hepatitis or measles may show lesion with collection of lymphocytes in interstitial tissue accompanied by monocytes and polymorphs. Rickettsial lesions are associated with vasculitis. The organism multiplies within the cell and produce muscle fragmentation and necrosis.

Diphtheria and other bacterial toxins are protoplasmic poisons that alter cellular respiration.

Endotoxins and Gram-negative bacteria produce fibrinoids in walls of coronary vessels and myocardial destruction. The changes resemble overwhelming intoxication due to epinephrine or the syndrome of traumatic shock.

Clinical Features

Myocarditis should be suspected in infants and young children if following are present:

Gallop rhythm, persistent tachycardia, cardiomegaly, cardiovascular collapse, congestive heart failure, dyspnea, hepatomegaly, characteristic ECG pattern or new appearance of a significant apical systolic murmur.

In isolated myocarditis there may be no preceding illness whatsoever. The child may suddenly become dyspneic in a few minutes. The majority have a gradual onset and follow a preceding URTI or pneumonia. Some begin with a history of vomiting once, twice or recurrent. In others the first sign of illness is a cough associated with mild irritability. In some there is simple failure to gain weight.

The infant with myocarditis is acutely ill with a respiratory rate between 60 and 120/minute, cyanosis and peripheral edema may occur.

In children over 1 year age the illness is less acute although they too may show cyanosis and collapse. There is tachycardia and heart rate is out of proportion to the temperature. Occasionally there is a soft systolic murmur at apex. The heart sounds may be normal or weak. A gallop rhythm is heard in majority. Gallop rhythm without murmur is highly suggestive of myocarditis. Apex beat is weak and diffuse and may be palpated in 5th space beyond nipple line.

X-ray shows cardiomegaly, marked in majority of cases. The ESR is usually elevated but may be normal. WBC count is variable, slightly elevated as a rule but may be normal and occasionally in range of 20 thousand.

ECG

Tachycardia is the rule. Conduction defects are common with varying degrees of heart block up to complete AV dissociation. The most diagnostic features are:

1. Lowering of QRS voltage in standard leads.
2. Flattening or inversion of T-wave of standard leads.

The QRS voltage is considered depressed when it is <5 mm in each of standard leads. The R-wave in V1 in right precordium is frequently <4 mm and often <2 mm. In left precordium R wave is considered depressed if <6 mm in V6. The S-waves are larger in comparison.

The normal T-wave in V6 usually approximates 3 mm in height and may be as high as 5–6 mm, rarely <2 mm after 6 months of age. In first 6 months of life it may be between 1 and 2 mm, exceptionally. Elevation of ST segment occurs in 5% of patients with acute myocarditis and a few cases of chronic. This is due to diffuse fibrosis of ventricular wall or localized necrosis of myocardium.

Q-wave in lead V6 is absent in 74% of cases. 0.5–1 mm in 12% and >1 mm in 14% cases.

85% of normal infants or children have Q-wave in V6 of 1 mm or more. A finding of Q-wave, if low voltage QRS and T-wave abnormalities persist after patient has recovered fully, it means that there is some degree of myocardial fibrosis. This does not interfere with a normal active life but occasionally may lead to heart failure.

DIAGNOSIS

Based on evidence of clinical and lab signs of myocarditis and exclusion of other form of heart disease. Myocarditis is usually indicated by a gallop rhythm, cardiomegaly, tachycardia, CHF, circulatory collapse, absence of murmurs, ECG abnormalities and the identification of etiological factors that precipitate myocarditis.

The echocardiogram shows large poorly contracting LV with a reduced ejection fraction and velocity of circumferential fiber shortening is seen. The LA is usually also enlarged.

In newborn echo may be normal.

Differential Diagnosis

1. Rheumatic fever
2. Infectious diseases
3. Toxins
4. Drugs
5. Congenital heart diseases.
6. *Pericarditis*: There may be enlarged heart shadow, tachycardia and T-wave abnormalities in ECG. The friction rub is present. The change in size of heart shadow occurs rapidly, a return to normal size may occur in pericarditis in 1–4 weeks, a feature that is unusual in myocarditis. Paracentesis will settle the problem with withdrawal of fluid. Echocardiography is a sensitive method for confirming the diagnosis. It should be remembered that pericarditis and myocarditis may occur together. In doubt digitalis should be administered.
7. *Endocardial fibroelastosis*: CHF is associated. Murmurs are absent or insignificant. Gallop rhythm is common.

Response to digitalis is good. Differentiation from myocarditis is hence difficult. However, a specific etiological agent may be identified that is commonly associated with myocarditis, e.g. coxsackievirus, diphtheria, encephalomyocarditis virus, pneumonia, influenza.

A coxsackievirus infection in first week or second week of life is more likely to cause myocarditis. Later it is unlikely to do so. A history of pleurodynia or pyrexial illness in mother a week or so before delivery suggests the possibility of coxsackie infection. The onset of endocardial fibroelastosis is usually in first 8 months of life. Myocarditis, apart from in newborn period due to coxsackievirus, occurs in only 30% of cases in first 8 months of life.

ECG gives the most useful differentiating feature. The majority of cases of endocardial fibroelastosis have an increased QRS voltage with LV loading pattern in certain precordial leads. 93% of myocarditis cases show decreased voltage in same precordial leads. The T-waves are inverted in endocardial fibroelastosis also but 50% of these cases have a significant Q-wave in V5 or V6, a finding which is rare in myocarditis unless a myocardial infarction is present.

T-wave in V5, V6 in myocarditis is characteristically flat or very slightly inverted but in endocardial fibroelastosis it may be inverted to a depth of 4–5 mm and in very high percentage of cases >1 mm.

The mumps antigen skin test is positive in endocardial fibroelastosis and unlikely in myocarditis especially under 4–5 years age group.

8. *Glycogen storage diseases of heart*: There is usually cardiomegaly with biventricular hypertrophy. Thickening of ventricular septum may take form of infundibular obstruction with characteristic finding of infundibular stenosis of LV.

ECG has a short PR interval, high QRS voltage and upright T-waves over right precordium and inverted T-waves over left. The T-waves show considerable voltage whether upright or inverted which differentiates these conditions from myocarditis. CHF is a terminal event. A family history is present.

When the heart is involved in glycogen storage diseases, there is likelihood of involvement of muscles throughout the body. The biopsy and histopathological analysis shows excess deposition of glycogen. The buffy coat of centrifugal blood may show unusual amount of glycogen. 76% die in first 6 months. Only 6% survive after infancy.

9. *Aberrant left coronary artery arising from pulmonary artery*: LV loading pattern and inverted T-waves over left precordium in ECG are a rule. Cardiomegaly without cardiac murmur. There is tachycardia and CHF. The echocardiogram shows large dilated LV with poor function. Angiocardiography reveals a huge LV and a small RV, compressed by a deviated septum. Aortogram demonstrates an RCA coming out of aorta in normal fashion but no LCA from aorta. ECG permits an accurate differentiation from other conditions in most instances since babies with an aberrant LCA off pulmonary show an anterior myocardial infarction pattern affirming the underlying pathology. The age of baby, course of illness, operative findings and or ultimate death with subsequent autopsy findings reveals the correct diagnosis and allows time to distinguish the anomaly from endocardial fibroelastosis and myocarditis. Myocardial perfusion scanning using thallium is a reliable new method of demonstrating ischemic zone and differentiating from other forms of cardiomyopathy.

10. *Medial necrosis of coronary artery*: The pulmonary and renal arteries are also involved and there may be signs of renal disease. Onset is usually in first 3 months of life. Although tachycardia is present it is usually not associated with CHF.

COXSACKIEVIRUS MYOCARDITIS

Commonly involves the neonate. Groups of cases may appear in epidemic fashion. Mother has a coxsackievirus infection with fever and/or pleurodynia in last week of pregnancy. A week after birth the infant develops same infection with damaging effect on heart muscles. While the disease is a generalized one and affects brain also, it is only myocarditis that leads to high mortality. This may be related to extra burden the heart is called upon to bear in circulatory adjustment in newborn.

Symptoms are generalized: Off feeds, feeding difficulty, breathlessness, severe dyspnea are present in majority. Fever and red throat are seen. Hepatomegaly occurs if CHF supervenes. Encephalitis may be evident.

Signs are tachycardia, dyspnea, hepatomegaly and cardio-megaly. ECG will confirm in all cases.

There is patchy necrosis of muscle tissue, different from a diffuse reaction associated with other forms of myocarditis. The neonate is acutely ill for a few days or weeks. Majority die after a short course of illness. If recovery occurs, it occurs rapidly over the next week or two. ECG changes may persist for 1–2 months. Digitalis, antibiotics, oxygen and other supportive measures are life-saving.

Poliomyelitis

32% cases develop focal myocarditis. The lesion usually consists of histiocytes, polymorphs, a few lymphocytes.

ECG abnormalities are found is 14% cases: Tachycardia, extrasystole, tall P waves, long PR interval, slurring of QRS, LAD, flat, diphasic or inverted T-waves.

Hypertension occurs in majority of patients from 3rd to 7th day of illness, after that BP subsides steadily and comes to normal by end of 2 weeks. It is more common in paralytic group. The cause of hypertension is not clear. Renal origin is suggested. Hypoxia has been mentioned as the cause in some cases since the use of oxygen lowers BP. Involvement of hypothalamus in bulbar poliomyelitis may cause hypertension. Retina shows spasm of arterioles in such cases.

In fatal bulbar poliomyelitis peripheral collapse and hypotension may occur. Such collapse is irreversible.

Heart failure is rare in poliomyelitis, however, pulmonary edema may occur as a terminal event.

Treatment

Digitalis: In infants and children who are desperately ill, this should be given IV. Starting with 1/4 of digitalizing dose, giving another fourth an hour later and giving rest of the digitalizing dose IV or orally.

Oxygen, antibiotics and diuretics should be used. Digitalis should be continued until all signs of heart disease have completely disappeared and the patient is entirely recovered. 3 months is minimum. Relapses are common. Before digitalis is stopped the ECG should be normal, no cardiomegaly, no CHF and health should be good. This may entail giving digitalis for 1–2 years or more. Digitalis should be discontinued gradually in step doses and patient observed for returning signs of myocarditis or heart failure.

ACTH and steroids have been shown to have a beneficial value. Cardiac arrhythmias are common complications of myocarditis.

3
Endocardial Fibroelastosis

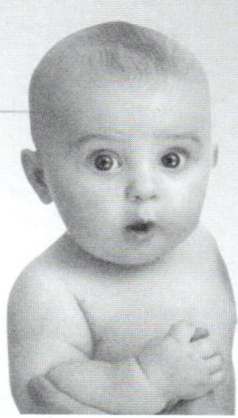

CLASSIFICATION

1. EF of LV, LA, RV and RA
2. Aortic, mitral, pulmonary or tricuspid.
3. *Associated CHD*: Coarctation of aorta, PDA, congenital heart block, WPW syndrome, anomalous LCA from pulmonary artery, aortic atresia and mitral stenosis.

EF occurs characteristically in LV. LA is also affected in 60% of cases. RV in 20% cases. RA is rarely involved.

LV is enlarged and dilated. In a few cases it is contracted, then it is associated with aortic or mitral valve stenosis.

75% cases have complicated form associated with CHD.

25% cases are isolated or uncomplicated by CHD.

17% of children with CHD have EF.

Longer than affected babies survive in the first year of life, the more likely they are to have a more extensive form of EF and more chambers involved.

Pathology

Cardiomegaly is considerable. Heart weight being 2 to 4 times the normal for the age. The endocardium on left side of heart is involved in 98% cases. Right and left both in 16% cases. Only left side is involved in 86% cases.

The characteristic lesion is a thickened layer of pearly whiteness covering the inner wall of LV and LA. It is stiff and rubbery and is spread diffusely over the endocardium of both LV and LA.

Valvular deformities are present in 34–51% cases. Aortic and mitral valves are most commonly involved. Microscopically there is hyperplasia of fibrous and elastic tissue of endocardium. The subendocardial myocardial junction shows a few degenerating muscle fibers, diffuse round cell infiltration and vacuolation. Occasionally an associated myocarditis is present.

The hypoplastic LV is a special group between primary EF without valvular lesion on one hand and aortic atresia on the other. In such cases the aortic valve ring is hypoplastic and aortic valve is small but normal. These children have a small LV cavity surrounded by a massively hypertrophied ventricular wall. In spite of the gross ventricular hypertrophy the heart is unable to maintain the circulation.

Etiology

1. *Inflammation*: EF following infectious mononucleosis and coxsackievirus are reported.
2. *Congenital developmental defect*: Elastic tissue is known to be influenced by a variety of factors during embryonic period.
3. *Hypoxia*: Premature closure of foramen ovale before birth might lead to LV and LA stasis and anoxia.
4. *Deposition of fibrin*: The surface layer is composed of fibers indistinguishable from fibrin.
5. *Hereditary defect*: The condition is autosomal dominant.
6. Nonspecific reaction due to ventricular dilatation. Interstitial myocarditis and obstructive lesions cause marked ventricular dilatation. This increase in endocardial tension in a physical way causes the development of EF.

Clinical Features

60% cases of aortic atresia are associated with EF, 4% of coarctation of aorta and 1% of PDA and in 50% of aortic stenosis who develop CHF in first year of life.

Many babies of EF without other anomalies develop normally and appear healthy and well nourished until there is a sudden onset of signs and symptoms.

In chronic cases anorexia and failure to gain weight are common features. Irritability is also frequent.

1. *Dyspnea*: Occurs in 91% cases, characterized by increase in respiratory rate which varies from 40 to 100/minute. There may be associated grunting or crow like sound. In chronic cases there is wheezing. Cough occurs in 40% cases and is most commonly due to CHF and associated respiratory infection.

2. *Cyanosis*: Unusual in EF, except in neonates who die in first week of life. When present cyanosis is associated with severe CHF or a terminal event. Oximetery suggests that it is peripheral in origin. Some cases may be due to pulmonary congestion.

3. *Gallop rhythm*: Occurs in 80% cases with CHF.

4. *Valvular involvement and heart murmur*: 34% cases. MV first AO second. 18% of primary EF cases have Bicuspid aortic valve.

Radiology

Cardiomegaly is universal. Average CT ratio is 69%. On echocardiography left atrial enlargement, left ventricular enlargement and reduced cardiac action are seen. Except during CHF the lung fields appear normal. LAE may at times be simulated by hypertrophied LV pressing back against the esophagus. This sign may also be present in cases of aberrant LCA arising from pulmonary artery.

ECG

Sinus rhythm is the rule but heart block complete or intermittent may occur in terminal stages. PR interval is within normal limits. Duration of P-wave averages 0.05 second. Only in rare occasions prolonged to 0.1 second. Amplitude of P-wave averages 2 mm. QRS interval is beyond normal limits in terminal cases. The T-wave deflection in V5–V6 is flat or inverted. Mean electrical axis ranges from –10 to +110°. Most significant aspect of ECG tracing is the presence of left loading pattern associated with increased voltage in LV precordial leads. 80% cases have LVH pattern as an isolated phenomenon. Characteristic tracing may show a tall R in precordial lead V6 and deep S in V1. Occasionally RVH is reported and then it is associated with a tall R or a QR pattern in V1 and deep S in V6.

RVH may occur in EF in the following circumstances:

1. Early weeks of life when RV pattern dominates.
2. Four chamber enlargement in EF.
3. EF with other CHD associated, e.g. preductal coarctation.
4. Acute failure with deep S in V6 suggesting RVH due to dilated heart. This S-wave disappears with treatment of CHF with digitalis and high voltage pattern of LVH predominates.

Diagnosis

A syndrome in neonates and infants with CHF and ECG signs of LVH and flattening or inversion of T-wave in V6 and V5. There are two primary groups of EF. First with an associated CHD. Second without CHD.

In the first group diagnosis is difficult before autopsy. It may be suspected in aortic atresia since 60% cases are associated with EF. An occasional case of coarctation of aorta may reveal a greater degree of LVH in ECG than one would expect. The associated cardiac anomaly is dominant and controls the prognosis. The characteristic features of EF are CHF, cardiomegaly, no murmur and a distinctive ECG pattern of LV load. The differential diagnosis involves conditions that simulate these features: Anomalous LCA arising from pulmonary artery, coronary calcinosis, glycogen storage diseases of heart, medial necrosis of coronary arteries, coarctation of aorta, aortic stenosis and mitral insufficiency. Many of these are associated with secondary EF reaction.

Recently echocardiography has been used in differential diagnosis of EF from hypertrophic cardiomyopathy. In EF LV diameter and LV outflow width is twice as large as control. Septal thickness and MV systolic motion are normal. In Hypertrophic cardiomyopathy there is marked narrowing of

LVOT, LV diameter diminished slightly and abnormal systolic motion of anterior leaflet of MV.

Nuclear medicine is invaluable in noninvasive assessment of cardiac function and performance in EF. Radionuclide angiography and gated blood pool studies are used for this purpose.

Myocardial perfusion and viability are assessed using radionuclides which accumulate routinely maximally in normal myocardium as is the case with thallium 201.

Coarctation of aorta is ruled out by determination of BP in arms and legs. When both coarctation and EF coexist, the ECG shows an LV strain pattern that is unusual in coarctation of aorta alone. PDA has the characteristic continuous murmur. When such murmur is not present, the more marked LVH pattern in ECG plus LAE may distinguish EF.

Babies with tricuspid atresia have much more cyanosis as a rule than babies with EF. The cyanosis shows an increase with crying. The heart shape is characteristic in TA, whereas in EF the heart shows generalized enlargement.

ECG shows horizontal heart in TA and T-waves in left precordial leads are upright.

In aortopulmonary septal defect there is less evidence of LVH, the hilar shadows are more engorged and may be pulsating. Angiogram and catheterization are diagnostic.

Aortic stenosis may show similar clinical picture but a loud murmur is heard in aortic area accompanied by thrill. Occasionally AS murmur is heard down LSE. In such cases LV pressure curve is obtained by Bjork needle through LA or via the trachea into LA. AS and EF may coexist.

Differential Diagnosis

1. *Anomalous LCA*: Most cases present in first 4 months of life. Onset with CHF, dyspnea, hepatomegaly and screaming or crying as if the infant were in pain. ECG shows an ischemic pattern of myocardial infarction with LV overloading pattern that produces a deep S-wave in V1 rather than a tall R in V6. There are deep Q-waves in lead 1, aVL, V5 and V6. ST

segment in V5 and V6 is elevated in majority. The pattern is that of anterolateral myocardial infarction. Myocardial imaging using thallium 201 shows defective uptake of radionuclide in infarcted myocardium. An aortogram with tip of the catheter in the region of the coronary arteries will reveal a large completely filled RCA arising from aorta and absent LCA indicating its anomalous presence elsewhere. The cases always die in infancy. A number of cases of anomalous LCA have mild degree of EF of LV at autopsy, which is a secondary lesion.

2. *Calcification of coronary arteries*: There is widespread calcification of arteries throughout body and may involve renal and thyroid arteries and arteries of numerous other vital organs. CHF may occur and produce ECG changes suggestive of EF. The condition is rare, uniformly fatal and does not respond to digitalis. X-ray of various portions of body may reveal calcifications in arteries.

3. *Glycogen storage disease of heart*: Fatal disease. Death occurs in first 8 months of life. ECG shows LVH and T-wave inversion in V6 and short PR interval. There is evidence of generalized muscular weakness since birth. The children have macroglossia. Biopsy is diagnostic.

4. *Myocarditis*: Coxsackie myocarditis when it occurs in mother during the end of pregnancy is likely to produce same infection in newborn baby. After 1 month of life the incidence of coxsackie myocarditis falls precipitously. In EF the onset is maximum in first 8 months of life. In myocarditis except coxsackievirus infection only 30% cases have their onset in first 8 months of life. The ECG in EF and myocarditis show differences of diagnostic significance. The voltage of R-wave in V6 or S-wave in V1 is abnormally high in EF. It is rarely increased in myocarditis. A pattern of myocardial infarction may be seen in 10% cases of myocarditis but it is very rare in EF. Q-wave in V6 of 1 mm or greater is seen in 60–70% cases of EF but a Q-wave in V6 is uncommon in myocarditis unless a pattern of myocardial infarction is present. 85% cases of EF have a left loading pattern and 93% of these have an

increase in voltage in leads pertaining to LV. In myocarditis only 7% show an increase in voltage in same leads. Punch biopsy of endocardium is diagnostic in atypical clinical presentation.

5. *EF associated with valvular involvement*: The combination of mural endocardial fibroelastic reaction and pearly white thickening of MV was regarded as primary EF by Kelley and Anderson in 1956. The majority of EF with valvular involvement show LV loading pattern in ECG. The presence of EF may be suspected in a baby with CHF in first year of life with a systolic murmur and inverted T-waves over left precordium with or without increased voltage of R in V6 or S in V1. Isolated AS or large intracardiac left to right shunt also give similar findings. Mumps antigen skin test is diagnostic in 91% cases under the age of 2 years. This test is less useful over 2 year age because of increased incidence of positive in controls. The test is nonspecific.

Treatment

1. Digitalis should be administered promptly. In desperately ill infants it is given IV. 1/4 of digitalizing dose state. 1/4 after 1 hour. Rest of the dose IV or orally in next a few hours.
2. Oxygen is needed when cyanosis is present. Antibiotics are useful since it is difficult to tell whether pulmonary signs are due to infection or failure.
3. Sedative should be given for restlessness.

   Digitalis should be continued until all signs of disease have disappeared and ECG shows normal tracing. In the light of present knowledge it should be for 2–3 years, preferably until both heart size and ECG are normal. Early therapy is important before heart has reached excessive proportions, to prevent death. A long-term prognosis of primary EF appears good in those cases whose heart size and ECG become normal. Deaths are due to CHF.

4

Heart in Rubella Syndrome

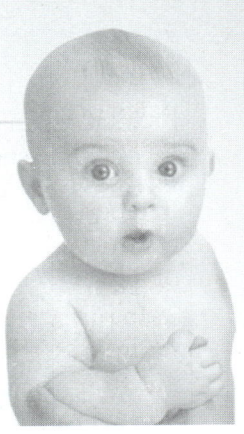

Rubella first described in 1752 in German literature as a variety of measles, Scarlet fever or a hybrid form of the two. Subsequently identified as a separate disease by Englishman in 1815 and named Rubella by a Scot. An ophthalmologist in 1941 recognized that a bunching of cases in congenital cataract could be explained by an epidemic of Rubella that occurred in eastern Australia in spring of 1940.

Pathology

Examination of aborted products of conception during first trimester of pregnancy shows patchy changes of necrotic nature in the endothelium of blood vessels in the chorion, brain and subendocardial myocardium of the atria. There is no evidence of inflammation. There is delay in development of cardiac septa. A wide variety of intracardiac malformations have been encountered in the live births including TGV, truncus arteriosus, atresia of AV valves, atrioventricular communis and TOF. TOF is the most common. These defects, are responsible for 5–10% of rubella CVS disease. Simple defects, such as ASD and VSD account for 5% of total cases affected. Small atrial defects due to stretching of foramen ovale flap due to L > R shunt are commoner, though impossible to detect clinically but confirmed by catheterization. Valvular lesions are noted on autopsy. These are nodular and distributed on leaflets of all four valves. Changes in myocardium are reported in both fetal and postnatal material. The affected myocardium forms a grey patch or brown patch over the ventricle. Microscopically there is swelling of myocardial fibrils that have loss of cross striation or pleomorphic nuclei. There is no evidence of inflammation. In blood vessels patchy necrotic changes are distributed in large conducting arteries, muscular arteries and in smaller vessels of systemic and pulmonary circuits.

In pulmonary circulation the MPA division may be small in infants. In older children thickening of vessels wall is evident and there is narrowing at the bifurcation of MPA. There is intimal thickening with irregular arrangements of elastic fibers in the media. Where the elastic tissue is distorted or fragmented intimal proliferation is maximal. Poststenotic dilatation of vessels may occur with thinning of vessels wall. Occlusive changes in arterioles are reported.

In aorta there is considerable thickening of entire vessel. Mostly in descending aorta but also immediately above the aortic valve in infants. Lesions are fibromuscular proliferation from below endothelium.

In ductus arteriosus elastic tissue tends to be absent and there is no myointimal heaping. Muscular wall is defective with an increased amount of collagen between smooth muscle cells. Focal changes are reported in many systemic arteries including those to abdominal organs, lung, heart, brain. There is intimal thickening and deficiency of elastic tissue. Endothelial swelling produces obstruction to flow of blood to critical areas of brain and abdomen which may be responsible for mental retardation and atretic malformations of gut.

Etiology

Viremia occurs in mothers before rash appears and placenta becomes infected. The fetus becomes involved through endothelial shedding from placenta or through the passage of infected white cells. A curious immunologic situation follows in which antibodies are formed but the virus remains alive. Breaks in chromosomal structure are reported. The cells replication is slowed. The total number in live born infants is considerably reduced. Some cytopathic damage also occurs. Growth may be sufficiently disturbed from very early infection to induce teratogenetic effects in growing organs, while later infection produces damage to the fetus of a much subtle variety. Susceptibility of adult female is less than 15%. Even during epidemics not all exposed gravida become infected. In addition the risk of damage to fetus declines with progressive fetal age at the time of maternal illness.

Hemodynamics

Changes in hemodynamics will be appropriate for individual malformations. Of more interest is detection of valvular lesions, of pulmonary arterial stenosis and of lesions in a systemic circulation.

Clinical Features

Postnatal rubella is a mild and self-limiting disease of children but fetal infection produces a series of clinical manifestations that are known together as Rubella syndrome. The most severe abnormalities include CHD, hearing loss, cataract, glaucoma, psychomotor retardation and neonatal purpura. Profound heart failure has been reported in babies with myocardial necrosis and large PDA.

Older children may be referred to cardiologist because of detection of a murmur. Most often this is a murmur of pulmonary artery stenosis with characteristic transmission from precordium to axilla and back.

Clues to rubella background are suggested by a low birth weight for gestational age, the birth between October and March or by testing for minor abnormalities of hearing and vision. Occasionally a child presents with systemic hypertension due to renal artery stenosis. Cases are also detected in screening program for hearing and speech defect, for eye dysfunction and for diabetes.

Radiology

In young infants with congenital rubella syndrome, particularly those severely ill in newborn period, the appearance of chest X-ray may be extremely variable. In older children and in those with left to right shunt cardiomegaly with pulmonary plethora is indicative of large left to right shunt through PDA.

ECG

In complex anomalies the ECG is helpful in directing attention to chamber hypertrophy. In older children with simple defects, such as PAS and PDA, the ECG changes are not striking though they are in expected directions. In very young infant particularly in newborn period appearance of frank infarction pattern in ECG must be looked for. A high incidence of unusually oriented frontal plane QRS axis suspicious of involvement of left bundle is reported.

Diagnosis

Easy in epidemic form. The ability to separate patients with rubella from those with other types of severe intrauterine infection is available through culture of virus and demonstration of the appropriate antibodies. Virus shedding may continue for many months even in infants who appear normal. Most infants with congenital rubella cease excreting virus and have normal immunoglobulin levels at age one year. The diagnosis of myocardial necrosis of extensive nature, PDA, PAS or combinations, as well as more complicated intracardiac malformations follows a fairly standard approach. It is difficult to map the extent of arterial damage in both circulations with certainty particularly on the systemic side. Possibility of involvement throughout the body must be remembered and periodic follow-up examinations should be done because changes in vascular system appear with passage of time.

Prognosis

There is a fairly high mortality in florid form of disease (e.g. with neonatal thrombocytopenic purpura). Cardiac contribution to death has been in those with massive ductal shunts or with extensive myocardial necrosis. 30% of survivors have cardiovascular abnormalities in long-term follow-up. Demonstration of arterial disease in coronay, cerebral, adrenal, pancreatic and mesenteric vessels may have implications of occlusive vascular disease of these organs. Bowel and myocardial infarction together with strokes and subarachnoid hemorrhage may be implicated from this source. Patients with TOF develop severe RVOT obstruction with marked PAS. Prognosis in them is bad. Where PAS is a major CVS manifestation, there is a little surgical attempt at therapy.

5

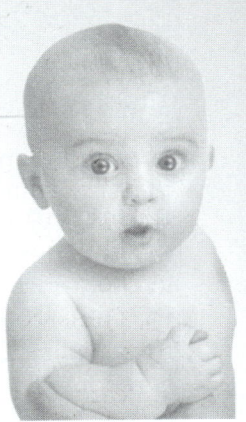

Heart in Acute Glomerulonephritis

Acute nephritis occurs as a result of a hemolytic streptococcal infection types 4 and 12. Some evidence of cardiac involvement is not uncommon in acute nephritis, it would precede hypertensive encephalopathy and uremia (9 and 4% respectively).

Clinical Features

1. **Heart size:** Slight increase in heart size may be related to increased blood volume or retention of fluid in myocardium rather than myocardial disease itself. Cardiac enlargement occurs in 58% cases of acute nephritis.
2. **ECG changes:** Low flat or inverted T1 and T2 in standard leads, alteration of ST segment and lengthening of QRS interval. Tachycardia, bradycardia, minor alterations in QT interval and the arrhythmias are occasionally seen.
3. **CHF:** Indicates the degree of myocardial involvement. Signs suggestive of CHF in nephritis are edema, dyspnea, hepatomegaly and cardiomegaly with pulmonary congestion. Crepitations are heard at lung bases. Pulmonary edema with copious sputum may develop. Indirect signs of CHF are tachycardia, gallop rhythm, apical systolic murmur, cardiomegaly and ECG abnormalities. CHF does not occur in absence of cardiomegaly. CHF is usually accompanied by hypertension. Contributing factors are sodium retention and hydremia.

Treatment

1. Adequate penicillin therapy to eradicate streptococcal infection, for 10 days.

2. In circulatory congestion fluid balance should be maintained. Fluid intake restricted. Lasix used. Serum potassium should be monitored carefully.

3. Hypertension should be treated with ACE inhibitors.

4. *Digitalis*: If features of true heart failure develop like cardiomegaly and hepatomegaly, digitalis must be given. In oliguria digitalis doses should be scaled down.

6
Heart in Collagen Diseases

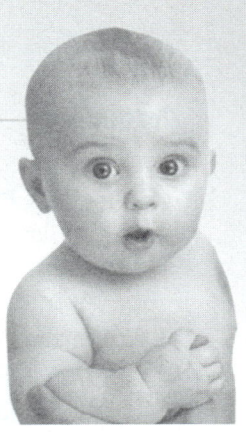

The term collagen diseases was first suggested in 1941 by Klemperer who showed that the lesions of SLE and diffuse scleroderma were the result of changes in collagenous tissues. The connective tissue of body is composed of cells and intercellular substances. Its structure differs according to local requirements. The cells are fibroblasts and intercellular substance consists of fibers (collagen, elastic, reticulum) and a homogenous ground substance composed of mucoproteins.

Fibrinoid degeneration of connective tissue of body is the most characteristic pathologic change but proliferation and inflammation may also occur in varying degrees. In rheumatic fever proliferation (heart valves) and inflammation (joints) predominate, although necrosis does occur in center of Aschoff nodule. In periarteritis nodosa lesions are limited to small and medium size arteries with proliferation and inflammation prominent. In SLE fibrinoid degeneration of connective tissue dominates with involvement of skin, joint capsule, serous membranes, blood vessels, endocardium, lymph nodes, etc. while proliferation and inflammation are minimum. In scleroderma lesions are essentially proliferative with thickening and sclerosis of collagen tissue of blood vessels, alimentary tract, lungs and skeletal muscles but fibrinoid changes have also been noticed. As to the etiology since fibrinoid degeneration is present, these diseases have an autoimmune origin.

DERMATOMYOSITIS

First described by Wagner in 1887. Features are muscular weakness and involvement of skin and subcutaneous tissues. Muscles of trunk and extremities, respiration and those of swallowing are affected. Pain and tenderness with progressive muscular weakness makes the patient bed ridden. Calcinosis of muscles and other tissues is found in advanced cases. Involvement of skin and subcutaneous tissues is shown in a dermatitis with indurated tissues of trunk and extremities. Facial skin lesions, periorbital swelling or generalized edema are seen. Involvement of skin over joints may lead to contractures.

Pathology

Skeletal muscles and skin are predominantly affected. Earliest lesions show edema of subendothelial connective tissue with collection of inflammatory cells in skin and muscles. Vascular changes are found with a hyalinized material in media of arterioles and inflammatory reaction around the vessel. Myocardium may show loss of striation, fragmentation and vascularization of muscle fibers. Interstitial edema occurs. Pericardium is usually spared.

CVS Involvement

Most common finding is a tachycardia out of proportion to the age of child. ECG shows flattening or inversion of T-waves due to myocardial involvement. Arrhythmias are reported. Heart murmurs may be heard. Edema is part of disease process of skin and tissues. Rarely it is due to heart failure. Dyspnea is of respiratory failure and not of myocardial origin. Raynaud's phenomenon in fingers and toes may occur.

SYSTEMIC LUPUS ERYTHEMATOSUS

First described by Kapozi in 1872 and is characterized by an erythematous skin rash involving the face particularly with a butterfly type of malar flush. It is associated with varying degrees of arthralgea, arthritis, polyserositis, lymphad-enopathy, splenomegaly, leukopenia, anemia and CNS manifestations. Onset is usually in second decade of life but seen in children between 5 and 10 years of age. The diagnosis is based on demonstration of LE cells in blood (found in 75% cases at some time).

Pathology

There is fibrinoid degeneration of connective tissue, in arteries of various organs. The epicardium and pericardium of heart are involved. The myocardium may show degeneration and fibrosis. Verrucae are seen on all valves particularly tricuspid. Renal vascular disease is common and associated with renal damage in 2/3 of cases. Hypertension secondary to renal cause is frequently noted.

CVS Involvement

Pericardial friction rub and pericardial effusion are noted. Heart murmurs may be heard on any area of precordium depending upon the valve affected. Endocarditis may be present without heart murmurs and heart murmurs may occur in absence of valve damage. ECG may reveal evidence of myocarditis with flattened or inverted T-waves. Cardiomegaly is common. CHF occurs in 25% cases. Severe valvular dysfunction is uncommon despite the frequent finding of noninfective Libman Sacks endocardial lesions at necropsy.

Raynaud's phenomenon due to interference with circulation of hands and toes is noted in 1/4 cases.

CNS involvement secondary to CVS changes is common and associated with convulsions.

Pancreatitis secondary to vascular changes is reported. Arteritis may be found in any organ system of body and thus bizarre signs and symptoms are to be expected in diffuse irregular patterns.

Treatment

The skin and joint manifestations are controlled by cortisone, ACTH or newer steroids. Myocardial function may also improve. Renal involvement may be improved by steroids and immunosuppressive drugs.

Hypertension and CHF are common after steroid therapy. Libman Sacks endocardial lesions are smaller and fewer in number in steroids treated cases as compared to nonsteroids treated patients. Increase in myocardial fat is seen. Corticosteroids while vital to the management of lupus erythematosus have an overall deleterious effect on heart. Coronary atherosclerosis may seem accelerated. Monoclonal antibodies are new modes of therapy.

PERIARTERITIS NODOSA

First described in 1866 by Kussmaul and Maier. Defined as a form of necrotizing inflammatory panarteritis affecting small and medium size arteries, throughout the body, characterized by signs of systemic infection and focal signs and symptoms due to scattered arterial lesions with local circulatory disturbances varying from relative ischemia to gross infarction.

Etiology

Periarteritis is caused by an allergic response to a variety of allergens: Bacterial and nonbacterial, e.g. sulphonamides, arsenical, DOCA. Rich in 1945 produced acute necrotizing arteritis with acute carditis and acute glomerulonephritis by repeated injections of foreign serum in rabbits.

Pathology

The lesions are limited to small and medium sized arteries of muscular type which are affected segmentally. The adventitia and media are involved in a proliferative reaction that is accompanied by edema and infiltration of inflammatory cells, polymorphonuclear cells and eosinophils. There is extensive necrosis of media with resultant aneurysms. Inflammation extends to intima with destruction of endothelium and thrombosis. Fibrinoid degeneration is found in ground substance of media and intima followed by fibroblastic proliferation and narrowing of vessels. The renal vessels are most susceptible followed by coronary, adrenal, pancreatic, mesenteric, hepatic, splenic and cerebral vessels.

Clinical Features

Multiplicity of manifestations. Onset is insidious. Several systems are involved. Initially protracted fever with pronounced tachycardia without obvious cause. High ESR and anemia are constant features. Vague symptoms include arthralgia abdominal distress, weight loss, lethargy, malaise, weakness and headache. Kidneys are involved in 90% cases. Urinary changes, such as albuminuria, cast and hematuria are found in 2/3 cases. Hypertension eventually develops in 2/3 of cases. There may be evidence of renal failure and associated changes in ocular fundi. Pain may be an important feature due to mesenteric vessels involvement, arthritis, polyneuritis, polymyositis, peripheral ischemia of Raynaud type or visceral infarctions. There may be painful subcutaneous nodules.

Edema occurs in 50% cases. Cause is nephropathy, CHF or polymyositis. A high leukocyte count is common but significant eosinophilia occurs in only 20% of cases.

Peripheral neuritis may be manifested by weakness, wasting, paresthesia and reflex changes.

CNS involvement may lead to convulsions, coma and death. Involvement of mesenteric arteries may lead to abdominal pain, nausea, vomiting, diarrhea or GIT hemorrhage. Perforation of bowel with peritonitis may occur.

Myocardial Involvement

This is usually secondary to coronary disease, augmented by hypertension. Occasionally a myocardial infarction may occur. CHF may develop as a terminal event. Cardiomegaly on X-ray and infarction pattern on ECG are seen. There may be evidence of pericarditis and myocarditis on ECG. LVH may be exhibited in presence of severe hypertension. Systolic murmurs may appear and are related to pathologic changes at valve margins. Percarditis may occur uncommonly with friction rub.

Diagnosis

By exclusion. By diffuse nature of the disease with eosinophilia and leucocytosis. Urinary findings and reversal of AG ratio may be of help. Biopsy confirms by showing characteristic changes in arterial wall.

Recently an acute febrile mucocutaneous syndrome has been described in infants by Kawasaki in 1967. Mucocutaneous involvement is accompanied by swelling of cervical lymph nodes.

The principal symptoms include:
- Fever of 1 to 2 weeks not responding to antibiotics.
- Congestion of conjunctivae.
- Changes in lips and oral cavity including dryness, redness, fissuring of lips, protuberance of tongue papillae and reddening of oral and pharyngeal mucosa.
- Changes of peripheral extremities characterized by initially reddening of palms and soles with an induration erythema and followed by membranous desquamation from finger tips.
- Polymorphous exanthema of trunk.
- Acute nonsuppurative cervical lymphadenopathy.

Kawasaki in 1967 described 50 cases. Sudden death due to acute cardiac failure has been reported. Autopsy reveal coronary aneurysm.

Infantile Periarteritis nodosa is a rare disease with poor prognosis.

Kawasaki disease is a self-limiting disease with excellent prognosis.

Treatment

Cortisone, digitalis provide varying degree of relief.

7

Heart in Neuromuscular Diseases

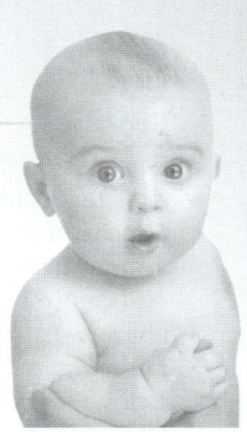

FRIEDREICH ATAXIA

A hereditary neurologic disorder characterized by a degeneration of optic nerves, cerebellum, olive and lateral and posterior columns of spinal cord. Usually caused by a recessive gene. Microscopically there is parenchymal atrophy and gliosis. In heart marked eccenteric hypertrophy of both ventricles is seen. Histology shows gross fibrosis separating hypertrophied muscle fibers in all cardiac chambers. Minor left atrial fibroelastosis and occasional thrombi are found. Subintimal fibrosis of coronary vessels occurs. Heart involvement in Friedreich ataxia may be pronounced in childhood.

Etiology

The basic cause of neurologic degeneration in Friedreich ataxia is unknown. Heart disease is associated with severe and diffuse neurologic disease. The cases with a positive family history have a more severe heart involvement than those without a family history of neurologic disease.

Pathogenesis of Cardiac Involvement

An ischemic cause secondary to small coronary vessels disease, neurologic dysfunction, and the suggestion that common genetic basis is there for both neurologic and cardiac disorders.

Clinical Features

Onset during childhood is gradual with gait disturbance being first feature. Upper limb involvement and dysarthria then appear. In fully developed case tendon reflexes and position and vibration sense are lost and nystagmus is present. Plantar response is extensor early in disease. Secondary skeletal changes as pes cavus and scoliosis are found in majority. Disease is progressive. There may be no symptoms referrable to CVS in patients with Friedreich ataxia even when extensive CVS involvement is present in childhood. In older patients exertional dyspnea and palpitation may be presenting symptoms of cardiac involvement. Clinically heart may be of normal size or enlarged. Gallop rhythm, PAT, AF or extrasystoles may be found. Soft systolic murmur is heard in pulmonary or mitral area, may be regurgitant. Diastolic murmurs after exercise may occur due to dilatation of heart. CHF is a terminal manifestation.

Radiology

Heart size is normal. Apex is down pointing and suggestive of LVH.

ECG

T inversion is seen in lead 1, 2, 3, avf and V5, V6. Normalisation of T-waves occurs after exercise in 80% of cases who have resting T-waves abnormalities. Sinus tachycardia is common. Dysarrhythmia with exercise have been observed. QRS axis is usually normal or deviated to right. QRS voltage is reduced is standard leads. 50% cases have evidence of ventricular hypertrophy.

Cardiac Catheterization

In severely affected patients RAP is elevated and RVEDP, CO is reduced. Hypertrophic LV cardiomyopathy with or without obstructive features have been described.

Echocardiography shows septal/posterior LV wall thickness ratio of 1.43–1.89. Systolic anterior movement of anterior mitral leaflet is seen.

Diagnosis

Positive family history is useful pointer. Early stages of Friedreich ataxia may be confused with chorea, cerebellar tumor, rheumatic heart disease, myocarditis or myoendocardial disease. ECG pattern is so consistent as to be an important confirmatory aid in diagnosis.

Prognosis

Majority of cases survive childhood. CHF is chief cardiac cause of death. Sudden death may occur due to gross coronary insufficiency either due to disease process or development of cardiac arrhythmias.

Treatment

Therapy of CHF and arrhythmia is done. In such instances improvement may be noted but is temporary. Prognosis poor with this complication.

PROGRESSIVE MUSCULAR DYSTROPHY

A hereditary disease of unknown etiology characterized by weakness and wasting of striated muscle groups.

There are 3 main types of clinical presentation:

Duchenne (pseudohypertrophic) form starts in early childhood in boys exclusively. The condition is rapidly progressive. Death occurring from respiratory tract infection or CHF before the age of 20 years. In 90% cases the disorder is transmitted as sex linked recessive. In 10% cases it is autosomal recessive.

The limb girdle form starts in second decade of life affecting both sexes and leading to severe disability by middle life. Inherited as autosomal recessive trait. Cardiac involvement is uncommon. Facioscapular humeral form may begin at any age and affects both sexes. Facial and shoulder girdle muscles are affected first. Transmission is autosomal dominant. Normal life span is possible. Pathologically there is atrophy of muscle cells with fatty and fibrous tissue replacement in skeletal as well as cardiac muscle. LV is thicker than RV. Large coronary arteries are normal. Small coronary arteries particularly supplying nodal tissue show degenerative changes.

Clinical Features

The onset is insidious. There is delay in acquisition of physical milestones, easy fatigability and difficulty in climbing stairs. A waddling gait and difficulty in rising from lying position is common. Weakness and wasting of shoulder and pelvic girdle develop. The thigh muscles are wasted but calf muscles are disproportionately large. The knee jerks are diminished or absent. Tachycardia is the earliest sign of cardiac involvement. Arrhythmia have been reported. Soft mitral first heart sound is noted. Ejection murmur in pulmonary area is heard. Third and fourth heart sounds are common. CHF is terminal.

Cardiomegaly on X-ray is uncommon but always present when CHF coexists. Scoliosis, a common sequelae of the disease may influence cardiac position and contour so that heart may appear abnormal.

ECG

Tachycardia, RVH, short PR interval, flat or negative T-waves in left chest leads, Q-wave abnormalities in left chest leads and avL (myopathic pattern, Wahi 1963). 50% of young patients have normal ECG tracings. ECG changes are most prominent in Duchenne type.

Cardiac catheterization shows normal right heart pressure at rest and on exercise.

Diagnosis

Electromyography, muscle biopsy, serum creatinine kinase. Most carriers have elevated creatinine kinase. The value of combining histochemical techniques with electron microscopy as a better marker for different myopathies is becoming increasingly apparent.

Systolic time indices appear to be sensitive means of discovering cardiac involvement in PMD.

8

Incidence of Congenital Heart Disease in Families

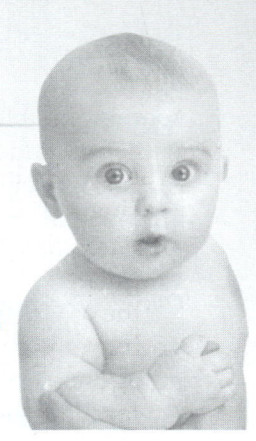

After one case of CHD has appeared in family there is approximately a 2% chance of a similar event in subsequent pregnancies.

Nora and associates have demonstrated that the risk of recurrence of a congenital heart defect in another child in a family varies with the frequency a lesion is found in the general population and the type of lesion in the first affected child. Thus if the child has a VSD the chance of his sibling having some form of CHD is approximately 4.4% or 1 in 22. With PDA 3.4%, TOF 2.7%, ASD 3.2%, PS 2.9%, AS 2.2%, coarctation 1.8%, TGA 1.9%, TA 1%, Ebstein anomaly 1.1%, Truncus 1.2% and pulmonary atresia which is a less commonly encountered lesion carries a much lower risk of 1.3% or 1 in 77.

FAMILIAL OCCURRENCE OF CHD

Clustering within certain families suggest that the cause of the abnormal development of heart can best be explained by a genetic predisposition made evident in appropriate prenatal environment. On the other hand, many instances of cardiac malformations can be traced strictly to environmental insults. Concentration within the families could be explained by the presence of same gene, similar prenatal environment or merely fortuitous occurrence of a very common abnormality. But the most probable explanation takes into consideration a combination of all these factors.

ENVIRONMENTAL FACTORS

The key to intrinsic problem lies in maternal stress mainly during first trimester of pregnancy:

1. *Parental age*: An increase in maternal age suggests the presence of some physiological disturbance associated with the aging process best illustrated by the striking correlation between chromosomal nondysjunction and late maternal age. Some association with late maternal age is suggested for VSD and TOF by Campbell who found more affected children born to mothers over 35 years and 40 years of age respectively. Mothers over 39 years of age have increased risk of producing children with CHD was demonstrated by Renwick in 1964. A correlation between a malformation and father's age implies a genetic event resulting from mutation, e.g. Achondroplasia where an increased incidence with paternal age has been demonstrated.

2. *Birth order*: There is higher incidence of PDA among the first births. Fetal distress is a possible cause (Moss 1964).

3. *Teratogenic agents*: Rubella infection in first trimester can result in a constellation of birth defects among which is PDA. A few cases of pulmonary stenosis following rubella are also reported. Positive correlation between mumps virus and endocardial fibroelastosis was found by St Geme in 1966.

   Coxsackievirus causes a variety of cardiac malformations. *Drugs*: Thalidomide caused ASD. Appetite suppressants, anticonvulsants and hormones taken during first trimester produce cardiac malformations.

   Diabetes in mother occurs 11 times more frequently in children with CHD then in mothers in general population.

   Vitamin A deficiency has been shown to cause abnormalities of aortic arch and heart.

4. *Hypoxia*: Chronic exposure to lower oxygen tension at high altitude may result in persistent PDA.

5. *Placental circulation*: In CHD discordance appears to be rule among monozygotic twins. Since the majority of these twins develop within a single chorionic sac and share a common vascular circulation competition between the fetuses could

not result in an imbalance to the disadvantage of one twin. This mechanism could also account for excess of monozygotic twins among multiple births with one or both members affected and for differences found in cardiac status of conjoined twins. Even in single pregnancies disturbances in placental circulation at a crucial time could cause malformation of heart.

TWIN STUDIES

Since MZ twins are genetically identical any variation between them must be environmentally determined. On the other hand, an increased frequency of concordance among MZ twins compared with DZ twins suggests presence of genetic determinants. The concordance rate for MZ twins is low (17%) although somewhat higher than for DZ twins (3.5%).

GENETIC FACTORS

1. *Single gene inheritance*: A genetic predisposition is frequently present. Mode of transmission appears to be autosomal dominant in some and autosomal recessive in others. Most convincing evidence is available for supravalvular aortic stenosis (AD inheritance). Dominant transmission for ASD also is suggested. Other cardiac malformations with AD inheritance are familial cardiomyopathy, familial ASD with prolonged AV conduction and hereditary prolongation of QT interval.
2. *Autosomal recessive inheritance*: There is an increased frequency of consanguinity among the parents of patients with dextrocardia (Lamy 1957). The familial nature of endocardial fibroelastosis does not fit either single gene or polygene inheritance. The cause of familial occurrence may be an infection, a mutagenic agent, a gene or a chromosome defect.

Polygenic Inheritance

Clustering of similar heart defects suggests the transmission of similar genes in presence of similar environmental factors.

A continuum of both genetic and nongenetic variables is intrinsic in polygenic traits and the appearance of an abnormality depends upon whether or not the combination of these variables exceeds a certain threshold.

The evidence indicates that though susceptibility to heart defects may be genetically determined environmental influences are the stronger components.

9

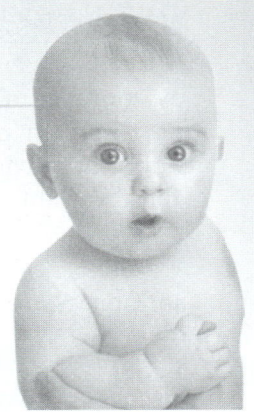

Gene Determined Syndromes with Congenital Heart Disease

A. Heart defects frequent

1. Ellis-van Creveld: ASD.
   Autosomal recessive.
2. Forney: Mitral insufficiency.
   Autosomal dominant.
3. Holt Oram: ASD.
   Autosomal dominant.
4. Hurler: Valvular defects.
   Autosomal recessive.
5. Idiopathic hypercalcemia: Supravalvular aortic stenosis.
   Autosomal recesssive.
6. Kartagener: Dextrocardia.
   Autosomal recessive.
7. Leopard (multiple lentigines): Pulmonary stenosis.
   Autosomal dominant.
8. Noonan: Pulmonary stenosis.
   Autosomal dominant.

B. Heart defects occasional

1. Acrocephalosyndactyly (Carpenter): PDA
   Autosomal recessive.

2. Apert: VSD, TOF.
   Autosomal dominant.
3. Cerebrohepatorenal (Zellweger).
   PDA, VSD.
   Autosomal recessive.
4. Cornelia de Lange: VSD.
   Autosomal recessive.
5. Fanconi pancytopenia: PDA.
   Autosomal recessive.
6. Focal dermal hypoplasia (Goltz):
   ASD. X-Linked dominant.
7. Incontinentia Pigmenti (block Sulzberger) : PDA.
   X-linked dominant.
8. Klippel Feil: VSD.
   Autosomal dominant.
9. Laurence-Moon-Biedl: Variable cardiac defects.
   Autosomal recessive.
10. Lissencephaly: PDA.
    Autosomal recessive.
11. Oculoauriculovertebral dysplasia (Goldenhar): PDA, TOF.
    Autosomal recessive.
12. Pierre Robin: Variable cardiac defects.
    Autosomal dominant.
13. Radial aplasia thrombocytopenia: TOF, ASD.
    Autosomal recessive.
14. Rubinstein-Taybi: PDA.
    Autosomal recessive.
15. Smith Lepli Opitz: ASD, TOF.
    Autosomal recessive.

10

Hereditary Disorders and Syndromes with Congenital Heart Disease

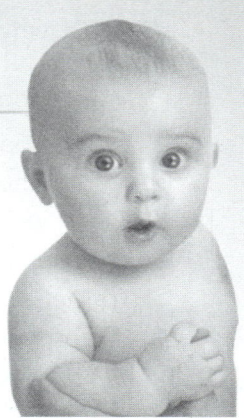

These can be grouped in the following manner:

1. Hereditary disorders with normal chromosomes in which congenital heart disease is common but is only one of the many abnormalities present.
2. Syndromes with abnormal chromosomes in which congenital heart disease is common but is only one of the abnormalities present.

The type of cardiac defect that can be encountered in above can be summarized into following:

1. Aortic regurgitation and/or mitral regurgitation which can be found in any of the following syndromes:
   Marphan
   Hurler
   Hunter
   Marquio Ulrich
   Scheie
   Marotequz Lamy
   Osteogenesis imperfecta
   Forney.
2. Atrial septal defect:
   Holt Oram
   Focal dermal hypoplasia
   Smith Lemli Opitz
   Radial aplasia thrombocytopenia
   Ellis-van Creveld

3. Patent ductus arteriosus:
   Acrocephalosyndactyly
   Cerebrohepatorenal
   Fanconi pancytopenia
   Lissencephaly
   Incontinentia pigmenti
4. Tetralogy of Fallot:
   Oculoauriculovertebral dysplasia
   Radial aplasia thrombocytopenia
   Smith Lemli Opitz
5. Ventricular septal defect
   Apert
   Cornelia de Lange
   Klippel Feil
6. Cardiomyopathy:
   Tuberous sclerosis
   Glycogen storage disease
7. Pulmonary artery stenosis:
   Cutis Laxa
   Leopard
   Neurofibromatosis
8. Pulmonary valve stenosis:
   Noonan
9. Supravalvular aortic stenosis:
   Idiopathic hypercalcemia
10. Aneurysms:
    Marphan
    Ehlers Danlos
11. Aortic stenosis:
    Alkaptonuria
12. Dextrocardia:
    Kartagener
13. Pulmonary arteriovenous fistula:
    Osler-Rendu-Weber
14. Systemic hypertension:
    Riley-Day
15. Conduction anomalies:
    Refsum
    Surdo cardiac

11

Clinic in Congenital Heart Disease

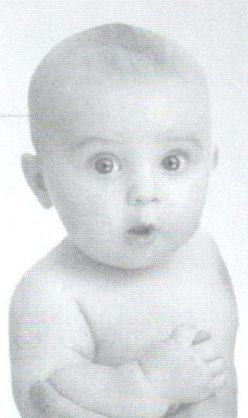

HISTORY TAKING

An age oriented or chronological approach to history is desirable.

1. Antenatal History

- Rubella, coxsackievirus infection.
- Threatened abortion.
- Previous stillbirths.
- Medication.
- Radiation.
- Vaccination with live virus vaccine.
- Hormonal treatment by diethylstilbestrol.

2. Natal and Neonatal History

- Weight.
- Weeks of gestation.
- Whether term or preterm.
- Length of labor.
- Resuscitation of baby at birth.
- Cyanosis at birth.
- Breathlessness.
- Grunting.
- Wheezing.
- Feeding difficulty.
- Apgar score.

3. Postnatal History

- Weight gain.
- Physical development.
- Appetite.
- Feeding difficulty.
- Developmental milestones.
- Lack of energy.
- Early tiredness.

4. Preschool and School Age

- Activity.
- Tiredness and breathlessness during activity.
- Difficulty climbing stairs.
- Joint pains.
- Fever of unexplained origin.
- Sore throat.
- Fatigue.
- Loss of appetite.
- Arthritis.

5. In Cyanotic Heart Disease

- Squatting.
- Need to stop and rest frequently.
- Dizziness.
- Episodes of unconsciousness.

6. Family History

- Heart defects.
- Hypertension.
- Myocardial infarction occurring in first degree relatives before the age of fifty years. In these cases there may be family tendency for elevated cholesterol.
- Diabetes.

PHYSICAL EXAMINATION

1. Child is acutely or chronically ill or essentially well.
2. Height and weight give degree of normal development.

3. Abnormalities of face and figure may allow identification of syndromes, e.g. Down, Marphan, Holt Oram, Turner.

4. Other congenital anomaly, e.g. cleft lip palate, clubbed foot, microcephaly, hypertelorism.

5. Evidence of Rubella syndrome, e.g. cataracts, deafness, cardiac murmur.

6. Presence of cyanosis. The child should be made to cry or exercised if cyanosis is inapparent. Conjunctival vessels are prominent in cyanotic children.

7. Tonsillar enlargement, enough to cause obstruction may cause intermittent hypoxia and pulmonary hypertension.

8. Arterial pulsations in neck. A continuous murmur may be due to arteriovenous fistula.

9. Lungs should be auscultated. Respiratory rate, dyspnea, grunting, dullness on percussion, diminished breath sounds, rhonci, atelectasis, consolidation and passive lungs congestion.

10. Abdomen should be palpated. Normally liver is palpable up to 3 cm in infants. It is enlarged in CCF up to 8 cm and may be felt to pulsate in TR with RVH. With digoxin liver size recedes rapidly and is measure of success of therapy.

     Palpable spleen, ascitis, prominently palpable aorta suggest an aneurysm or systemic hypertension.

11. Extremities should be examined. Clubbing of fingers with cyanosis is associated with congenital cyanotic heart disease, chronic cor pulmonale, arteriovenous fistula in lungs, cirrhosis of liver, infective endocarditis, polycythemia or hereditary anomaly. In cyanotic heart disease hands are warm and flushed and the nailbed at site of clubbing is shiny. Absent femorals suggest coarctation of aorta. Varying pulse strength indicates premature beats or arrhythmias. Bounding pulsations in both radial and femoral arteries occurs in aortic regurgitation, large PDA or thyrotoxicosis.

CARDIOFACIAL SYNDROME (ASYMMETRIC CRY)

First described by Parmalee in 1931 as a partial seventh cranial nerve palsy.

Cayler in 1969 first related the presence of congenital heart disease in this syndrome in 14 infants.

Pape and Pickering in 1972 published largest series of 44 cases varying in age from day 1 to 16 years with a variety of other anomalies associated with this syndrome.

The 7th CN palsy is not evident on smiling. The child must be made to cry vigorously.

Left side facial weakness occurs in 55% and right side weakness in 45% cases.

50% of these children have congenital cardiovascular abnormalities followed closely by abnormalities of head and neck and musculoskeletal system.

Other abnormalities in decreasing order of frequency are genitourinary, CNS, GIT and respiratory.

22% cases with asymmetric cry had no abnormalities. The cause of localized facial muscle weakness is not birth trauma or intrauterine posture or moulding, neither facial nerve palsy since electromyography shows intact nerve but absent facial muscle response.

Nelson and Eng in 1972 defined the condition as congenital hypoplasia of depressor anguli oris muscle, thus differentiating it from congenital facial palsy.

The asymmetric cry persists with passage of time as late as up to 15 years of age.

There is no cosmetic problem and individual is able to smile normally. It is only when the lips are widely contracted as in crying or an excessive grimace that the failure of lower corner of mouth becomes apparent.

The heart defects found in this syndrome are TOF, PDA, TA, VSD, ASD, single ventricle, bicuspid aortic valve, double aortic arch, truncus arteriosus and aortic stenosis.

CONGENITAL HEART DISEASE AND SCOLIOSIS

It occurs from 1 to 19% of cases of congenital heart disease. Overall incidence is 12%. It is 3 times more common in cyanotic CHD. Maximum incidence is 45%, between 4 and 9 years. 18% above 9 years.

Scoliosis occurs earlier in cyanotic CHD than it does when scoliosis is an isolated phenomenon.

Incidence of scoliosis in general population is 0.03 to 6%. Thoracic curve occurs in 50% cases. Thoracolumbar in 12%. Lumbar in 20%.

Congenital anomalies associated with scoliosis and CHD are club foot, cleft palate, Down syndrome, mental retardation and tracheoesophageal fistula.

Cardiac lesions most commonly associated with scoliosis are TOF, VSD, ASD, PDA and coarctation of aorta.

Congenital scoliosis occurs as result of abnormalities of vertebrae. This could be wedge shape body or hemivertebrae or failure of segmentation. Sometimes a boney bar joining nearby ribs. Abnormalities can be seen on chest X-ray.

Scoliosis congenital or idiopathic may be recognized in early years of life. Majority are static throughout growth period of child. If the curvature is progressive it can be corrected surgically with a Milwaukee brace, Harrington rod or Dwyer cable instrumentation. Surgical fusion can be done to prevent further spinal deviation.

HEART SOUNDS

- Pitch is the frequency of vibrations per second.
  - Intensity is the magnitude of sound wave.
  - Harmonics and overtones modify the quality of sound.
- Duration of heart sound determines whether it is recognized as a click, snap, tone or murmur.
  - The click is shortest and murmur longest.
  - Human ear is unable to detect some sounds immediately after hearing some loud sounds. This is fatigue phenomenon or masking.

– The closest splitting that can be appreciated by the ear is that of clicks at an interval of 0.02 second apart.

FIRST HEART SOUND

The first component is inaudible. It is a minor vibration that appears to be related to the muscle bundles of LV and the initial change is the shape of that chamber during systole. This is named zero component. First segment of higher frequency occurs during the early phase of the rise of LV pressure and of its first derivative. It is caused by tension of LV structures with acceleration of the walls and deceleration of blood within chamber.

Second component of higher frequency occurs at time of opening of aortic valve and coincides with an indentation or a second peak of first derivative of LV curve. This sound is related to sudden acceleration of blood and deceleration of structures that occur immediately after opening of aortic valve. C component appears at time of first peak of aortic pulse when it changes from a very rapid to less rapid rise in pressure. It coincides with peak of first derivative of aortic pulse. This component is believed to be caused by vibrations of infundibulum of LV, in walls of aorta and blood contained in these chambers. There may be a D component which occurs with maximal expansion of aortic wall and is therefore a vascular vibration. This interpretation recognizes exclusive importance of LV in causing first heart sound.

The first component occurs at first third of LV pressure rise. The second component occurs at opening of aortic valve. Third component occurs at point at which the still rising aortic pressure curve shows a change towards horizontal.

An alternative explanation suggests that both left and right heart events contribute to production of first heart sound. First component is related to atrial contraction—atrial component of first heart sound. This sound is absent whenever QRS complex is not preceded by a P-wave. It coincides with or occurs just after Q-waves. It is probably due to ventricular filling and can be audible in some healthy people.

Second low frequency component which is inaudible occurs at time of crossover of LV and LA pressures and could be due to coaptation of mitral valve leaflets.

Third component a higher frequency sound and first major audible component occurs coincident with LA 'C' wave and with point of maximal posterior motion of anterior mitral valve leaflet as seen in echocardiogram. This is thought to be due to tensing of chordae tendinae and mitral valve.

Fourth component and second easily audible component occurs coincident with right atrial 'C' wave and also with point of closure of tricuspid valve as shown on the echocardiogram. Factors delaying tricuspid valve closure delay this component. A few audible after vibrations may follow this last component. There is a relation between first heart sound and rapidity of LV contraction.

First heart sound is increased in amplitude in hyper-thyroidism or with administration of drugs that stimulate myocardium directly or indirectly, e.g. epinephrine and amyl nitrite. First heart sound may be decreased in amplitude when there is weakness of LV contraction.

First heart sound varies in complete AV block. This is related to timing of atrial contraction in relation to ventricular contraction. First heart sound varies with length of PR interval in acute rheumatic fever in children with or without mitral insufficiency. First heart sound is soft or almost absent when the conduction time in a child is between 0.18 and 0.24 seconds.

Splitting of first Heart Sound

There are two high frequency components of first heart sound. Mitral and tricuspid, attributable to closure or tension of two AV valves. Tricuspid valve closure follows mitral valve closure. In normal Phonocardiogram splitting of first heart sound is evident in components A and B. Separation of these two components may be very close and not audible by human ear.

Increased Intensity of First Heart Sound

This occurs when there is rapid ventricular upstroke, increased atrioventricular flow as in left to right shunt or in high cardiac output. Shortening of atrial ventricular filling time as in tachycardia due to any cause also causes increased intensity of first heart sound.

An increased intensity of first heart sound also occurs in presence of short PR interval.

Loud first heart sound in mitral stenosis is always associated with a loud opening snap.

Reduced intensity of first heart sound: Due to poor conduction through chest wall, prolonged PR interval or a myocardial disease with slow rise of ventricular pressure pulse.

Systolic Sounds

Early systolic ejection sounds may be divided into aortic and pulmonary.

Aortic ejection sounds result from aortic valve disease. Aortic stenosis, aortic regurgitation or bicuspid aortic valve. They also occur as a result of dilated aorta which may be found in marked pulmonary stenosis with a VSD or pulmonary atresia with a VSD or in systemic hypertension or in idiopathic dilatation of aorta. The sound also occurs in syphilitic and atheromatous aortas. Aortic ejection sound occurs 0.06 seconds after chief components of first heart sound. This ejection sound is well heard in mitral area but is usually best heard in fourth left intercostal space and less well at apex.

Aortic ejection sounds occur later than pulmonary ejection sound and do not vary much during respiration as do pulmonary ejection sounds.

Pulmonary ejection sounds occur in pulmonary valve stenosis and pulmonary artery dilatation. Pulmonary artery dilatation may be due to pulmonary hypertension as in Eisenmenger syndrome or it may be idiopathic. Pulmonary ejection sounds can usually be identified down the left sternal border particularly in third and fourth intercostal space but they are poorly transmitted to apex. Sounds diminish or disappear during inspiration. There is usually some dilatation of pulmonary artery in ASD but a pulmonary ejection sound is not heard until after the repair and then be related to dilated but slack pulmonary artery.

An aneurysm of membranous portion of ventricular septum may be associated with VSD. A click may occur 120 mili second after Q-waves of ECG and is highly indicative of the pathology.

Post Ejection Clicks

These sounds occur after rapid upstroke and after the rapid ejection phase is over. They occur in mid or late systole, heard by stetho. They can occur in normal children but most commonly are associated with mitral valve prolapse and are usually accompanied by systolic murmur honking in type and best heard at apex.

SECOND HEART SOUND

Aortic valve closure is louder of the two components of second heart sound in all areas including pulmonary area in normal heart and is sole component heard in mitral area. Pulmonary valve closure is softer and confined to pulmonary area chiefly. It is best identified on inspiration that prolongs right ventricular systole. Splitting of second sound in pulmonary area is not audible on expiration in 98% of children. Thus a single sound on expiration is normal finding in children. On inspiration two components of second sound are separated by an interval varying from 0.02 to 0.06 sec. A greater separation can be achieved by slow deep respiration in reclining posture. An inaudibility of P2 is rare at any age but is usually due to low intensity rather than fusion with A2. This occurs when hyperinflation of lungs is present.

Second Sound In Heart Abnormalities

Wide splitting of second heart sound may occur in right bundle branch block (RBBB), ASD, anomalous venous return, PS, RVF and myocarditis.

In RBBB there is delayed rise in RV pressure resulting in late pulmonary valve closure. Some variation with respiration can be identified.

In ASD there is increased width of splitting due to large stroke volume and a measure of RBBB. In presence of a large defect splitting is fixed and does not vary significantly with phases of respiration. However after surgery splitting may continue but will vary with inspiration.

With anomalous venous return there is invariably a large ASD. There issue wide fixed splitting of two components of second heart sound in pulmonary area.

In pulmonary valve stenosis with intact ventricular septum pulmonary component is soft and greatly delayed. In severe stenosis pulmonary valve closure is not audible. In pulmonary stenosis with VSD pulmonary second sound is absent due to markedly diminished pulmonary blood flow and pressure in pulmonary artery. But if there is a relatively large pulmonary blood flow and configuration of valve suitable a pulmonary closure sound may be audible. It may occasionally be heard after a successful Blalock operation.

In VSD with left to right shunt splitting of second heart sound may be of normal degree and pulmonary component of normal intensity. This is because most VSD are small and heart is functionally normal. When shunt is increased without increasing pulmonary vascular resistance splitting of second sound may be increased in width but not fixed because large VSD may have both systolic and diastolic loading of both ventricles. Splitting of second sound in significant VSD does not vary more than 0.1–0.2 sec with inspiration and in such cases diastolic shunting accounts for a substantial amount of blood flow and this tends to damp normal respiratory variation while not completely abolishing it. As pulmonary vascular resistance rises over several years in children proceeding to Eisenmenger syndrome degree of splitting between A2 and P2 is gradually reduced until they become fused. Thus a single fused second sound is characteristic of VSD with high pulmonary vascular resistance.

Splitting of second sound in pulmonary area may occur in pulmonary arterial hypertension when there is delay in pulmonary component due to right heart failure. Pulmonary second sound may also be delayed in systolic overloading of RV due to RBBB.

Reverse Splitting of Second Heart Sound

This occurs when pulmonary valve closure is completed before aortic valve closure. It may be found in LBBB and WPW syndrome when early RV activation may take place.

Reverse splitting is also found in aortic stenosis, systolic hypertension, LVF and myocarditis.

Single Second Heart Sound

This may occur in TOF with pulmonary atresia or severe pulmonary stenosis. It may occur in Eisenmenger syndrome with VSD. Or it may be found in single ventricle with pulmonary atresia or with high pulmonary vascular resistance. Uncommonly a single second sound may be considered to be present when pulmonary and aortic component is inaudible.

Diastolic Sounds

There are three causes of early diastolic valve opening sounds:
1. Atrioventricular valve opening snap occurs in mitral stenosis.
2. Atrioventricular valve abnormalities without stenosis, such as occurs in Ebstein anomaly.
3. Increased atrioventricular flow which is a common phenomenon in left to right shunt in children but may also occur in acute rheumatic fever and at times in normal child.

In mitral stenosis it occurs as a result of fused cusps somewhat thickened carried by rapid ventricular inflow into LV which produces a sharp sound.

In CHD a mid-diastolic murmur is frequently result of a left to right shunt than it is due to MS.

THIRD HEART SOUND

Rapid ventricular filling causes vibrations that are sufficiently intense to be audible as third heart sound occurring 0.15 sec after second heart sound.

Third heart sound occurs in some healthy children. Its low pitch is more readily audible by bell rather than diaphragm of stethoscope. It is best heard at apex after inspiration when child is turned on his side. Third heart sound is heard in 8% of normal children and 50% of children with RHD. Occasionally third heart sound may appear to have some duration because of fusion of asynchronous filling sounds from each ventricle. This can mimic a mild diastolic rumble.

FOURTH HEART SOUND

Normally atrial contraction is inaudible. A large A-wave coupled with atrial sound is a useful measure of ventricular abnormalities. It is more audible in childhood when there is a summation of atrial sound and ventricular filling sound as occurs in gallop rhythm.

HEART MURMURS

Leatham classified heart murmurs due to three main factors:

1. High flow through a normal or abnormal valve.
2. Forward flow through a constricted or abnormal valve into a dilated vessel or heart chamber.
3. Regurgitant flow through an incompetent valve or a congenital anomaly, e.g. PDA or VSD.

CLASSIFICATION OF MURMURS

A. Systolic Ejection and Systolic Regurgitant Murmurs

1. Left ventricular outflow tract murmurs:
   a. Valvar: Aortic stenosis.
   b. Subvalvar: Discrete subvalvular aortic stenosis.
   c. Supravalvar: Narrowing of ascending aorta.
2. Left ventricular inflow tract murmurs:
   a. Valvar: Mitral regurgitation.
3. Right ventricular outflow tract murmurs:
   a. Valvar: Pulmonary stenosis.

b. Subvalvar: Infundibular stenosis.

c. Supravalvar: Supravalvar pulmonary stenosis.

4. Right ventricular inflow tract murmurs:

a. Tricuspid regurgitation.

B. Diastolic Murmurs

1. Regurgitation across semilunar valves:

a. Aortic regurgitation.

b. Pulmonary regurgitation.

2. Increased flow across atrioventricular valves:

a. Increased flow across mitral valves:

– PDA.

– VSD.

– Austin Flint murmurs.

b. Increased flow across tricuspid valves:

– Atrial septal defect.

– Mitral regurgitation.

– Tricuspid regurgitation.

– Aortic regurgitation.

– Ebstein anomaly.

3. Obstruction at atrioventricular valve:

a. Mitral stenosis.

b. Parachute mitral valve.

c. Tricuspid stenosis.

d. Intracardiac tumors.

C. Continuous Murmurs

- Patent ductus arteriosus.
- Blalock shunt.
- Arteriovenous aneurysm of lung.
- Large collateral to pulmonary artery from bronchial artery.
- Aortic septal defect.
- Coronary artery aneurysm or fistula.
- Total anomalous pulmonary venous return.
- Communication of aneurysm of aortic sinus with pulmonary artery, right atrium or right ventricle.

- Traumatic arteriovenous fistula of thorax.
- Congenital arteriovenous fistula in chest wall.
- Anomalous coronary artery entering pulmonary artery.
- Coarctation of pulmonary artery.
- Dissecting aneurysm with fistula communicating with right atrium.

SYSTOLIC EJECTION MURMURS

A mid systolic ejection murmur may occur as a result of valvar or infundibular obstruction of the right or left ventricular outflow tract or it may be due to an increased rate of ejection through an otherwise normal valve or slightly irregular valve without narrowing or simply due to dilatation of pulmonary artery or aorta beyond a normal valve.

A murmur from such a cause is usually described as diamond shaped and begins after closure of atrioventricular valves and stops before semilunar valve closure.

An ejection murmur from right heart may be diamond shape with a peak occurring little later than left heart since the pressure in right ventricle is usually less than left ventricle. When there is marked ventricular obstruction the systolic murmur is prolonged and more rounded in shape when recorded. Intensity of aortic ejection or closure sounds is related to valve mobility and not primarily to severity of narrowing of valve. In differential diagnosis of left ventricular outflow tract obstruction one needs to consider valvar, subvalvar and supravalvar origin as well as that due to idiopathic hypertrophic subaortic stenosis. Acquired aortic stenosis is uncommon in children.

Murmur significant of LVOT obstruction is best heard in first and second right intercostal space and second and third left intercostal space. It radiates into neck. Murmur may be well heard at apex.

Right ventricular outflow tract obstruction may occur as isolated valvar or infundibular pulmonary narrowing with intact ventricular septum but more commonly it occurs with ventricular septal defect as in tetralogy of Fallot.

Pure valvar pulmonary stenosis causes ejection phase to lengthen as obstruction becomes more severe. Pulmonary closure sound is therefore progressively delayed and splitting of second heart sound widens. At the same time pulmonary closure sound becomes fainter and finally disappears. Aortic closure sound is masked by prolonged systolic murmur.

In presence of infundibular obstruction pulmonary ejection sound or click is never encountered and pulmonary closure sound is not audible except in mildest cases.

When stenosis is at valve click is present. When pressure gradient is less than 80 cm of Hg splitting of second sound is wider than one would expect with infundibular stenosis. Mechanism of respiratory variation in intensity of pulmonary ejection sound or click.

During expiration sound becomes louder and later with longer interval between it and first heart sound. During inspiration there is decrease in pulmonary end diastolic pressure that parallels change in intrathoracic pressure. In contrast there is absolute increase in right ventricular end diastolic pressure with equalization during atrial filling phase. This is due to increased venous return during inspiration augmenting right ventricular end diastolic volume. This leads to early opening of pulmonary valve prior to right ventricular systole and when right ventricular systole does occur movement of dome of valve is minimal or absent. During expiration pulmonary end diastolic pressure increases and exceeds right ventricular end diastolic pressure and pulmonary valve remains in closed position in diastole. With onset of right ventricular systole sudden ascent of dome of valve produces loud ejection sound.

In tetralogy of Fallot very clear aortic closure sound is heard but pulmonary valve closure is inaudible. This differentiates tetralogy of Fallot from isolated pulmonary stenosis. In branch stenosis of pulmonary artery there is ejection systolic murmur at upper left and right sternal borders that is widely transmitted to right chest and back and often to axilla. Systolic murmur may become continuous particularly with more peripheral pulmonary artery stenosis. There may be loud often palpable pulmonary closure sound accompanied by late ejection click in Eisenmenger's syndrome associated with ventricular septal defect. There may be short faint systolic murmur and pulmonary diastolic murmur as pulmonary vascular disease progresses in severity.

Increased flow across pulmonary valve, e.g. in atrial septal defect may produce systolic ejection murmur.

Flow murmur can also occur in anemia, hyperthyroidism, fever, anxiety, exercise and excitement.

In straight back syndrome in which there is loss of normal thoracic kyphosis of spine in young people benign ejection systolic murmur is heard. Murmur may be associated with wide splitting of heart sounds and pulmonary ejection sound that varies with respiration. Diagnosis is by lateral X-ray of spine which demonstrates lack of normal thoracic kyphosis.

SYSTOLIC REGURGITANT MURMURS

There is flow of blood in retrograde fashion from one chamber or vessel of higher pressure to a chamber or vessel of lower pressure during systole, e.g. mitral regurgitation.

In mitral regurgitation at the onset of left ventricular contraction pressure rises in ventricle and closes mitral valve. A murmur then begins with or immediately after the first heart sound. In rheumatic heart disease with mitral regurgitation, atrioventricular conduction time is prolonged and this permits the mitral and tricuspid valves to assume a closed or nearly closed position before onset of ventricular systole. This has effect of softening first heart sound. When regurgitation is marked there is a large reservoir of blood at beginning of ventricular diastole in left atrium and this gives rise to rapid ventricular filling sound that is recognized as a short diastolic rumble at the beginning of diastole. This is a common finding in children with considerable mitral regurgitation, tricuspid regurgitation, atrial septal defect and ventricular septal defect.

In tricuspid insufficiency during inspiration there is decrease in intrathoracic pressure which results in increased venous return to right atrium. This in turn increases blood flow through right side of heart and intensifies tricuspid murmur. Murmur of tricuspid regurgitation is best heard in lower left sternal border area. Murmur increases with inspiration and decreases with expiration.

In ventricular septal defect a pansystolic murmur is heard in lower precordium often with a thrill. In infant and young children in whom murmur is decreasing in size the murmur may become shorter and fainter, while it may begin with onset of systole it may disappear before end of systole as defect becomes progressively smaller before ultimately closing completely. A midsystolic murmur may occur in mitral regurgitation due to papillary muscle dysfunction. Inadequate tension of papillary muscle may cause prolapse of part of mitral valve which produces some mitral regurgitation and midsystolic murmur. Fibrotic or scarred papillary muscle may hold down leaflet during ventricular contraction and produce systolic murmur. Dilated ventricle may displace papillary muscles and prevent proper coaptation of valve leaflets during systole and produce murmur.

When systolic murmur of mitral regurgitation is due to prolapse of anterior leaflet of mitral valve the flow is directed over posterior leaflet. The murmur is then usually best heard at apex and transmitted to axilla. When prolapse occurs in posterior leaflet of mitral valve with flow being directed at anterior leaflet murmur is more likely to be directed to base of heart or to left of sternum. Abnormal prolapse of mitral valve leaflet usually involves posterior cusp and anomaly may be related to minor papillary muscle dysfunction. Systolic murmur is often accompanied by click or snapping sound. A variety of physical or physiological maneuvers, exercising patient or administration of drugs may alter intensity and timing of murmur and click.

Systolic honking, whooping or musical noises are produced by transvenous pacemaker catheters situated across tricuspid valve. In hypertrophic obstructive cardiomyopathy which is associated with left ventricular outflow tract obstruction and mitral regurgitation there is diminished compliance in hypertrophied portion of left ventricle muscle. This produces prominent 'A' wave and audible atrial gallop sound. Pathological problem is eccentric hypertrophy of septum which is progressive and associated with abnormal contraction of papillary muscles that leads to anterior displacement of anterior leaflet of mitral valve. Thus during systole there is an initial period in which there is no significant obstruction of left ventricular outflow tract but with progression of contraction of ventricle the septum deviates and bulges to left thus, the anterior leaflet of mitral valve is in apposition with it producing obstruction to outflow tract of left ventricle. Initially there is an ejection systolic murmur without gradient. However, as contraction proceeds gradient develops in outflow tract and second murmur of mitral regurgitation occurs. In summary there is early rapid ejection period followed by rapid upstroke of carotid pressure and flow murmur occurs in early systole. Thereafter a significant pressure gradient develops with flow diminishing through obstructive outflow tract as it narrows. This period is followed by late systolic murmur due to mitral regurgitation. In diastole there is atrial diastolic gallop associated with decreasing compliance of left ventricle. If there is distension or increased volume of left ventricle muscular obstruction of outflow tract may be diminished and thus alter murmurs. Such agents as isoproterenol and digoxin increase obstruction and beta adrenergic blockers decrease obstruction. Straining phase of Valsalva maneuver decrease diastolic volume and therefore increases obstruction. Vasopressor agents may diminish intensity of murmur by increasing afterload. Intensity of murmur parallels the gradient, getting louder with more severe obstruction and fainter with diminution of gradient.

DIASTOLIC MURMURS

They are commonly produced by increased flow across tricuspid or mitral valves or due to a regurgitant valve either pulmonary or aortic, only occasionally in children narrowing or obstruction of atrioventricular valve produces a diastolic murmur as in mitral stenosis.

AORTIC VALVE REGURGITATION

Murmur is best heard down left sternal edge using diaphragm of stethoscope, more easily found at end of expiration with breath held or with patient sitting up and leaning forward. Murmur begins after aortic component or second and usually fades away as first sound is approached.

Aortic regurgitation may also produce diastolic murmur at apex referred to as Austin Flint murmur which is due to vibration of mitral valve because of aortic regurgitant flow back into left ventricle and augmented by vibrations due to atrial systole.

PULMONARY VALVE REGURGITATION

This is commonly heard in postoperative period in patients who have undergone total correction of tetralogy of Fallot. Pulmonary regurgitation may also occur in Eisenmenger syndrome, congenital anomaly of pulmonary valve and infective endocarditis.

INCREASED FLOW ACROSS TRICUSPID VALVE

In presence of atrial septal defect or shunt from left atrium to right atrium flow through tricuspid valve may be two to three times that of mitral valve. Right ventricle is enlarged and at onset of diastole there is rush of blood into dilated ventricle that causes diastolic murmur. Similar murmur may be heard in tricuspid regurgitation due to overloading of right atrium. It is also heard in Ebstein disease, hyperthyroidism and severe anemia. In presence of left to right shunt at aortic level or ventricular septal level there is increased flow across mitral valve which produces an inflow diastolic murmur and usually indicates that a considerable shunt is present.

ATRIOVENTRICULAR VALVE NARROWING OR STENOSIS

Diastolic murmur of mitral stenosis is due to blood propelled at stenotic orifice of valve. Part of murmur is inflow diastolic and occurs early in diastole. Second part is associated with atrial systole and is often referred to as presystolic. In presence of atrial fibrillation presystolic accentuation disappears and only mid diastolic murmur persists.

CONTINUOUS MURMUR

This means murmur begins in systole and goes into diastole. Murmur need not be through entire cardiac cycle. Classical continuous murmur is heard with patent ductus arteriosus. Murmur begins just after second sound, reaches its peak with rise of aortic pressure and subsides during diastole but may go right up to next first heart sound depending upon pressure gradient between aorta and pulmonary artery. If pressure in pulmonary artery rises it shortens diastolic component of murmur. If pressure in pulmonary artery equals that in aorta murmur may disappear entirely or may simply be heard as short systolic murmur.

In newborn because of high pulmonary artery pressure a faint murmur or no murmur at all may be present and murmur may become continuous as pressure in pulmonary artery falls. Murmur disappears as ductus closes.

Similar murmur may be heard from large collaterals from bronchial artery to pulmonary artery.

When there is an anomalous coronary artery entering pulmonary artery murmur is usually absent but when present it is fainter than that heard in patent ductus arteriosus. Coronary artery aneurysm or fistula may give continuous murmur but this is heard louder over lower precordium than in pulmonary area.

Murmur of congenital arteriovenous fistula may be similar. Narrowing in coarctation of pulmonary artery may give a similar continuous murmur but such murmur is more likely to be distributed out into chest and is softer than patent ductus arteriosus murmur since narrowing of pulmonary artery is usually not extreme.

Venous hum may be heard over upper precordium in many normal children due to flow of blood into large collecting veins at entrance to right atrium. Such murmurs are often heard above or below right or left clavicle. They may vary with respiration and can often be obliterated or diminished by turning head to one side or another.

Murmur of coarctation of aorta may rarely be heard as continuous murmur. It is recognized as systolic murmur usually in pulmonary area and referred through to back. In spite of stethoscope impression of systolic murmur a sound tracing shows that murmur extends into early diastole.

FUNCTIONAL CARDIAC MURMURS

Approximately half of normal children have systolic murmur of some degree in some portion of precordium.

The criteria for benign murmurs of heart are:
1. Relatively low intensity.
2. Limited to small area.
3. Short duration.
4. Coarse vibratory quality.
5. Lack of other evidence of heart disease.

Short systolic murmur appearing at tachycardia and disappearing when heart rate slows to normal are functional. Such murmurs may appear with fever, anxiety, exercise and infection and disappear during resting state.

Murmurs that disappear during inspiration are usually functional.

There are two common types of functional murmurs that cause difficulty in diagnosis in infancy and childhood:
1. **Venous hum:** Best heard in aortic area conducted to neck. Also occasionally heard in pulmonary area. This is continuous murmur and since it varies in intensity it simulates patent ductus arteriosus. Its softness and lack of machinery like quality help to distinguish it from patent ductus arteriosus. It has diastolic accentuation in contrast to systolic accentuation characteristic of patent ductus arteriosus. Slightly louder with inspiration.
   Venous hum has its origin in jugular vein as it joins subclavian. It is more readily heard with patient sitting up

and head slightly extended and turned to left. Pressure on jugular vein diminish or obliterate murmur entirely.

Graf and associates in 1947 found venous hum in 50% children under 9 years age and in 30% between 12 and 15 years age.

2. Lower precordial murmur between apex and sternum

It is coarse, low pitched, vibratory or twanging string type murmur. It may encroach upon mitral area thus suggesting possibility of rheumatic origin. However, it is best heard to right of apex and not over it. It is shorter in duration than murmur of mitral regurgitation and has coarser scratchy quality. Soft first heart sound may also occur with this functional murmur. However, this functional murmur is not transmitted to axilla.

REGULATION OF BLOOD PRESSURE

CAROTID SINUS REFLEX SYSTEM

This is mediated through pressor receptors located in walls of internal carotid arteries and aorta. If arterial pressure increases, walls of these vessels are stretched and impulses flow to medullary portion of brain where they inhibit sympathetic nervous system and excite parasympathetic. This leads to decrease in activity of heart and dilatation of peripheral arterioles. Action of parasympathetic nerves further decrease cardiac activity and blood pressure is reduced. This mechanism is brought into play in few seconds resulting in readjustment of circulation. Delay in this response leads to fainting.

CNS AND ISCHEMIC RESPONSE

This is not initiated until blood pressure falls to 20 mm Hg. It is activated by severe shock or marked elevation of CSF pressure or a tumor of brain compressing vasomotor center. It may also be initiated in severe cyanotic congenital heart disease. It contributes at times to initial slightly elevated blood pressure seen in newborn in first few minutes of life.

ABILITY OF SMOOTH MUSCLES OF VEINS AND ARTERIES

Relaxation and contraction depends upon volume they enclose. Major response lies in veins which can accommodate to markedly increased blood volume in 15 to 30 minutes. This mechanism appears to be effective after cord is tied in newborn baby as adjustment of excess blood from placenta takes place. It is probably a helpful adjustment in first 6 hours of life when there is increase in circulating blood volume.

ABILITY OF CAPILLARIES

Capillaries shunt or shift fluid in and out of tissues permitting more adequate adjustment to large blood transfusion or excessive blood loss.

HEMODYNAMIC RESPONSE OF KIDNEYS

This acts slowly and is dependent on renal blood flow and pressure with excretion or retention of fluid and salt.

HORMONAL ACTIVITY

This alters renal arterial pressure through release of glomerulotropin from brain cells thus affecting secretion of aldosteron which in turn acts on renal tubular epithelium and causes absorption of sodium and retention of water. A normal healthy newborn has an average blood pressure of 80 mm Hg. This falls to a level between 60 to 65 mm Hg and then gradually rises over a period of days and weeks until it stabilizes between 90 to 100 mm Hg at 5 months.

Premature babies have mean level 40 to 60 mm Hg.

Newborn with respiratory distress syndrome have lower systolic blood pressure during first 3 weeks of life. Elevated blood pressure in early moments of life appears to be due to sympathetic stimulation associated with trauma of birth. In difficult delivery there may be added factor of ischemic response.

Width of be Cuff

Premature 3 cm
Newborn to 2 years 4.5 cm

2 to 4 years 7 cm
5 to 9 years 10 cm
10 to 14 years 13 cm
15 cm for larger children with obese arms and legs

Methods

1. *Auscultation*: Systolic pressure is that point at which initial Korotkoff sounds are heard. Muffling of sounds is the best index of diastolic pressure.
2. Palpation
3. *Flush technique*: A suitable size cuff is placed around arm. Baby's arm is elevated and hand grasped firmly so that as large an area as possible is blanched. Pressure is maintained while cuff pressure is elevated. Cuff is slowly deflated and hand observed for signs of flushing. Point at which flush first appears in blanched area is taken as blood pressure. This method can show a pressure differential between arm and leg in coarctation of aorta.
4. *Oscillometer*: Pressure changes are transmitted through arterial wall to pressure cuff and hence to oscillometer where they are magnified to observer.
5. *Doppler ultrasound technique*: Arterial wall oscillations cause major components of Korotkoff sounds. Properly placed Doppler ultrasound transducer is more sensitive in directly detecting arterial wall oscillations than stethoscope.

   Determination of blood pressure in infants and children is useful in coarctation of aorta, aortic insufficiency, aortic stenosis, patent ductus arteriosus, poliomyelitis, acute and chronic nephritis, hypertension, pheochromocytoma, head injuries, brain tumor, vasovagal syncope, myocarditis and shock.

CHEST X-RAY IN CONGENITAL HEART DISEASE

PULMONARY VASCULAR PATTERN

The vessels may be normal, increased or decreased in size. If increased vascular disorder may involve arteries predominantly as in left to right shunt or bidirectional shunt or veins secondary to left side obstructive lesions.

A shunt and obstruction may coexist.

During first few days of life there is persistence of high pulmonary vascular resistance of fetal circulation and in some instances vessels may remain small due to hypoxic vasoconstriction. Normal pulmonary arteries are seen extending out from hila and taper gradually toward lung periphery. Intrapulmonary arteries in lower lobes are usually larger in caliber than those in upper lobes. Vessels margins are distinct. An end on pulmonary artery branch and companion air containing bronchus are visible in perihilar area. Normally these are of equal size. Enlarged pulmonary artery and pulmonary vein occur as a result of left to right shunt. In perihilar area end on artery and bronchus are visible and artery will be larger than bronchus. Vessels extend further in periphery than normal. Enlargement of pulmonary artery is not apparent radiologically when there is left to right shunt with pulmonary to systemic flow ratio of < 2 : 1.

Engorgement of pulmonary artery when due to left to right shunt at ventricular or great artery level is usually a manifestation of both increased blood flow and increased pressure in pulmonary vascular bed. Patients with large left to right shunt may develop left heart failure due to left side volume overloading. In mild form pulmonary artery is enlarged and lungs are clear. In severe form dilated arteries in perihilar region lose their distinct margins and become blurred due to leakage of fluid in interstitial perivascular sheath. There may be associated clouding of lungs due to pulmonary edema. Pleural effusion may develop.

In infants lungs in this situation are hyperinflated and diaphragm flattened.

Pulmonary venous hypertension may be due to left side obstructive lesions or primary left ventricular disorders that result in left ventricular failure. The changes are manifest by a redistribution of blood flow such that vascular pattern in upper lobes is greater than that in lower lobes.

As venous pressure rises there is leakage of fluid in interstitial tissue and alveoli producing a reticular pattern that extends out to lung periphery with varying degree of interstitial veiling. In lateral film clear definitions of all vessels margins in hila are lost and airways are indistinct due to enlarged vessels and perivascular and peribronchial edema. Thickened interlobar septa are visible as short horizontal lines abutting on pleura in costophrenic angles (Kerley B lines).

Decreased pulmonary vascularity occurs with right to left shunt as in tetralogy of Fallot. Diameter of pulmonary artery is reduced. Pulmonary arteries extend to lung fields in periphery only to junction of inner and middle third. Main pulmonary artery is small. In lateral films pulmonary artery small and hila appear empty. Proximal bronchi and distal trachea are visualized clearly. Pulmonary vascular obstruction in its most severe form, e.g. pulmonary atresia may present disorganized vascular pattern. Small stringy vessels representing an intermingled bronchial and pulmonary arteries are visible producing a reticular appearance throughout lung. Normal pulmonary trunk is not present and hila are small.

Unilateral pulmonary atresia or severe stenosis of main pulmonary artery branch can be recognized by decreased vascular pattern in one lung. Affected lung is usually small. Vascularity in unaffected lung is increased.

Prominence of main pulmonary artery may be observed as normal phenomenon in normal individual particularly in female in pediatric age group and is often termed idiopathic. Similar appearance is observed with pulmonary valve stenosis. Differentiation of these may be difficult radiologically. With pulmonary stenosis, however, dilatation of left main branch is also present and there is evidence of right ventricular enlargement. Aneurysmal dilatation of pulmonary artery may occur with tetralogy of Fallot and absent pulmonary valve or as an isolated lesion. Main pulmonary artery is grossly enlarged and there is dilatation of one branch more commonly right. Peripheral pulmonary vessels are either normal or slightly dilated. Enlargement of main pulmonary artery may obstruct a bronchus partially with development of emphysema.

High course of left pulmonary artery is described as diagnostic feature of truncus arteriosus.

HEART SIZE AND SHAPE

In neonate CT ratio of > 58% on supine film made at 403 focal film distance in inspiration can be considered to be abnormal. During first year ratio gradually decreases to be 50% on normal 6 feet focal film distance.

Interpretation of cardiac size may be complicated by thymic silhouette in neonate and young child up to 2 years age. In lateral film thymus is present anteriorly or a subtle notch is visible separating thymic shadow lower margin from heart. Should thymus merge imperceptibly with heart impressions of anterior rib may cause scalloping of apparent heart border. This when present is diagnostic of thymic tissue. Disappearance of thymus shadow occurs after one week therapy with oral steroid hormone administration.

In infancy and early childhood individual chamber enlargement is difficult to assess and one chamber, such as left ventricle may enlarge and displace right ventricle so simulate right side enlargement.

Cardiac Shapes in Congenital Heart Disease

Pulmonary vascularity increased
1. Egg shape: Complete D transposition of great arteries.
2. Snowman (figure of 8): Total anomalous pulmonary venous drainage to left vertical vein.
3. Triangle (no visible right superior vena cava): Atrial septal defect (secundum)
4. Discreet convex bulge at left upper cardiac border: Single ventricle with ventricular inversion, absent right ventricle sinus, left juxtaposition of atrial appendages.

Pulmonary Vascularity Increased or Normal

1. Long convex left superior mediastinal contour: Congenitally corrected L transposition of great arteries.
2. Prominent main pulmonary artery and left branch: Pulmonary stenosis.

Pulmonary Vascularity Normal

Scimitar syndrome: Hypoplasia right lung with anomalous pulmonary venous return.

Pulmonary Vascularity Decreased

Couer en Sabot: Tetralogy of Fallot.

AORTA

The contour of aorta and side of arch are diagnostic.

In infancy aorta is difficult to recognize because of thymus. Ascending aorta in children is usually not visible on posteroanterior film and when seen or if there is localized dilatation a diagnosis of aortic stenosis, aortic regurgitation or coarctation of aorta is suspected.

Upper descending aorta is usually clearly outlined particularly on a overpenetrated posteroanterior film. Left lateral margin is normally smooth. However, if it is notched a coarctation of aorta usually exists (so called '3' sign). Corroborative evidence may be obtained with barium esophagogram. Barium column in this case is indented on left both at level of aortic arch and just inferior to this by poststenotic dilated segment. Intervening protrusion of barium between two concavities representing coarctation site (so called 'E' sign).

Aortic arch or knob may be prominent often due to dilatation of root of subclavian artery, small in presence of a long segment preductal coarctation or not clearly visible as it is obscured by a dilated left subclavian artery.

Position of aortic arch when not clearly visible can be identified by deviation and indentation of trachea.

Although usually left side a right aortic arch in presence of levocardia is a strong evidence that congenital heart disease exists. Incidence of right aortic arch in congenital heart disease:

- Tetralogy of Fallot – 31%.
- Truncus arteriosus – 31%.
- Double outlet right ventricle – 20%.
- Tricuspid atresia – 5%.

- Isolated ventricular septal defect – 2.3%.
- Complete D transposition of great arteries – 2.3%.
- Congenitally corrected L transposition of great arteries – 1%.

POSITIONAL ANOMALIES OF HEART

Cardiac malposition may occur due to:

1. Secondary to anomalies of lung, diaphragm and skeleton. Atelectasis, hyperinflation of lung, elevation of hemidiaphragm or skeletal anomalies are easily recognized. Hypoplasia of lung due to absent one pulmonary artery or anomalous pulmonary venous connection (Scimitar syndrome) are difficult to recognize.

2. In association with asplenia or polysplenia. In normal individual with situs solitus of heart and abdominal viscera, aortic arch, stomach bubble and spleen are situated on left and liver on right. Left atrium is located on side of stomach and aortic arch is on left side. Position of cardiac apex is variable and although commonly left side (levocardia) it may be on right side (dextrocardia).

With situs inversus aortic arch, stomach and spleen are on right and liver on left side. Left atrium on right side. Cardiac apex is on right side. In presence of asplenia or polysplenia visceral situs may be indeterminate. Liver extends to both sides of midline and stomach bubble is central. When this relationship is present position of left atrium cannot be determined and complex cardiac disease should be suspected.

With visceral situs inversus, right aortic arch and dextrocardia incidence of severe cardiac disease is low. If there is dextrocardia with visceral situs solitus and left aortic arch or levocardia with visceral situs inversus and right aortic arch incidence of severe cardiac anomalies is high.

BONY THORAX

With clinical and radiologic stigmata of Down syndrome atrioventricular canal defect or ventricular septal defect are suspected.

Bone changes described are manubrium sterni with two separate ossification centers, absence of twelfth ribs and an abnormal configuration of lumbar vertebrae.

In rubella syndrome proximal end of humeri are irregular and show poor mineralization of growth plate with linear or ovoid lucencies that alter trabecular pattern in metaphysis. Patent ductus arteriosus and peripheral pulmonary artery branch stenosis are common.

Premature sternal segment fusion is well known with congenital heart disease both cyanotic and acyanotic. It appears to be more frequent in cyanotic congenital heart disease and more in females than males.

Pectus carinatum is more common in cyanotic congenital heart disease than acyanotic congenital heart disease.

Rib notching is a valuable sign in diagnosis of coarctation of aorta. It is not seen before 6 years of age. Most commonly 4th to 8th ribs are involved. If notching is unilateral coarctation site may be proximal to either left subclavian artery or an aberrant right subclavian artery. In former notching is confined to right ribs in later left ribs.

Patients with straight back syndrome may exhibit murmur simulating heart disease. Spine is straight and anteroposterior diameter is diminished in chest. Heart may appear enlarged and pulmonary artery prominent simulating pulmonary valve stenosis.

12

Embryology of Congenital Heart Disease

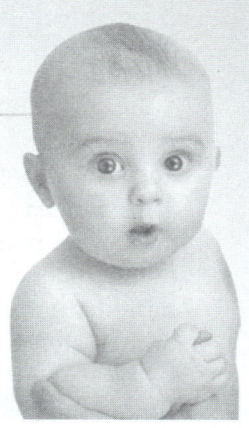

Heart develops from progressive fusion of pair of vessels that arise in mesoderm covering ventral aspect of foregut. Directly ventral to these vessels lies primitive pericardial cavity which has arisen from a split in mesoderm in this area and directly caudal lies septum transversum, a sheet of mesoderm lying between primitive thoracic and abdominal cavities.

Heart tube gradually invaginates dorsal wall of pericardial cavity so it comes to lie suspended in cavity by thin dorsal mesocardium.

Rapid growth of heart tube leads to development of marked flexure which has its convex aspect facing ventrally and also to breakdown of dorsal mesocardium leaving visceral layer of pericardium surrounding heart tube in continuity with parietal pericardium, lining fibrous pericardium only at its arterial and venous ends.

A series of dilatations now begin to appear in heart tube. These form from cephalic to caudal. Bulbus cordis and ventricle lying on ventrocephalic side and atrium on dorsocaudal side. Atrium and ventricle are connected by constricted portion of tube called atrioventricular canal.

Bulbus cordis is connected at its cephalic end to truncus arteriosus from which ventral aortae and 6 aortic arches arise. At caudal end sinus venosus which receives whole of venous drainage from embryo except that from lung buds opens into dorsal part of atrium. During 4th week of development bulboventricular loop twists to right carrying truncus arteriosus with it.

Bulbus cordis now joins right extremity of ventricle at sharp angle before passing up on ventral aspect of heart.

Turning of ventricle to right produces spiral twist in long-axis of both bulbus cordis and truncus arteriosus which is partially responsible for spiral course of aorticopulmonary and bulbar septa.

FORMATION OF SINUS VENOSUS AND ITS INCORPORATION INTO RIGHT ATRIUM

Early venous drainage of embryo consists of the following veins:
1. Right and left anterior and posterior cardinal veins which chain corresponding anterior and posterior half of embryo.
2. Right and left vitelline veins which drain yolk sac and primitive gut.
3. Right and left umbilical veins which drain blood from developing placenta.

Anterior and posterior cardinal veins on each side unite to form common cardinal veins which enter dorsal part of septum transversum and are here joined by right and left umbilical and vitelline veins to form right and left horns of sinus venosus. Subsequent changes due to growth of liver and development of cross anastomosis cut down number of veins entering sinus. Right horn of sinus venosus receives right common cardinal vein which becomes terminal part of superior vena cava and terminal part of right vitelline (hepatic) which becomes terminal part of inferior vena cava.

Left horn of sinus venosus which becomes coronary sinus loses all its extracardiac tributaries and persists because bulk of venous drainage of heart itself returns via this route.

Left common cardinal vein (left superior vena cava) disappears except for a thin fibrous strand passing down from last inch of left superior intercostal vein in front of root of left lung to join oblique vein of left atrium. This strand also indicates path taken by persistent left superior vena cava. Sinus venosus itself is gradually absorbed during 7th and 8th weeks into posterior part of right atrium.

Cephalic part of right valve of sinus venosus becomes incorporated into crista terminalis while caudal part forms valve of inferior vena cava and valve of coronary sinus. Left valve of sinus venosus becomes absorbed into interatrial septum and disappears.

Failure of sinus venosus to be absorbed in right atrium results in persistence of sinus venosus. In this condition right and left horns of sinus enlarge to form a chamber that lies posterior to right and left atria. This chamber receives right superior and inferior vena cava and frequently a persistent left superior vena cava as well. It communicates with posterior part of right atrium through an elliptic opening guarded by remains of right and left valves of sinus venosus.

During 4th week a single pulmonary vein arises from a capillary plexus that lies on ventral aspect of lung buds. This vein runs ventrally to enter venous mesocardium and penetrate posterior aspect of left atrium immediately to left of septum primum. It is subsequently absorbed into left atrium together with its tributaries right and left pulmonary veins. These two veins are gradually taken into atrium. Finally absorption continues until upper and lower tributaries of two pulmonary veins are reached so that it is usual to find an upper and lower vein entering left atrium on each side.

Early pulmonary venous plexus communicates freely with posterior and common cardinal veins. Terminal part of posterior cardinal vein becomes on right side arch of vena azygose and on left side part of left superior intercostal vein that lies on left side of arch of aorta. Occasionally one or more of pulmonary veins drain by way of channels derived from their early connections with cardinal system. In such cases they may drain directly into either azygose vein or into right atrium on right side or into an enlarged left superior intercostal vein, persistent left superior vena cava or coronary sinus on left side.

A greater or lesser amount of blood from lungs depends upon number of pulmonary veins that follow these abnormal routes is thus discharged into right atrium.

FORMATION OF CARDIAC SEPTA

There are four principle septa which develop to bring about formation of 4 chambered heart from original single tube. These are:

1. Interatrial septum.
2. Septum of atrioventricular canal.
3. Interventricular septum.
4. Bulbar septum.

INTERATRIAL SEPTUM

A compound septum made-up of two developmentally separate septa.

Septum primum develops during 5th week of intrauterine life as a sickle shape fold in dorsocephalic wall of primitive atrium, just to left of left valve of sinus venosus. Free margin of this fold grows ventrocaudally toward septum of atrioventricular canal which at this stage is formed by two mesodermal outgrowths, anterior and posterior endocardial cushions.

Passage between growing margin of septum primum and endocardial cushions of atrioventricular canal forms foramen primum of interatrial septum.

Finally during 6th week cephalic part of septum primum breaks down to form ostium secondum and lower margin of septum primum fuses with left edge of atrial surface of septum of atrioventricular canal.

Septum secondum appears during 6th week as thick crescentic fold on ventrocephalic wall of atrium between left valve of sinus venosus and septum primum. This septum grows in dorsocaudal direction gradually overlapping ostium secondum in septum primum and at same time incorporating left valve of sinus venosus into dorsal part of its right side.

Septum secondum ceases to grow just after its crescentic margin has overlapped foramen secundum.

Part of foramen primum not covered by septum secundum forms floor of fossa ovalis and lies opposite opening of inferior vena cava with result that blood entering right atrium by this route pushes thin septum primum to left and passes below thick margin of septum secundum and through foramen secundum into left atrium.

Aperture formed by boundary of lower margin of septum secundum and lower margin of foramen secundum forms foramen ovale.

Anterior part of septum secundum fuses with septum of atrioventricular canal immediately to right of septum primum.

Defect in normal growth pattern result in abnormalities:

1. Septum primum and septum secundum may fail to develop so that no separation of two atria occurs.

2. Septum primum and anterior part of septum secundum may fail to fuse with septum of atrioventricular canal giving rise to persistent foramen primum which may be either a single or fenestrated aperture. Foramen secundum may be normal or absent.

3. When there is delay in breakdown of septum secundum to form foramen secundum septum primum may be displaced into left atrium by increasing blood flow and fuse across its cavity. This results in left atrium being divided into a posterior chamber receiving pulmonary veins and an anterior chamber communicating with left auricular appendage, left ventricle and sometimes right atrium. A small foramen primum usually connects anterior and posterior chambers. Septum secundum may grow down to separate atria or it may be defective, leaving a communication between either right atrium and posterior chamber through a late forming foramen secundum or right atrium and anterior chamber below its crescentic lower margin. Floor of fossa ovalis being absent due to displaced foramen primum.

4. Septum secundum may fail to develop at all leaving a large patent foramen secundum.

5. Septum secundum may only partially overlap foramen ovale giving rise to various degrees of patent foramen ovale.

FORMATION OF SEPTUM OF ATRIOVENTRICULAR CANAL

During 5th week of intrauterine life two septa which are referred to as cushions because of their appearance begin to grow from dorsal and ventral aspects of atrioventricular canal. These broad septa are derived from mesenchyme of subendocardial region. As growth proceeds fusion between two septa occurs first on right side and then gradually extends across toward left leading to formation of a broad partition. It is with cephalic side of left side of this partition that atrial septa fuse.

Shortly after appearance of dorsal and ventral septa two lateral septa one on each side grow into canal to complete boundaries of primitive tricuspid and mitral valves. It is from mesenchymatous tissues of margins of these orifices that valve cusps develop. Defect in normal growth pattern of septa of atrioventricular canal may result in abnormalities:

1. Dorsal and ventral septa may fail to fuse so that there is no division of atrioventricular canal although a large dorsal and ventral valve usually develops along unfused margins of these septa.
2. Dorsal and ventral septa may arise and fuse more to one side or other of atrioventricular canal leading to greater or lesser degree of stenosis of mitral or tricuspid valve. This is more liable to occur on right side because this orifice becomes closely related to right bulbar ridge as it passes down to join ventricular septum.
3. Dorsal and ventral septa may fuse incompletely and as fusion normally occurs first on right side usually results in bifid or double anterior cusp to mitral valve.

INTERVENTRICULAR SEPTUM AND BULBAR SEPTUM

Division of common ventricle into right and left ventricles is intimately associated with division of bulbus cordis. This is to be expected since bulbus cordis will be gradually incorporated into right and left ventricles to form infundibulum and aortic vestibule respectively and for this reason bulbar defects are often associated with interventricular septal defects.

During 4th week there is a sharp flexure at junction of bulbus cordis with ventricle. During 5th – 6th week depth of this flexure is gradually reduced which considerably shortens length of posterior wall of bulbus cordis and eventually results in its disappearance thus bringing aortic valve ring in contact with ventral aspect of fused endocardial cushions. This disappearance of posterior wall of bulbus cordis as result of reduction of bulboventricular sulcus also means that there will be no muscle in posterior wall of bulbus cordis. Whether this part of outflow tract lies in contact with mitral or tricuspid valve area of endocardial cushions or is entirely separate from them with muscle intervening depends upon degree of reduction of bulboventricular sulcus together with right or left torsion of bulboventricular loop. In addition in abnormal dextro or levo torsion with normal reduction of bulboventricular sulcus whichever valve ring lies posteriorly will come to lie in contact with endocardial cushions. At same time as these changes are appearing in bulbus cordis a low crescentic ridge appears in common ventricle near its apex. Dorsal horn of this ridge reaches dorsal cushion of atrioventricular canal near its right margin while ventral horn extends to ventral cushion near its left margin. Free edge of this ridge thus lies obliquely across caudal aspect of broad atrioventricular canal septum and between two streams of blood entering ventricle through right and left atrioventricular orifices. These streams of blood are probably one of factors responsible for bulging of ventricle on either side of ridge to form right and left ventricle and for gradual increase in height of septum. There is still a free communication between two ventricles above septum. This gap forms primary interventricular foramen which is bounded by free margin of ridge ventrally and fused atrioventricular cushions dorsally.

Closure of communication between two ventricles: Two ridges right and left composed of mesenchymal tissue grow into cavity of bulbus cordis dividing it into an infundibular portion in front and an aortic vestibule behind. As left ridge extends caudally it passes more ventrally and finally meets and fuses with ventral end of free edge of interventricular septum along which it extends in a dorsal direction. Right ridge passes more dorsally and thus comes into relation with ventral aspect of tricuspid orifice where it meets ventricular cushion of atrioventricular canal. It passes directly across to reach free edge of septum a short distance behind attachment of left bulbar ridge with which it fuses. Greater part of communication between ventricles is thus cut off by fusion of bulbar ridges with ventral four fifth of free edge of interventricular septum. There is still a small foramen remaining bounded by fused atrioventricular cushions, dorsal margin of right bulbar ridge and most posterior part of free edge of interventricular septum. This secondary interventricular foramen which is the last part to close is finally cut off by extension of mesenchymatous tissue from right side of fused interventricular cushions during 7th week of intrauterine life. Portion of interventricular foramen closed by extension of tissue from fused atrioventricular cushions becomes fibrous and forms membranous septum.

Anterior interventricular branch of left coronary artery develops in subepicardial tissue in direct relation to attached margin of ventral end of muscular interventricular septum while inferior interventricular branch of right coronary artery is correspondingly related to attached margin of dorsal end. These vessels are thus in a position to supply both muscular septum and walls of ventricles and throughout life accurately outline on surface of heart position of peripheral margin of muscular interventricular septum. With final closure of secondary interventricular foramen aortic vestibule is bounded by fused bulbar ridges in front, membranous septum on right, fused atrioventricular cushions behind while on left side it communicates with rest of left ventricle through primary interventricular foramen.

Defects in normal development of interventricular septum may result in any of following abnormalities:

1. Membranous septum may fail to develop. This is commonest type of ventricular septal defect and is frequently associated

with bulbar defect due to incomplete absorption of bulboventricular angle which keeps bulbus cordis too far to the right of ventricular septum.

2. Right and left bulbar ridges may fail to fuse leading to a communication between infundibulum and aortic vestibule. This is situated close to pulmonary valve.

3. Interventricular septum may be perforated at one or more places due to the fact that tissue between early muscular trabeculae of septum has given way.

DEVELOPMENT OF INFUNDIBULUM AND AORTIC VESTIBULE

During 5th week in addition to right and left bulbar ridges which are developing to divide bulbus cordis into aortic vestibule and infundibulum to further ridges of mesenchymal tissue form one along ventral wall and one along dorsal wall with result that during 6th week bulbus cordis is largely filled with tissue derived from this source.

During 5th week outline of pulmonary valve becomes demarcated at apex of infundibulum and of aortic valve at apex of aortic vestibule as result of absorption of excess mesenchymal tissue, above and below these points, with result that valve cusps project into cavities as fleshy little elevations.

In 7th week absorption of tissues has extended throughout greater part of infundibulum and aortic vestibule and constriction between lower end of infundibulum and right ventricle has begin to disappear.

By 8th week fleshy elevations of pulmonary and aortic valves have been modeled into delicate cusps and sinuses above valves are well formed. Constriction between right ventricle and bulbus cordis has completely disappeared and all excess mesenchymal tissue has been absorbed.

Defects occurring in development of infundibulum and aortic vestibule may result in following abnormalities:

1. Absorption of mesenchymatous tissue in infundibulum may fail entirely with result that during later stages of intrauterine life this tissue is converted into dense fibrous tissue that runs throughout length of infundibulum thus leading to both a valvular and infundibular stenosis.

2. Absorption may extend for a short distance below valve cusps so that actual valve may develop normally but absorption in rest of infundibulum is incomplete and leads to greater or lesser infundibular stenosis.

3. Absorption in infundibulum is almost complete but constriction between infundibular half of bulbus cordis and ventricle fails to disappear leading to formation of lower bulbar stenosis in which right ventricle and infundibulum are separated by thin constriction at point just above anterior papillary muscle.

4. Infundibulum may form normally but margins of cusps of pulmonary valve may remain adherent giving rise to valvular pulmonary stenosis.

5. Absorption of mesenchymatous tissue in aortic vestibule fails to take place leading to subaortic stenosis in which aortic valve and aortic vestibule are fused to a greater or lesser extent. Owing to reduction of depth of bulboventricular angle and disappearance of greater part of posterior wall of bulbus cordis length of stenosed portion is much shorter than that found in complete infundibular stenosis.

Disorders resulting from abnormal development of bulbo-ventricular region of heart:

Disorders are due to:

1. Incomplete reduction of bulboventricular sulcus.

2. Reduced dextrotorsion or reduced levotorsion of bulboventricular loop.

3. Combination of incomplete reduction of bulboventricular sulcus and reduced dextrotorsion or reduced levotorsion of bulboventricular loop.

If bulboventricular angle fails to undergo reduction bulbus cordis will be either too far to right (dextrotorsion) or too far to left (levotorsion) of muscular part of interventricular septum. This will result in outflow tract of both great arteries arising from morphologic right ventricle and in ventricular septal defect due to inability of bulbar part of septum to join up with membranous and muscular part of septum. If there is reduction in amount of dextrotorsion or levotorsion as well the relationship of outflow tracts of both great arteries to each other will also be altered and muscle will be found separating posterior vessel from endocardial cushions, e.g. where there is 180° reduction in amount of torsion aorta will arise from right ventricle anterior and to right of pulmonary artery. While with a reduction of 125° in amount of torsion pulmonary and aortic outflow tracts will be side by side and there will be right and left muscular infundibulum.

1. Normal and reduced dextrotorsion of bulboventricular loop with failure of reduction of bulboventricular sulcus and situs solitus of atria:
   - Right atrium will discharge into right sided right ventricle.
   - Left atrium will discharge into left sided left ventricle.
   - Aorta and pulmonary artery will both arise from right ventricle.
   - Membranous ventricular septal defect.
   - Bulbar septum will end in right ventricle with a free lower border that lies to the right of interventricular septum.

2. Normal and reduced dextrotorsion of bulboventricular loop with failure of reduction of bulboventricular sulcus and situs inversus of atria:
   - A morphologic right atrium will lie on left side and discharge into a morphologic left ventricle.
   - A morphologic left atrium will lie on right side and discharge into a morphologic right ventricle.
   - Membranous ventricular septal defect.
   - Bulbar septum will end in morphologic right ventricle with a free lower border lying to right of ventricular septal defect.
   - Aorta and pulmonary artery will both arise from right ventricle.

3. Normal and reduced levotorsion of bulboventricular loop with failure of reduction of bulboventricular sulcus and situs solitus of atria:
   - On right side a morphologic right atrium will discharge into a morphologic left ventricle.

- On left side a morphologic left atrium will discharge into a morphologic right ventricle.
- Ventricular septal defect.
- Bulbar septum will end into morphologic right ventricle with a free lower border on left of ventricular septal defect.
- Aorta and pulmonary artery will both arise from left sided morphologic right ventricle.
4. Normal and reduced levotorsion of bulboventricular loop with failure of reduction of bulboventricular sulcus and situs inversus of aorta:
   - On left side a morphologic right atrium will discharge into a morphologic right ventricle.
   - On right side a morphologic left atrium will discharge into morphologic left ventricle.
   - Ventricular septal defect.
   - Bulbar septum will end in morphologic right ventricle to left of ventricular septal defect.
   - Aorta and pulmonary artery will both arise from left sided morphologic right ventricle.
5. Normal and reduced dextrotorsion of bulboventricular loop with normal reduction of bulboventricular sulcus and situs solitus of atria:
   - Atria and ventricles are oriented as in normal heart.
   - In 180° reduced dextrotorsion aorta arises from infundibulum of right ventricle, pulmonary artery arises from pulmonary vestibule of left ventricle and there is complete uncorrected transposition.
6. Normal and reduced dextrotorsion of bulboventricular loop with normal reduction of bulboventricular sulcus and situs inversus of atria:
   - On right side a morphologic left atrium will discharge into morphologic right ventricle.
   - On left side a morphologic right atrium will discharge into morphologic left ventricle.
7. Normal and reduced levotorsion of bulboventricular loop with normal reduction of bulboventricular sulcus and situs solitus of atria:

– On right side a morphologic right atrium will discharge into morphologic left ventricle.
– On left side a morphologic left atrium will discharge into morphologic right ventricle.
8. Normal and reduced levotorsion of bulboventricular loop with normal reduction of bulboventricular sulcus and situs inversus of atria:
– On right side a morphologic left atrium will discharge into morphologic left ventricle.
– On left side a morphologic right atrium will discharge into morphologic right ventricle.

Generally when there is reduction of 180° in amount of torsion a ventricular septal defect is unlikely unless membranous septum does not fail.

Ventricular septal defect is likely with lesser degree of torsion because the alignment of bulbar septum and interventricular septum are not in same plane with result that various components necessary for closure of secondary interventricular foramen are unable to link up.

DIVISION OF TRUNCUS ARTERIOSUS

Truncus arteriosus is short arterial stem that connects bulbus cordis to caudal ends of ventral aortae and 6 aortic arches.

Ventral aortae arise from ventral aspect of truncus while 6 aortic arches arise from dorsal aspect.

Separation of these two sets of vessels is brought about by growth of mesenchymatous tissue into lumen of truncus. As these ridges pass toward bulbus cordis they take spiral course so that right truncal ridge first passes onto dorsal wall and then onto left wall while left truncal ridge first passes to ventral wall and then to right wall. They are thus in position to join right and left bulbar septa at a point just above pulmonary and aortic valves. These ridges in truncus finally meet and fuse leading to formation of aorticopulmonary septum.

Defects in formation of truncus may lead to abnormalities:

1. Septum may fail to develop leading to condition of persistent truncus arteriosus. If present as an isolated defect pulmonary

arteries arise from cephalic end of a common channel. In true common truncus arteriosus aortic and pulmonary valves are normal. Most cases of common truncus in addition to defect in truncus have either a defect in aortic and pulmonary valves which are developed from bulbar ridges or are cases of aortic or pulmonary atresia.

2. Septum may only partially form leading to formation of aorticopulmonary fistula.

DEVELOPMENT OF AORTIC ARCHES

Paired ventral aortae arise from ventral aspect of apex of truncus arteriosus and extend cephalically ventrolateral to primitive pharynx. From these vessels 5 pairs of aortic arches develop in series and pass around pharynx in corresponding pharyngeal arch to join paired dorsal aortae lying dorsolateral to pharynx. A 6th pair of aortic arches develops from dorsal aspect of apex of truncus arteriosus itself and passes around pharynx to join dorsal aortae also.

Caudal to pharyngeal part of gut tube dorsal aortae fuse dorsal to gut tube to form a single midline vessel.

Subsequent fate of these vessels is as follows:

1. First two pairs of aortic arches degenerate.
2. Fifth aortic arches are very rudimentary and degenerate.
3. Right ventral aorta becomes brachiocephalic artery and right common carotid artery. Left ventral aorta becomes left common carotid artery.
4. Right and left third arches and dorsal aortae cephalic to these arches become right and left internal carotid arteries and extend to cranial cavity to supply greater part of forebrain and its outgrowths.
5. Right and left external carotid arteries arise from point where third arches leave ventral aortae and extend cephalically ventrolateral to pharynx to supply whole of inside and outside of skull and face except brain.
6. Left ventral aorta forms that part of adult arch of aorta that lies between origin of innominate artery and origin of left common carotid artery.

7. Right fourth arch forms that part of right subclavian artery that lies between its origin and origin of vertebral arteries.
8. Left fourth arch forms that part of arch of adult aorta that lies between origin of left common carotid artery and origin of left subclavian artery.
9. Ventral part of right sixth arch forms commencement of right pulmonary artery. Dorsal part disappears.
10. Ventral part of left sixth arch forms commencement of left pulmonary artery. Its dorsal part forms ductus arteriosus in embryo and fetus and ligamentum arteriosum after birth.
11. Dorsal aortae between third and fourth arches disappears.
12. Right dorsal aorta between origin of seventh intersegmental artery and its point of fusion with left dorsal aorta disappears together with dorsal part of sixth arch which is linked to it.

Abnormalities in normal pattern give rise to:

1. Right dorsal aorta caudal to fourth arch may fail to degenerate giving rise to double aortic arch that completely encircles trachea and esophagus.
2. Right dorsal aorta between right fourth arch and its point of fusion with left dorsal aorta may persist, whereas left dorsal aorta between origin of left subclavian and ductus arteriosus disappears. In this type of right aortic arch persistence of left ductus arteriosus draws right dorsal aorta behind trachea and esophagus to left side so that it descends on left side of vertebral column until it reaches midline again at level of 12th thoracic vertebra. If, however, left ductus disappears as well as left dorsal aorta beyond left subclavian artery and right ductus persists then right dorsal aorta will descend on right side of vertebral column to reach midline at 12th thoracic vertebra.
3. Right fourth arch may disappear and right dorsal aorta from its point of fusion with left up to origin of 7th intersegmental branch may persist to form first part of right subclavian artery. Left ductus in these cases draws persisting part of right dorsal aorta behind esophagus to left side of vertebral column so that subclavian artery thus arises from adult arch of aorta just beyond left ductus and passes behind esophagus to reach right side.

4. Very rarely remains of fifth aortic arch may be present and form a small channel leaving and joining concave aspect of arch of aorta proximal to attachment of ligamentum arteriosum.

COARCTATION OF AORTA

In this condition there is constriction of dorsal aorta either at aortic isthmus between origin of left subclavian artery and ductus arteriosus or else in immediate vicinity of attachment of ligamentum arteriosum.

In first type of constriction which is in form of diffuse narrowing or obliteration probably develops early in intrauterine life due to fact that a large amount of blood is removed from aorta by brachiocephalic, left common carotid and left subclavian arteries. This leaves a much diminished flow through portion between origin of left subclavian artery and point where caudally directed stream from ductus arteriosus enters it. There is thus no adequate stimulus in way of blood flow to bring about enlargement of this portion of dorsal aorta.

Any additional congenital defect in heart that diminishes aortic blood flow will further aggravate this tendency to remain narrow and may even lead to obliteration.

In those conditions where constriction is in vicinity of ductus arteriosus exact etiology is less clear. Various factors have bearing on this condition:

1. Fibrosis and contraction of ductus arteriosus affects arterial wall at its attachment either by involving wall directly or by exerting traction at wall causing kink at this point.

2. Recurrent laryngeal nerve encircles aorta immediately beyond attachment of ductus arteriosus and exerts pressure on wall as it is being dragged caudally. Early disappearance of right ductus arteriosus is due to twisting of heart as whole to left and persistence of right vitelline vein which holds right side of heart at lower level including right pulmonary artery. This means that right recurrent laryngeal nerve will exert greater traction on right ductus arteriosus then left recurrent laryngeal nerve does on left ductus arteriosus.

13

Nerve Supply of Heart

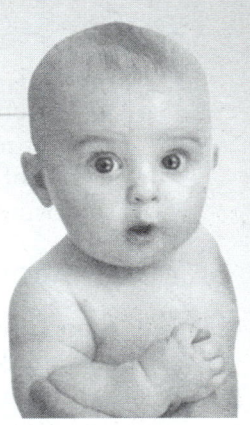

Heart receives its nerve supply from parasympathetic and sympathetic divisions of autonomic nervous system.

Parasympathetic fibers arise from dorsal nucleus of vagus nerve and leave main trunk of vagus nerve as superior and inferior cervical cardiac branches and as two or more thoracic branches. On right side cervical branches pass inferiorly behind subclavian and brachiocephalic arteries to reach deep cardiac plexus which lies on bifurcation of trachea. Thoracic branches pass forward on side of trachea and also enter deep plexus. On left side superior cervical cardiac branch passes inferiorly behind left common carotid artery and joining with thoracic branches enters deep cardiac plexus. Inferior cervical branch passes forward across lateral aspect of arch of aorta and enters superficial cardiac plexus which lies on front of ligamentum arteriosum. After reaching deep cardiac plexus parasympathetic fibers pass through it and reach heart via venous mesocardium and terminate on ganglion cells situated in subepicardial tissue at cavoauricular junction and in posterior part of atrioventricular groove. Postganglionic fibers are distributed to specialized muscles of sinoatrial and atrioventricular nodes and to coronary vessels. Those reaching superficial cardiac plexus relay in this plexus and are distributed to smaller branches of coronary arteries via arterial mesocardium. Sympathetic fibers arise as preganglionic and postganglionic neurons from superior, middle and inferior cervical ganglia and upper five thoracic ganglia of sympathetic trunks. On right side they enter deep cardiac plexus. On left side superior cervical branch reaches superficial cardiac plexus while those from middle, inferior and all thoracic ganglia enter deep cardiac plexus. Sympathetic fibers enter heart via venous and arterial mesocardium and are distributed to nodes and larger coronary vessels. Afferent fibers travel in all of cardiac branches of vagus nerve, their cell bodies situated in inferior ganglion. Sympathetic cardiac branches all carry afferent fibers except branches from superior cervical ganglion which are purely efferent.

Action of vagus is slowing of rate of contractions and diminution of their force due to effect on specialized conduction tissue. Excessive vagal stimulation may bring out missed beats or cardiac arrest. Vagal fibers to coronary arteries cause vasoconstriction. Sympathetic fibers bring about an increase in rate and force of contractions and dilatation of coronary arteries. Excessive sympathetic stimulation especially in absence of vagal control may bring about ventricular fibrillation.

14

Atrial Septal Defect

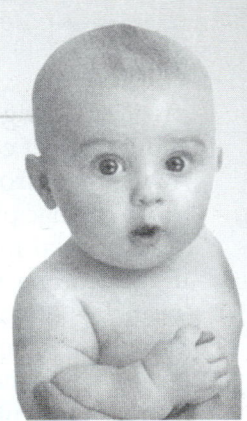

OSTIUM SECUNDUM

This defect can be subdivided into:
1. Normal atrial septum, patent foramen ovale.
2. Central fossa ovalis defect: 75% of ostium secundum.
3. Inferior caval defect: 25% of ostium secundum.
4. Large inferior venacaval defect.
5. Superior caval defect: Anomalous right upper and middle pulmonary veins.
6. Atrioventricular defect.

OSTIUM PRIMUM

There is an opening in lower portion of septum that may be either large or small. Lower margin of this opening is valve tissue at point of meeting of mitral and tricuspid valves. There is usually a cleft in mitral valve. Developmentally this category is described as partial endocardial cushion defect.

Atrioventricularis Communis (Common Atrioventricular Canal)

This consists of an opening in lower portion of atrial septum as in ostium primum but is associated with failure of fusion of valve tissue at center of atrioventricular canal resulting in variety of atrial and ventricular septal defects and mitral and tricuspid valve defects.

Other types of combination of atrial septal defect may be found: There may be multiple openings in septum, complete absence of interatrial septum or combinations and degrees of ostium secundum and ostium primum.

Congenital anomalies of heart associated with atrial septal defect or a pathologic degree of patency of foramen ovale:

1. *Acyanotic group*: Ventricular septal defect, patent ductus arteriosus, coarctation of aorta and defects of mitral valve.
2. *Cyanotic group*: Pulmonary stenosis, pulmonary valve atresia, tricuspid atresia, transposition of great vessels, tetralogy of Fallot, anomalous pulmonary veins (partial or complete) and Ebstein disease.

Patent foramen ovale closes functionally shortly after birth but may maintain a slot like opening for life. It may be forced open by other defects, such as pulmonary stenosis, tricuspid atresia and Ebstein anomaly and then it contributes to functional pathology of anomaly concerned.

PREVALENCE

Atrial septal defect is most common congenital cardiac anomaly (17% of total congenital heart diseases).

- Ostium secundum 53% of total atrial septal defects.
- Ostium primum 18%.
- Atrioventricularis communis 25%.

FAMILIAL OCCURRENCE

1. **Ostium secundum and prolonged atrioventricular conduction time:** Syndrome of atrial septal defect with prolonged PR interval is manifestation of single mutant autosomal gene with high degree of penetrance. Usual type of atrial septal defect is sporadic with little likelihood of recurrence in subsequent sibling or children. However, when defect is accompanied by prolonged PR interval genetic prognosis is dramatically changed and risk is almost 50% that condition will recur in subsequent siblings or children of affected persons.

2. **Familial atrial septal defect of atrioventricular canal variety:** 19% of cases of atrial septal defect have one or more relatives with congenital heart disease.

3. **Holt-Oram syndrome:** Anomalies of osseous system occurring in conjunction with atrial septal defect. This disorder is transmitted as autosomal dominant. These children can have their atrial septal defect corrected in usual manner however a number of rhythm abnormalities are reported in these patients.

PATHOLOGY

Ostium Secundum

Heart is generally enlarged. Right atrium is distended. Right ventricle is enlarged cavity. Right ventricle wall is hypertrophied moderately. Pulmonary artery is larger than aorta. In infants and children defect varies from 2 to 4 mm up to 15–17 mm in size. When opening is 2 cm by 2 cm or more atria are considered to be functioning as common atrium. Defect may simply be failure of valve of foramen ovale with broadening of opening. It may take form of fenestration of septum. Occasionally opening may be high up near entrance of superior vena cava. This is associated with partial anomalous pulmonary venous drainage with one or both pulmonary veins entering right atrium or superior vena cava. It is probable that anomalous veins maintained an abnormal atrial opening in upper portion of septum during embryologic development and resulted in its continued patency during postnatal life. Ostium secundum may occur with great variety of other malformations of heart. Most important of these is prolapse of mitral valve. Polysplenia may coexist. Calcification of tricuspid valve is reported.

Endocardial Cushion Defects

Anomalies (ostium primum and atrioventricularis communis) resulting from abnormal development of endocardial cushion. Partial form is called ostium primum and consist of opening in lower portion of atrial septum that may be either large or small.

Lower margin of this opening is valve tissue at point of meeting of tricuspid and mitral valve. Cleft in anterior leaflet of mitral valve is commonly present but tricuspid valve and ventricular septum are usually intact. More severe form of endocardial cushion defect is atrioventricularis communis, also called common atrioventricular canal which is characterized by defect in lower part of atrial septum and an associated defect in proximal part of ventricular septum with abnormalities of atrioventricular valves. Most common arrangement is to have both atrial and ventricular septal defect with cleft tricuspid and cleft mitral valve. Next in frequency is intact tricuspid valve associated with atrial septal defect and ventricular septal defect and cleft mitral valve. Next in order is ventricular septal defect but no atrial septal defect and cleft mitral but intact tricuspid valve. There may be an atrial septal defect but no ventricular septal defect and intact tricuspid valve with mitral valve cleft. Rarely there is left ventricle to right atrium defect with cleft tricuspid but normal mitral valve. Pulmonary artery is larger than aorta. Right ventricle capacity is increased. Its was is thicker than left ventricle. All cases show external fullness in region of infundibulum that can be recognized in X-ray of chest. Right atrium is large. Pulmonary artery branches are dilated. There is evidence of shunt from left atrium to right atrium with gross overloading of right side of heart and pulmonary circulation. Atrial septal defect is large in most instances in lower portion of septum with no tissue between defect and common mitral and tricuspid valve structure. There is usually a crescentic piece of tissue constituting remnant of atrial septum which protrudes down into heart from upper portion of atrium. There is usually communication between left ventricle and right ventricle over upper and anterior portion of ventricular septum. This opening is sometimes obstructed to some degree by meshwork of fine trabeculae proceeding from valve to septal margin. In some cases these trabeculae may be so short and so bound down to septum that defect is minimal and minimal passage of blood during systole may occur. In majority of cases there is smooth opening of considerable proportions that permits a large blood flow from left ventricle to right ventricle during each systole.

Down syndrome is associated with atrial septal defect.

HEMODYNAMICS

Shunt from left atrium to right atrium is recognized by increased oxygen saturation in right atrium over that of superior vena cava but is also recognized by angio-cardiography, indicator dilution curves or radionuclide angiography.

In presence of small atrial septal defect pressure difference between atria is not more than 3 mm Hg. With an opening of more than 2 sq cm two atria function as one and there is no pressure difference. In this circumstance characteristic shunt from left atrium to right atrium does not appear to be due to pressure difference and since there is common filling pressure for both ventricles relative receptiveness of ventricles must be decisive factor.

There is a tendency for percentage of patients with raised pulmonary vascular resistance to increase with advancing years, even in presence of relatively benign anomaly.

Oxygen administration is helpful in differentiating between various categories of response of pulmonary vasculature in atrial septal defect. Inhalation of oxygen will reduce pulmonary vascular resistance and thus pulmonary pressure in majority of children who have pulmonary hypertension due to this cause. Small shunt with low resistance show minimal response to oxygen. There are two categories of pulmonary vascular resistance. A functional one which responds to oxygen and an organic obstructive one which show a little or no response to oxygen. Pulmonary vascular resistance in atrial septal defect is usually within normal range: As long as right ventricle output is maintained cyanosis does not occur because systemic venous blood returning to heart is carried out continuously through pulmonary circulation. If right ventricle output fails as in congestive heart failure mixing of blood from two atria may occur and some of desaturated blood may enter systemic circulation. Pulmonary venous engorgement may be cause of unsaturated blood returning to left atrium.

Right ventricle failure is indicated by lowered right ventricle output, appearance of cyanosis or by distinct but less obvious fall in oxygen content of arterial blood. It may be brought on by excessive blood flow through right side of heart, marked increase in pulmonary vascular resistance or tricuspid regurgitation.

Left ventricle failure is indicated by further congestion of pulmonary vascular bed and systemic venous system and is more likely to occur when mitral regurgitation or mitral stenosis complicates atrial septal defect.

Digitalis increases cardiac output of right ventricle failure without altering venous pressure but with left ventricle failure digitalis reduces venous pressure while maintaining output.

Ratio of pulmonary to systemic blood flow is 2:1 or more in 90% cases of atrial septal defect in adults and 95% in children thus indicating that pulmonary pressure and resistance are characteristically low in this particular anomaly.

Development of pulmonary vascular obstruction is a slow process. When atrial defect is combined with other anomalies, e.g. ventricular septal defect, patent ductus arteriosus or both, arterial changes are more likely to occur in childhood and Eisenmenger syndrome with reversal of flow and cyanosis may occur in childhood. This syndrome is rare in children with simple ostium secundum.

CLINICAL FEATURES OF OSTIUM SECUNDUM

This is not recognized in early years of life.

60% are females and 40% males.

Some patients are thin, others have average physique. Average height is within normal limits. Thin emaciated appearance is not normally present. Failure to thrive occurs in 30% of cases of ostium secundum and 60–90% cases of endocardial cushion defect.

1. *Exercise tolerance* good in majority of children. Dyspnea on effort is common.

2. *Cyanosis* rare, except as a terminal event when heart failure supervenes or when a left superior vena cava is attached to left atrium. 50% children have a slight decrease in oxygen

saturation. Wood recorded incidence of Eisenmenger complex in this anomaly as 6%.

3. *Cardiac impulse* forceful apex beat is seen in 90% children. Best elicited by having them sit up and lean forward slightly, then with palm of hand over precordium in left parasternal area increased force of right ventricle can be appreciated through relatively thin chest wall. A thrill is present in pulmonary area in 2% of ostium secundum cases without pulmonary stenosis. When a thrill is present in pulmonary area pulmonary stenosis is associated with ostium secundum atrial septal defect.

4. *Heart murmur* in 20% cases cardiac murmur is not recognized until after infancy. 98% have murmur up left sternal border, being maximum in first to second intercostal spaces in 75% and second to third intercostal spaces in 25% on left side. Murmur is grade 2, moderate intensity, not widely distributed. Harsher murmurs are associated with pulmonary stenosis. Mid-diastolic murmur is heard between apex and sternum, common in patients with large defect. It is due to rapid inflow from right atrium to right ventricle during diastole. It is present in 85% cases of ostium secundum.

   Splitting of second heart sound can be recognized. Pulmonary component is always of normal or slightly increased intensity. Width of splitting is fixed and does not vary with respiration. Occasionally it varies with respiration in children with small defect with only a slight increase in pulmonary blood flow.

5. *Electrocardiogram* right ventricle hypertrophy with incomplete right bundle branch block. P-wave is elevated slightly. PR interval increased to 0.19 second. Left axis deviation may occur rarely in ostium secundum. Characteristic axis is between 90° and 150° (right axis deviation).

6. *X-ray chest* in infants and young children there may be equivocal cardiomegaly and relatively normal vascularity. Most patients with a large shunt show cardiomegaly, full

pulmonary artery segment and increased arterial markings in lungs. Aorta is of normal size and on left. Left atrium is not enlarged, an important distinguishing feature from post-tricuspid shunts with intact atrial septum. A vertical shadow on left side of mediastinum suggests association of left superior vena cava. An azygous continuation of superior vena cava or anomalously connected right pulmonary veins can be suspected by a prominence above superior vena cava right atrium junction.

7. *Echocardiography* enlarged right ventricle end diastolic dimensions may be sole feature. This in itself is not diagnostic. Septal motion may be normal, intermediate (type B) or reversed (type A). Septal motion tends to be related to size of shunt. It is type A in patients with largest shunt and large right ventricle dimensions. Echo also detects associated anomaly, e.g. mitral valve prolapse.

8. *Angiocardiography* to confirm that left to right shunt is occurring at atrial level and to obtain an indication of extremes of defect size, i.e. trivial versus absent atrial septum. Other applications include detection of pressure gradient across pulmonary valve or bifurcation of main pulmonary artery, examination of mitral valve and left ventricle anatomy and function. Anatomy of left and right pulmonary veins or superior vena cava and their connections can be clarified. Selective left atrial injection in left anterior oblique position will allow identification and localisation of defect. Contrast will spill over superior vena cava. To determine precise dimensions of defect a balloon catheter filled with contrast can be slowly drawn across the communication. This is repeated with increasing amount of contrast in balloon when a point of resistance and mild deformity is reached during traverse. Defect is roughly diameter of balloon inflated to that degree.

Contrast injection into main pulmonary artery with patient supine gives most consistent visualization of an atrial left to right shunt and allows indirect assessment of defect size. Tilted projections reveal branch stenosis.

Right ventricle injection shows abnormal pulmonary valve. Left ventricle injection in anteroposterio and right anterior oblique views clarify mitral anatomy particularly prolapse of mitral leaflets.

9. *Pulmonary hypertension*: Pulmonary hypertension with pulmonary artery pressure more than 50 mm Hg is present in 5% of children with ostium secundum, isolated defect. All of this group have significant cardiac symptoms. Occasional cases have cyanosis with effort. Intensity of pulmonary valve closure is increased and pulmonary valve closure is palpable. A few have pulmonary diastolic murmur down left sternal edge. Dominant 'a'-wave is observed in jugular venous pulsations. Cardiomegaly is present larger than other group. CT ratio >65%. Height of R-wave in V1 exceeds 16 mm in all cases. Incidence of pulmonary hypertension is higher when atrial septal defect secundum is complicated by other lesions, such as ventricular septal defect, partial anomalous pulmonary venous drainage or patent ductus arteriosus.

These children have higher incidence of respiratory infections.

Complicated Ostium Secundum Pulmonary Stenosis with Atrial Septal Defect with Left to Right Shunt

10% of ostium secundum.

40% patients have cyanosis on exertion.

Systolic thrill felt in pulmonary area. Closure of pulmonary valve delayed and soft. Mid-diastolic murmur is rare. Jugular venous pulse has prominent A-wave. Heart size is small. Left pulmonary artery is dilated in a few and its origin is usually high. Pulmonary vascular markings may be increased and pulsatile in a few but as a rule they appear normal. R-wave in V1 is >16 mm in 80% cases. Systolic gradient across pulmonary valve ranges from 20 to 70 mm Hg during cardiac catheterization. Moderate left to right shunt is present at atrial level but no right to left shunt can be detected under resting conditions. Surgical treatment of pulmonary stenosis is required in children with pressure gradient exceeding 50 mm Hg. In small gradient atrial septal defect is closed without dealing with pulmonary stenosis.

Atrial Septal Defect with Partial Anomalous Pulmonary Venous Drainage

Partial anomalous pulmonary venous drainage to right atrium is seen in 7% cases. Right pulmonary vein is anomalous. Atrial septal defect is small and located at entrance of superior vena cava (sinus venosus defect) in 50%. In other half atrial septal defect is at center of septum. Incidence of cyanosis with exertion and pulmonary hypertension is more. At cardiac catheterization pulmonary drainage into superior vena cava can be probed. Injection of contrast medium delineates pulmonary veins entering right atrium. Gradient across atrial septum in presence of large left to right shunt suggests a small atrial septal defect with partial anomalous pulmonary venous drainage.

Atrial Septal Defect with Mitral Valve Prolapse

Most common anomaly associated with ostium secundum. Degree of mitral valve prolapse is insignificant to produce physical findings until after correction of atrial septal defect. However, at times significant mitral regurgitation may be present producing pan systolic murmur at apex. In such cases differential diagnosis is from ostium primum defect with cleft mitral valve and atrial septal defect with rheumatic mitral valve incompetence. Electrocardiograph shows superior QRS axis in ostium primum. Echocardiogram is helpful in differentiating. Significant mitral regurgitation changes hemodynamics of atrial septal defect. Closure of atrial septal defect without appropriate treatment of mitral valve prolapse may cause postoperative congestive heart failure. Treatment is by valvuloplasty. Rheumatic mitral regurgitation may require valve replacement.

Atrial Septal Defect with Mitral Stenosis (Lutembacher's Syndrome)

Mitral valve involvement is usually congenital. Rarely rheumatic. Fatigue and dyspnea on exertion occur but congestive heart failure and atrial fibrillation are rare. First heart sound is markedly accentuated which is palpable at apex. Opening snap is not heard or recorded by phonocardiography. Left atrial hypertrophy is not seen. Cardiothoracic ratio exceeds 65% and prominent pulmonary conus is seen. Most cases of Lutembacher's syndrome are 30 years by the time they become symptomatic. This is true for acquired mitral stenosis. However, when mitral stenosis is congenital in origin symptoms may appear very early in life.

Atrial Septal Defect with Ventricular Septal Defect

Since disability is severe heart disease is recognized in first year of life. 50% develop congestive heart failure. 40% have cyanosis on crying. Physical findings are those of ventricular septal defect or pulmonary hypertension. Systolic thrill is felt in 75% cases. Cardiomegaly occurs. Left atrial enlargement is slight to moderate. Tall R-wave in V1 with combined ventricular hypertrophy is seen in electrocardiogram. QRS axis ranges between +60° and +150° in 75% cases. Left axis deviation is found in 25% cases. Cardiac catheterization reveals atrial septal defect with large left to right shunt. Systolic pressure in pulmonary artery or right ventricle is equal to systemic pressure. Angiocardiogram is helpful in delineating the anomaly present. A ventricular septal defect with tricuspid regurgitation gives similar catheter findings.

Isolated Ostium Primum Atrial Septal Defect

No physical signs of mitral regurgitation. Slight left atrial enlargement. No eletrocardiographic evidence of left atrial hypertrophy or left ventricular hypertrophy.

Ostium Primum with Cleft Mitral Valve

10% of total atrial septal defect group. Symptomatic cardiac disability is common. Dyspnea, easy fatigue, congestive heart failure and cyanosis on exertion with evidence of mitral regurgitation is present. Cardiothoracic ratio exceeds 65%. Left atrium size may be normal or slightly enlarged. QRS axis between –50° and –130°. Left ventricle hypertrophy combined with right ventricle hypertrophy is found in majority in eletrocardiography. At cardiac catheterization pulmonary hypertension is uncommon. An apical systolic murmur of mitral or tricuspid regurgitation is unlikely to be present. Second heart sound is narrowly split with marked accentuation of pulmonary component due to pulmonary hypertension. Significant cardiomegaly and dense hilar shadow is a rule. On echocardiography features of right ventricle volume overload are seen. Abnormal anterior displacement of mitral valve results in prolonged diastolic apposition of anterior mitral leaflet to septum. Left ventricle outflow tract appears narrow. Reduplication of systolic image of mitral valve is seen.

Common Atrium and Cleft Mitral Valve

Cyanosis at rest is unusual but may be apparent with exercise. Murmur of mitral regurgitation is usually not present. Commonly there is left axis deviation and counterclockwise vector. Right ventricle dominance is usually present but combined ventricle loading pattern may also occur.

Atrioventricularis Communis

Features appear in first or second year of life and failure to thrive is invariable. Cyanosis with crying is noted in majority. Congestive heart failure is an early event but may not appear in those who are dying in first year due to other causes. Second heart sound is closely split with accentuated pulmonary component. Heart is greatly enlarged with cardiothoracic ratio >65%. Right ventricle outflow tract is prominent. Left atrial enlargement is slight to moderate. Electrocardiograph shows combined left ventricle and right ventricle hypertrophy. Left atrial hypertrophy is seen in 10% cases. QRS axis is between –60° and –140°. In echocardiogram anterior leaflet of mitral and tricuspid valves are contiguous in plane of ventricular septum in diastole when septal echos appear deficient. Single leaflet appearing predominantly mitral may pass through septum and merge in tricuspid valve. Multiple systolic echoes are seen in mitral valve. Left ventricle outflow tract is narrow. Right ventricle enlargement occurs in 85%. Cardiac catheterization reveals pulmonary hypertension at or near systemic levels. Frontal angiocardiogram reveals anomalies. Right border of heart appears serrated or scalloped.

DIFFERENTIAL DIAGNOSIS

Electrocardiogram provides most reliable method in differentiating ostium secundum from ostium primum defect. In secundum mean axis and QRS complex lie between +60 and +150° and frontal vector rotates in clockwise manner. Left axis deviation and counterclockwise vector is characteristic of primum defect. When pulmonary hypertension is found with secundum defect associated cardiac lesion should be searched since incidence of combined lesions is greater when pulmonary hypertension is present. When pulmonary stenosis is associated with atrial septal defect and persistent left to right shunt, its presence may be suspected by systolic thrill and altered pulmonary component of second heart sound. Closure of pulmonary valve is delayed and soft. Cyanosis with exertion or dominant 'a'-wave in jugular venous pulse may be seen. Heart is smaller. Hilar shadows normal. R-wave in V1 exceeds 16 mm.

When mitral stenosis occurs with atrial septal defect it may be congenital or rheumatic in origin. Rheumatic mitral stenosis takes considerably longer time to develop. Hence, rare in childhood. Mid-diastolic murmur and presystolic murmur are louder and first heart sound accentuated at apex and axilla. Giant 'a'-wave may be seen in jugular venous pulse. Radiologically heart is significantly enlarged and pulmonary conus unusually prominent. QR pattern or dominant R-wave is seen in V1. When atrial septal defect is large signs of mitral stenosis are less impressive. When defect is small, signs of mitral stenosis are striking. Jugular venous pulse is normal and left atrium is enlarged in small atrial septal defect. In large atrial septal defect jugular venous pulse has prominent 'a'-wave and left atrium is normal in size on fluroscopy. When atrial septal defect is associated with ventricular septal defect severe disability, congestive heart failure and cyanosis on exertion are common in first year of life. Systolic murmur and thrill occur at left sternal edge. Heart is markedly enlarged. R-wave in V1 exceeds 16 mm. Evidence of left atrial hypertrophy and left ventricular hypertrophy may be present.

Common atrium resulting from complete absence of atrial septum should be considered when cyanosis is noticed at rest in patients with ostium primum defect. Marked left axis deviation of P-wave with relatively short PR interval is characteristic.

Atrioventricularis communis gives rise to severe disability, congestive heart failure and cyanosis in early infancy. Down syndrome is coexistant. Clinical signs suggest ventricular septal defect. Cardiomegaly on X-ray and biventricular hypertrophy on electrocardiograph.

Atrial septal defect with patent ductus arteriosus gives rise to right ventricular hypertrophy. Although continuous murmur of patent ductus arteriosus is heard, one may not suspect atrial septal defect. Hence, when atrial septal defect is associated with patent ductus arteriosus clinically it may be suspected by continuous murmur with right ventricular hypertrophy in ECG. Cardiac catheterization may be required to differentiate.

Coarctation of aorta may occur with atrial septal defect. Femoral pulses should be felt and blood pressure taken in all four limbs.

Prognosis

Death from ostium secundum in childhood is uncommon. Prognosis in major combined lesions is poor. Causes of death are congestive heart failure, hyperkinetic pulmonary hypertension, mitral stenosis or mitral regurgitation and atrial fibrillation, Eisenmenger complex or infection may supervene. Those that die in early life have associated anomalies, e.g.

ventricular septal defect, patent ductus arteriosus, mitral stenosis and coarctation of aorta.

Spontaneous closure of atrial septal defect has been described in 3% cases. Closure tends to occur in early years of life usually in first five years. Mechanism of closure is not known but it seems likely that foramen ovale was stretched open and subsequently hemodynamics of atria allowed less stretch and normal growth permitted functional closure.

Treatment

With cardiopulmonary bypass technique using pump oxygenation surgical closure of atrial septal defect has become very safe. Risks are lowest in first decade.

Selection of Cases for Surgery

Since spontaneous closure takes place in first five years surgery should be deferred beyond this age. In atrial septal defect secundum in asymptomatic child defect should be closed when pulmonary to systemic flow ratio is 2.5: 1 or more (Moss 1971). Ostium primum and atrioventricularis communis: Since associated lesions are multiple surgical techniques are directed toward repairing each anomalous segment as adequately as possible. Extracorporeal circulation is required. Since mortality is so high in babies with atrioventricularis communis those who present with signs and symptoms in first year of life should be considered for surgery. Respiratory infections are common in these babies and require antibiotics. If failure develops they need digitalis and other supportive therapy.

Arrhythmias

There are three main internodal tracts in right atrium. Anterior tract is shortest. Middle tract courses along limbus of fossa ovalis to atrioventricular node. Posterior is longest and follows crista terminalis through valve of inferior vena cava to atrioventricular node. At surgery these tracts can be damaged by either incision in auricle or septum or by placement of sutures. Thus, it is suggested that to preserve at least one internodal tract the atriotomy incision should be made parallel to crista terminalis.

Incidence of dysrhythmia or conduction defects is recorded as 52%. Right bundle branch block increase in 30% of these. Atrial fibrillation, atrial tachycardia, nodal rhythm may occur. Postoperative arrhythmias can be controlled by digitalis. When arrhythmia is endangering life or recovery of patient cardioversion countershock is indicated. Quinide may be given following countershock for a few weeks as a prophylactic measure.

15

Patent Ductus Arteriosus

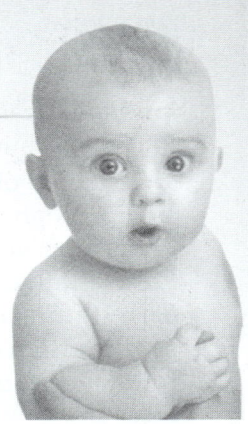

Ductus arteriosus is large vessel connecting distal portion of main pulmonary artery to ventrolateral aspect of aorta just distal to left subclavian artery or to brachiocephalic branches of aortic arch. Though a large structure in fetal life ductus is normally obliterated after birth and eventually becomes fibrous ligament.

ANATOMY

The angle of entrance of ductus into aorta is acute, about 32°. The degree not changing significantly at the time of constriction in neonatal period. During fetal life its diameter is equal to aorta and pulmonary artery. At the end of newborn period ductus is usually thick its lumen being much narrower. Later fibrosis converts ductus into ligamentum arteriosum. Calcification of ligamentum is relatively common in children. Normal closure begins at pulmonary artery end of ductus, hence there is a conical formation to persistently patent channel, aortic end forming mouth. In partial persistence of ductus, demonstrated angiographically the portion remaining open is at pulmonary artery end of duct. This variant is associated with pulmonary stenosis, tetralogy of Fallot and pulmonary artery stenosis. Aneurysmal changes are seen in children dying less than 2 months of age. Right sided ductus is rare.

Histologically ductus has thick intima, media with single elastic lamina, variable mucoid material and an intricate helicoid spiral muscular arrangement. Initial mounds appear in 6th month of fetal life and consist of smooth muscles fibers together with mucoid substance projecting through deficiency in elastic lamina. These developments are considered as prerequisite for ductal closure. Single elastic lamina shows point of rupture, reduplication and fragmentation as early as 4th month of fetal life. These changes precede formation of intimal mounds and together with signs of hyperplasia of smooth muscle cells in media at base of mound constitute evidence for view that mounding is a secondary recuperative processfor damage created in elastic layer during fetal existence.

A strong contraction of smooth muscles is main factor responsible for postnatal closure of ductus. Arrangement of muscle spirals in ductus is uniquely suitable for obliteration of lumen with very littleshortening of channel. In contracted state intimal mounds form longitudinal ridges, wall becomes thicker and muscle bundles in media and intima are separated by structureless material resembling mucoid degeneration. Subsequently a slower change involving cytolysis of dead cells and replacement of much of media with fibrous tissue occurs and eventually this itself shrinks to obliterate lumen.

Heart: Left ventricle, left atrium, aorta and pulmonary artery are enlarged as a result of abnormal left to right shunt. In rare type of malformation where reversal of shunt is predominant feature right ventricle hypertrophy and right atrium hypertrophy are seen alone.

Closure of Ductus

Latest data show that in healthy term babies significant left to right shunt through ductus stops by later part of first day of life. Initially closed ductus may reopen temporarily under usual conditions with a variety of thermal enviornments.

In low birth weight infants born prematurely, in late phase of respiratory distress or after episode of apnea normal circulatory transition including closure of ductus is delayed. Left to right shunt of variable size is a frequent complication. There is tendency for closure to occur at an age equivalent to term gestation.

ETIOLOGY

Delayed Closure of Ductus or Nonclosure

Prenatal factors

1. Familial aggregation of PDA suggests a genetic influence.
2. Recurrence of cardiac defect in later born siblings of patient with PDA is 2%.
3. Maternal rubella in first trimester is known to cause PDA in number of offsprings of such mothers. Actual amount of smooth muscles in ductus wall is reduced.
4. LBW premature babies have high incidence of PDA. Many have large left to right shunt. Hypoxia, fluid overload, enzyme deficiency, reduced smooth muscle bulk has been suggested as causes. The evidence now favors some maturational cause related to prostaglandin function or to final chain of initiation of smooth muscle contraction.
5. Ductus closure can be delayed in several congenital heart diseases, e.g. tetralogy of Fallot.

Postnatal factors

1. **Hypoxia:** Ductus sometimes reopens after initial functional closure. In naturally born partially asphyxiated state ductus constricts possibly due to effect of catecholamine release. If oxygenation is improved ductus dilates and finally constricts when oxygen saturation reaches 85%. Influence on ductal function after short exposure to hypoxia might prolong dilating response of more acute reaction. Relationship between reduced oxygen pressures of high altitude and PDA incidence is documented.

   Oxygen triggers duct constriction by increasing rate of oxidative phosphorylation within smooth muscle cells.
2. Noradrenalin, adrenalin, acetylcholine also cause isolated ductus to contract.
3. Bradykinin and acetylcholine augment hypoxia induced ductal constriction.
4. Prostaglandin E maintains patency of ductus. With exception of prostaglandin F2 alpha all prostaglandins relax smooth

muscles of fetal ductus arteriosus under low oxygen tension. Ductal sensitivity is most marked to PGE2 is maximal at beginning of last trimester of gestation and declines thereafter while contractile response to oxygen increases as term approaches. It is thought that fetal ductus is maintained open by continuous endogenous production of PGE2 acting on highly responsive ductal smooth muscle. When arterial oxygen rises at birth ductal sensitivity to PGE2 markedly reduced and ductus constricts. In cyanotic infants PaO_2 never rises high enough to cause complete loss of sensitivity to E2. Duct remains partially open. In premature infant prostaglandin responsiveness remains relatively dominant and although PaO_2 rises at birth the duct is still responsive to PGE2 in many infants and remains patent.

INCIDENCE

PDA in general population between 1:2500 to 1:5000. Isolated PDA accounts for 12% of all CHD. In term newborn 1:1881 live births. In preterm with RDS 15%.

PDA is more common in females that increases in summer months. About 2% of PDA incidence is explained on basis of rubella infection *in utero*.

HEMODYNAMICS

Before birth blood is directed from pulmonary artery through ductus into aorta due to high pulmonary vascular resistance. After birth there is alteration in relationship between pulmonary and systemic pressure resulting in left to right shunt through patent ductus. Factors that influence flow of blood through PDA are diameter of ductus and pressure relationship on either side although in newborn period vasomotor tone of ductus itself can contribute much more to pressure flow variations. In those with large ductus PVR becomes an important factor. In a small number with pronounced pulmonary hypertension and large ductus it is probable that there is not a normal fall in PVR after birth but that same alteration will occur allowing left to right shunt of small volume. Retention of a very high level of PVR in younger infants is related to a history of recurrent hypoxia usually from pulmonary disturbances.

Clinical Features

History

Congenital rubella, prematurity, especially associated with birth asphyxia or respiratory distress syndrome.

History of difficult delivery, asphyxia neonatorum, cesarean section and upper gastrointestinal abnormalities may be helpful in baby at term with clinical signs of PDA.

Significant disability in children is very occasional. But in infants serious disability occurs which is related to size of pulmonary blood flow. Congestive heart failure, failure to thrive and recurrent pulmonary infections are common.

Growth retardation occurs in one-third of patients. Preoperative congestive heart failure is associated with severe growth failure. Most chidren have growth acceleration after surgery if it is undertaken before 3 years of age.

Cardiovascular Examination

Cyanosis even transient is absent apart from a few cases of failure in infancy or with bidirectional flow through ductus from pulmonary hypertension.

Precordial thrill systolic, less often continuous or systodiastolic is palpable in pulmonary area. Thrills are less often detected in infants.

Femoral and radial pulses are equally brisk. Femoral pulse may be weaker than normal. Pulsation in suprasternal notch is frequently seen and thrill often extends to this area. 75% of older children and 95% of infants have pulse pressure exceeding 45 mm Hg. It also occurs in ventricular septal defect and mitral insufficiency.

On auscultation of heart 3 types of murmur are heard: Continuous murmur or machinery murmur in pulmonary area. It begins after commencement of first heart sound, persists through second heart sound and dies away gradually during the long pause. The murmur is rough and thrilling. It begins softly and increases in intensity so as to reach its acme just about or immediately after incidence of second heart sound and from that point gradually wanes into its termination. The second heart sound can be heard to be loud and clanging. The crescendo systolic element in pulmonary area is late in onset and this feature of timing is not present in other congenital defects that may have murmur maximal in this area. Occasionally continuous murmur in a young patient may alter from one examination to another or during same examination. A valve like structure is believed to be responsible for intermittent obliteration of shunt. Great variation in murmur can be produced by a variety of postural changes in an unusually long patent thin ductus due to kinking of channel in different body postures.

Spontaneous disappearance of continuous murmur is rare. It may occur with closure of ductus. This is noted in newborn infants especially premature. Otherwise disappearance of continuous murmur may be result of development of pulmonary hypertension secondary to severe pulmonary vascular resistance causing obstruction.

Abbreviated Murmur

This murmur is identical with continuous murmur until second heart sound after which it fades away quite abruptly. Intensity of this murmur is not different from classic murmur and eddy sounds which are common in high velocity situations of small to moderate size ductus are helpful in diagnosis.

Nonspecific Murmurs

Majority are low intensity, mid systolic ejection, maximal in pulmonary area. Soft ejection murmur is most frequently encountered. These features are confined to patients who have an extremely large duct or who have a trivial communication.

There is an overall relationship between presence of pulmonary hypertension and absence or shortening of diastolic murmur in PDA. At time when murmur may be only systolic or may even be absent a trivial flow through a greatly constricted ductus may be occurring.

When the murmur is soft or intermittent it may be more certainly recognized by addition of vasopressure drugs, such as phenylephrine or mephentamine. In patient with large volume left to right shunt an apical mid diastolic murmur is noted.

Second Heart Sound

There is slightly accentuated pulmonary valve closure, normal splitting. Eddy sounds are noted in pulmonary area in large shunts. With high pulmonary vascular resistance second heart sound becomes accentuated but not single and pulmonary ejection sounds become audible in advanced cases. Paradoxic splitting is confined to patients with large shunts.

Features in Very Young Infants

All newborn infants symptomatic and dying within a few days of life will be found to be having a widely patent ductus. Rarely newborns may present with pulmonary edema in first few days of life. More of newborn patients who present with respiratory difficulty and congestive heart failure have signs that support clinical diagnosis of PDA. Preterm babies have either continuous or abbreviated murmur. In term babies nonspecific murmurs are present in 17%. In 78% a ductal murmur can be identified in first year. The crackling crescendo nature of murmur in systole and short spillover into diastole should go in favor of making a diagnosis of PDA in infant without a frank continuous murmur. Presentation with these atypical signs is exceptional.

RADIOLOGICAL FEATURES

Heart size

Large ductus correlates well with cardiomegaly and left ventricular hypertrophy.

Heart Contour

Often normal in simple PDA. In large shunt or with pulmonary hypertension there is a pulmonary artery bulge in left mid border of heart and combined ventricular hypertrophy. Aorta is prominent and the angle between aortic knuckle and main pulmonary artery is filled in. Barium swallow confirms the size of left aortic arch and also can determine the degree of enlargement of left atrium. Left atrial enlargement is very common in children, is invariable in symptomatic infant group and permits exclusion of atrial septal defect.

Ductus Bump

A transient mass visible in chest X-ray of term infant in first day of life. Usually disappears by third day of life and is benign. Presence of calcification in region of ductus in children with congenital heart disease is evidence against patency of ductus.

Lung Vascularity

Increase in lung vascular marking is usual. Majority have grade 2 increase and in most this is evenly distributed throughout lung. In preterm infant with left to right ductal shunt pulmonary plethora in sequential radiographs is as reliable as echo-cardiography in establishing severity. Development of pulmonary vascular disease produces a disproportionately increased main pulmonary artery, slight enlargement of lobar and segmental arteries and reduction of peripheral vascularity. Calcification in pulmonary arteries may be seen where there is longstanding shunt reversal but actual calcification of duct is more likely to be associated with closure or aneurysm.

ELECTROCARDIOGRAM

A normal ECG is present in only a third of uncomplicated PDA. QRS: Left axis deviation is rare until adolescence but is present in 15% cases. Normal axis in 83%.

Atrial hypertrophy: 5% have left atrial hypertrophy as the sole abnormality in ECG. 5% show left atrial hypertrophy in association with left ventricular hypertrophy.

Ventricular hypertrophy: Slight left ventricular hypertrophy in older cases. Combined ventricular hypertrophy may be seen in less than 3 years of age.

Upward concavity of ST segment in lead ll, lll, avf, V5 and V6 is seen in patients over 1 year age. This is a useful diagnostic point since it is uncommon in other congenital heart diseases. Incomplete bundle branch block is an uncommon finding reported in 2 to 4% of cases.

Correlation of ECG with other features of PDA: Normal ECG has normal CT ratio. Large ducti are found in a few cases without ECG changes. Patients with left atrial hypertrophy as sole abnormality have small heart and small ducti. Cases with right ventricular hypertrophy show severe pulmonary hypertension. In infants in severe cases ducti are large and heart grossly enlarged. In infants under 6 months there is no good correlation between degree of right ventricular hypertrophy and level of mean pulmonary artery pressure or the degree of left ventricular hypertrophy and shunt size. In older children prompt postoperative reduction in voltage of Q and R in V6 has been noted.

ECHOCARDIOGRAM

Though not diagnostic it can give an indication of degree of hemodynamic disturbances. Varying degrees of left atrial and left ventricular enlargement will be found. There is good correlation between left atrial diameter and left to right shunt size. There has been considerable interest recently in using this technique for this purpose in respiratory distress syndrome of premature infants.

CARDIAC CATHETERIZATION

A rise of oxygen content of blood in pulmonary artery over that obtained from right ventricle. The flow through ductus averages 40% of left ventricle output. There is no change in pulmonary blood flow with effort except in cases with elevated left atrial pressure at rest when exercise decreases pulmonary blood flow. Pulmonary artery pressure is not raised significantly. Preoperative catheterization is of considerable value in infants with symptoms or in cases exhibiting the effects of pulmonary hypertension. Infant with symptoms, cardiomegaly, ECG evidence of left ventricle or combined ventricular hypertrophy show a large aortico pulmonary shunt and high pulmonary artery pressure. When the shunt is confined to pulmonary artery the question is whether there is aortic septal defect or PDA is present. This is solved by direct catheterization of ductus and descending aorta. Arterial oxygen saturation in usual case is normal. In cases with pulmonary hypertension or bidirectional flow or in infants with marked pulmonary hypertension there is lower oxygen saturation of blood from femoral artery than that obtained from brachial artery analysis. A difference that can be augmented when the patient breaths a mixture containing 10% oxygen.

PDA occupies a position intermediate between VSD and ASD with regard to development of pulmonary vascular disease in older children.

Measurable alterations of pulmonary vascular bed are not usually established until after infancy.

ANGIOCARDIOGRAPHY

It can define duct diameter. Contrast is injected from a catheter placed retrogradly near aortic isthmus from either umbilical or femoral arterial route.

Complications

1. *Congestive heart failure*: There is dyspnea, gallop rhythm and enlarged liver. There is some response to medical treatment but surgery is advised.
2. *Infective endocarditis*: Less common in young children and infants. The vegetations tend to proliferate at pulmonary end of ductus and in pulmonary artery. Embolization of lungs occurs. Thus, it may mimic tuberculosis or pneumonia. Patients with PDA having fever should get blood culture done. Penicillin therapy is preferred. Surgery is deferred until infection is subsided.
3. *Aneurysm of ductus*: Mycotic in nature. Many aneurysms are associated with infective endocarditis. Pressure effect from aneurysm may cause recurrent laryngeal nerve palsy, left lobar collapse due to compression of bronchus. Pressure in

pulmonary artery is a more important factor than actual size of vessel in producing a compression effect.

4. *Aortic embolism*: In pulmonary stenosis or atresia accompanying tetralogy of Fallot, tricuspid atresia, pulmonary atresia with intact ventricular septum or single ventricle, presence of PDA is of some benefit to patient. Closure of ductus is then contraindicated.

In some cases PDA poses additional hemodynamic problems on heart

1. *VSD*: There is classic continuous murmur in pulmonary area and pansystolic murmur with thrill in 3rd and 4th left intercostal space. In such cases VSD is small size. Pulmonary vasculature is normal. Pulmonary artery pressure and pulmonary vascular resistance is normal or only slightly elevated. The rare type 1 VSD where murmur is maximally heard in pulmonary area may be completely obscured by duct murmur. Difficulty in diagnosis of combination arises when there is substantial pulmonary hypertension. Murmur due to one or both defects become atypical. In these cases hemodynamic studies are required.

2. *Coarctation of aorta*: In young infants in congestive heart failure with coarctation of aorta signs of PDA may be lacking. Sometimes there is widespread continuous murmur over pulmonary area, axilla and back simulating PDA but created by passage of blood through coarctation itself. In older patients similar murmur may be produced by collateral vessels.

3. *Aortic stenosis*: Presence of ejection systolic murmur with thrill in aortic area and in neck with disproportionately enlarged left ventricle and aorta should arouse suspicion. Several patients with large flow isolated PDA have loud ejection systolic murmur in aortic area and a coarse thrill in carotid vessels due to high left ventricular stroke volume. Conversely ductus may be silent in association with aortic stenosis with severe pulmonary hypertension.

4. *Pulmonary stenosis and pulmonary artery stenosis*: The association can be suspected by presence of prominent

jugular 'a'-waves and right ventricular hypertrophy in ECG even though ejection systolic murmur of pulmonary stenosis is masked by loud continuous murmur of PDA. Association of pulmonary artery stenosis is very common in patients with rubella background.

5. *Mitral regurgitation*: All have large PDA and usually pulmonary hypertension.

PDA with Pulmonary Hypertension

In PDA there is usually an increase in pulmonary blood flow because of continuous left to right shunt through aortico pulmonary communication. Pulmonary circulation can accomodate considerable increase in blood volume without change in pressure.

Mechanism of Pulmonary Hypertension

1. Markedly increased pulmonary blood flow. Beyond a certain volume of flow in pulmonary circuit pulmonary artery pressure becomes elevated.

2. Increased pulmonary venous pressure. Left ventricular failure from any cause or any similar obstruction of flow in left heart, e.g. mitral stenosis, endocardial fibroelastosis and triatrial heart by increasing pressure in pulmonary veins will result in elevation of pulmonary artery pressure. In such cases pulmonary wedge pressure is abnormally high.

3. Increased pulmonary vascular resistance. This is due to two causes.

    a. Structural changes principally thickening of walls of arterioles and small muscular pulmonary arteries with associated intimal changes.

    b. Persistence of fetal stucture in pulmonary small vessels may be cause of pulmonary hypertension in some cases of PDA. Kinetic effect of pulmonary artery pressure pulse may promote degenerative changes in pulmonary small vessels.

A functional element exists. Effect is produced by varying vascular resistance with differing oxygen tension in inspired air.

Hyperkinetic Pulmonary Hypertension

The higher pulmonary artery pressure the less classic murmur and more serious symptoms. Most have congestive cardiac failure. Features are due to large volume left to right shunt. Abolition of shunt surgically leads to drop in pulmonary artery pressure to normal levels. Late development of pulmonary vascular disease is not reported.

PULMONARY VASCULAR DISEASE

Patients with clear evidence of acquired pulmonary vascular disease: Pulmonary hypertension absent or moderate in childhood and true increase in pulmonary vascular resistance occurs due to prolonged aortico pulmonary shunting. These cases initially have left to right shunt, then bidirectional and finally right to left shunt. In ECG serial tracings at first there will be normal tracing or left ventricular hypertrophy, changing at a later stage to combined hypertrophy and then right ventricular hypertrophy alone.

Patients without clear evidence of pulmonary vascular disease have a relatively high vascular tone due to predominant proportion of blood entering right atrium flowing through right ventricle and pulmonary artery during fetal life. Exertional dyspnea is a common symptom in these cases. Cyanosis may be early but does not often become generalized for many years. As it is confined to legs alone or left arm and legs a superficial examination may not disclose its presence. Clubbing is correspondingly a localized phenomenon when present. Murmurs are atypical. There is never a continuous murmur. Systolic, diastolic alone or both systolic and diastolic murmur are present. Second heart sound in pulmonary area is greatly accentuated, palpable and split. Pulmonary ejection click is invariably present. Congestive heart failure is a terminal complication. Sudden death, infective endocarditis and hemoptysis may occur. Heart is of normal size on X-ray. Cardiomegaly occurs with congestive heart failure. Pulmonary artery segment bulges greatly. Hilar vascularity is not remarkable. ECG shows right axis deviation and right ventricular hypertrophy. Cardiac catheterization demonstrates the malformation by direct probing of ductus. Pulmonary artery pressure exceeds systemic level. Shunt through ductus is right to left. Blood samples from right radial artery are more saturated with oxygen than femoral arterial samples. Calculated pulmonary vascular resistance is markedly elevated. Pulmonary arteriography shows opacification of descending aorta in these circumstances. Indicator dilutional techniques will reveal more strikingly the functional hemodynamics. At autopsy there are marked right ventricular hypertrophy with pulmonary artery dilatation and atheroma. Microscopic changes in pulmonary artery are invariable.

DIAGNOSIS

The uncomplicated case: A well child free of any symptom and cyanosis is found on routine examination to have a continuous machinery murmur in second left intercostal space. X-ray may show normal size heart or slight cardiac enlargement and lung vascularity is slightly increased. ECG shows no axis deviation and some degree of left ventricular hypertrophy. Continuous murmur is heard even in infants.

Differential diagnosis of continuous murmur

1. *Venous hum* common in young children. It may be heard over base of heart and be maximal to the right or left of sternum. Movement of neck to one side or jugular compression abolishes hum. Extension of neck increases its intensity. In PDA these maneuvers do not change the murmur. Second heart sound in pulmonary area is frequently accentuated in PDA.

2. *Pulmonary arteriovenous fistula* in very young children a fistula in left upper lobe may cause confusion. Cyanosis and clubbing are present in association with normal size heart and normal ECG.

3. *Aortico pulmonary window*: Typical continuous machinery murmur occurs in second left intercostal space in association with left ventricular hypertrophy. Cyanosis may be present. Aortography is best method for visualizing the defect. With this technique differentiation from PDA is possible in infants.

4. *Ruptured sinus of Valsalva*: Rare in children but may occur in course of infective endocarditis. A machinery murmur in sixth left intercostal space and left ventricular hypertrophy in ECG with left to right intracardiac shunt on catheterization.

5. Coronary arterial fistula, traumatic or congenital thoracic wall fistula, congenital or surgically created aortico pulmonary arterial anastomosis, mitral atresia, aortic regurgitation, coarctation of aorta, supracardiac form of total anomalous pulmonary venous return and pulmonary artery stenosis produce a continuous murmur over precordium.

Complicated Cases

Associated Defects

1. *Cyanotic cases*: Presence of continuous murmur in association with cyanotic congenital heart disease is an indication either of PDA or collateral circulation to lung through bronchial arteries. Some of these patients will only be slightly cyanosed if collateral flow is large but with exception of tricuspid atresia they show right ventricular hypertrophy in ECG. Rarely tetralogy of Fallot may be associated with such a large flow through the ductus that normal oxygen saturation is seen on exercise but heart is enlarged, pulmonary vascularity increased and combined ventricular hypertrophy is present in ECG.

2. *Noncyanotic cases*: PDA in association with aortic stenosis, coarctation of aorta, ventricular septal defect, atrial septal defect and ventricular septal defect with aortic regurgitation occasionally causes confusion but the to and fro murmur present in this anomaly with left ventricular hypertrophh in ECG and angiographic findings should allow its separation from PDA. One-third of symptomatic infants of PDA and considerable cardiac enlargement will have atypical murmurs. The problem in these patients is to separate isolated PDA from combined defects. Truncus arteriosus with pulmonary artery arising from common trunk may be difficult to differentiate in an infant. Usually the patients are noncyanotic. There is a harsh systolic

murmur over precordium and heart failure responsive to digitalis develops in early infancy. The second heart sound is loud and single. Early diastolic murmur of truncus valve incompetence is common. Pulse is bounding. ECG shows left ventricular hypertrophy or biventricular hypertrophy. Aortogram demonstrates filling of pulmonary artery with contrast material. A firm clinical diagnosis of PDA is impossible without accessory investigations in cases of PDA with severe pulmonary hypertension associated with high pulmonary vascular resistance. Occasionally a history of intermittent cyanosis of left arm and both legs is obtained or differential clubbing of these areas is seen. Cyanosis may be entirely absent clinically and murmur if present unhelpful. The only unequivocal feature on auscultation is loudness of pulmonary second sound indicative of marked pulmonary hypertension. When predominant reversal of ductal flow is present right ventricular hypertrophy is the rule. Such cases are clinically considered as ventricular septal defect, aortico pulmonary window, PDA with reversal of flow, primary pulmonary hypertension and transposition of great vessels complexes.

SPONTANEOUS CLOSURE OF DUCTUS

For practical purpose it is assumed that great majority of healthy babies will have no shunt through ductus within 24 hours after birth. However, delay in accomplishing the relatively mature pulmonary circulation in the first month is associated with a delay in normal closure of ductus. Spontaneous closure is likely to occur in premature infants with clinical evidence of PDA after first few days of life. More than 75% of ducts in premature infants will undergo spontaneous closure within 4 months of birth. Possibility of spontaneous closure in term infants is maximal in first two to three months. Earlier hypoxic episodes can cause delay.

Treatment

Medical Management

Prophylaxis: The suggestion of routine therapeutic abortion for mothers affected by rubella during first trimester of pregnancy remains controversial. Most important prophylactic step is administration of rubella vaccine to female children.

Therapy: Treatment of infective endocarditis both prophylactic and therapeutic with proviso that patients with large left to right shunt should be operated upon after control if they fail to progress satisfactorily.

Medical closure by noninvasive methods

1. *Increased ambient oxygen concentration*: In term infants response is variable. The explanation of different responses may lie in different action of duct muscles either because of predetermined anatomic alterations or effect of metabolic disturbance on normal action toward duct closure.
2. *Prostaglandin synthetase inhibitors*: In ventillator dependent infant with severe congestive heart failure secondary to large ductus indomethacin offers a dramatically successful alternative to surgical ligation. Transient but significant depression in urinary output occurs. It is not clear whether this results from decreased renal blood flow or from increased ADH production. Permanent renal damage is unlikely.

Surgical Management

Indications: In uncomplicated cases operation may be advised after 6 months of age and before child starts school. In preterm infant with respiratory distress and deteriorating pulmonary function who do not respond to anticongestive therapy and minimal ventilatory support the first step is to give prostaglandin synthetase inhibitors and only if that regime fails it is necessary to proceed to direct ligation of ductus. Infant with isolated PDA and hyperkinetic pulmonary hypertension should be operated after 6 months of age.

In patients with pulmonary hypertension and pulmonary vascular resistance surgery is deferred. The basis for nonoperation is that long-term prognosis in Eisenmenger's syndrome is at least superior to prospect of perioperative death or to early demise from unrelieved congestive heart failure after removal of escape mechanism provided by ductus arteriosus.

Such a course is inevitable at surgery for patients with pure right to left ductal shunts due to very high pulmonary vascular resistance. It is a distinct risk for patients with trivial shunts in either direction and may occur when the shunt is only left to right.

Patients with PDA tolerate closure better than those with VSD and similar degree of pulmonary hypertension and increased pulmonary vascular resistance.

In conclusion it is unwise to close ductus of patients with high calculated pulmonary vascular resistance and pulmonary to systemic flow ratio of less than 2:1 due to doubts about long-term benefits except perhaps in infancy.

Type of Operation

1. Gross 1939 first reported ligation of ductus.
2. Gross later in 1943 changed his technique to division of ductus.
3. Blalock in 1946 suggested modification of ligation method known as suture ligation.

In short, wide ductus division is preferable to ductus ligation. Controlled hypotension in subjects with pulmonary hypertension or friable ductus is a valuable adjunct to operative technique.

Immediate Results

1. Increase in systemic systolic and diastolic pressure.
2. Decrease in pulmonary artery pressure.
3. Patients with severe pulmonary vascular disease deteriorate immediately when duct is clamped.
4. Disappearance of continuous murmur and decrease in activity and volume of heart.

Late Results

1. Improvement in growth.
2. ECG reverts to normal.
3. Recurrence of shunt (with duct ligation).

16

Persistent Truncus Arteriosus

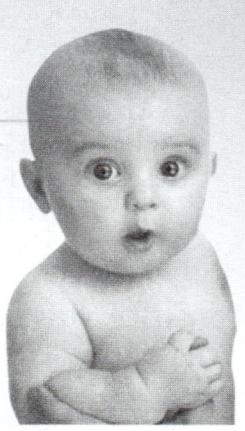

A condition in which all three circulations, systemic, pulmonary and coronary arise from a single vessel, leaving base of heart through single valve.

This definition excludes aortic atresia, pulmonary atresia and aortico pulmonary window.

ANATOMY

One large trunk leaves base of heart due to failure of truncal septum to develop and separate aorta from pulmonary artery. This failure may be complete when pulmonary artery branches arise directly from trunk or partial when there is main pulmonary artery arising from trunk. Semilunar valve is commonly tricuspid. Cusps are thick and polypoid and appear to threaten coronary ostia. These abnormal cusps are result of developmental arrest of local growth with persistence of fetal form. Truncal valve overrides ventricular septum. Its circumference equals that of normal semilunar valve. Coronary ostia are abnormal. Right or left coronary artery arise from non coronary cusps. VSD is large and due to under development or virtual absence of distal part of pulmonary infundibulum. Defect does not have upper border. Lower border is formed by septal band in proximal infundibulum. Defect is similar to that seen in TOF. Truncal valve is in fibrous continuity with mitral valve and also with tricuspid valve when septal band is not well developed. There is no subtruncal conus.

Variants in Pulmonary Artery

1. Aortopulmonary septum is partially formed so that while MPA is separate in its upper part septum is absent below so forming common truncus. Distal MPA gives rise to right and left pulmonary artery.
2. Aortopulmonary septum is entirely absent. There is no discreet MPA and both pulmonary artery branches arise from common trunk separately.
3. Right or left pulmonary artery may be absent. Respective lung being supplied by collaterals.
4. Fourth arch is poorly developed and sixth arch predominates. This results in small hypoplastic ascending aorta or coarctation or atresia of isthmus. In these cases there is large PDA which is continuous with descending aorta.

Associated Anomalies

PDA, coarctation of aorta, single ventricle and multiple congenital noncardiovascular anomalies.

Hemitruncus

Very rare condition in which one pulmonary artery arises normally from right ventricle while the other usually supplying the lung opposite to the side of aortic arch arises from ascending aorta. With low pulmonary vascular resistance and large artery lung may become overperfused and heart failure develops. In these cases banding of artery or implantation of artery into MPA may be necessary.

Pseudotruncus

In this condition the pulmonary circulation is supplied by descending aorta.

ANATOMIC CLASSIFICATION
Collett and Edwards (1949)

Type 1: Single pulmonary trunk and ascending aorta arising from common trunk.

Type 2: Left and right pulmonary arteries arising close together from dorsal wall of truncus.

Type 3: Right left or both pulmonary arteries arising independently from either side of truncus.

Type 4: No pulmonary arteries and apparent absence of sixth aortic arch. Lung being supplied by way of bronchial arteries.

Type 5: Aortopulmonary fenestration.

Anderson Classification (1957)

Type 1: Pulmonary arteries arising from trunk proximal to innominate arteries.

Type 2: Absence of one pulmonary artery.

Type 3: Absence of both pulmonary arteries.

Type 4: Partial truncus arteriosus.

Van Pragh Classification (1965)

Type A: Those with VSD.

Type B: Those without VSD.

A1: Same as Collett type 1.

A2: Same as Collett type 2, 3.

A3: Absence of one or other pulmonary artery branches. Respective lung being supplied by collaterals or bronchial arteries and hemitruncus.

A4: Poorly developed fourth arch with aortic isthmus displaying hypoplasia, coarctation, atresia or absence and with large PDA.

PHYSIOLOGIC CLASSIFICATION

Clinical picture and natural history of truncus arteriosus is largely determined by size of pulmonary blood flow. This in turn depends upon pulmonary vascular resistance or narrowing of pulmonary arteries.

Group 1: High PBF with low PVR. This is common picture in infancy and is associated with refractory cardiac failure. Cyanosis is not noted.

Group 2: Normal or slightly increased PBF due to increasing PVR. These children do not have failure but are cyanosed on exertion.

Group 3: Low PBF due to ostial narrowing or progressive pulmonary vascular disease. Cyanosis is marked.

High PBF in group 1 is responsible for absence or mildness of cyanosis. There is large pool of pulmonary venous blood returning to left atrium and being ejected from left ventricle into common trunk. Right ventricle is also contracting to systemic pressure and ejecting systemic venous return into common trunk. Large VSD allows free communication between right ventricle and left ventricle and resultant admixture of blood determines depth of cyanosis. Where pulmonary blood flow is large volume overload on heart is severe. Any coexisting insufficiency of truncal valves will make matters worse as a proportion of ejected stroke volume regurgitates into ventricles during diastole. Thus CHF is common and as LAP rises pulmonary edema and impairment of diffusion of oxygen from alveoli to capillaries may cause desaturation of pulmonary venous blood and increase cyanosis. When PVR starts to climb in group 2 and 3 pulmonary venous return declines although heart failure disappears and heart is smaller cyanosis will become more marked. Once PVR has risen to 1/3 to 1/2 systemic levels this Eisenmenger reaction is progressive even though surgical correction a high-risk in these patients may be successfully carried out.

CLINICAL FEATURES

Children with truncus present in early weeks of life. 68% infants die before reaching 3 months of age.

Infant presents with CHF with or without chest infection. Overriding impression of these children is that they have large left to right shunt since at this stage cyanosis is mild and clinical features are similar to a child with VSD or PDA in CHF. What mild cyanosis is present could be ascribed to pulmonary edema.

1. *Failure to thrive*: Failure to gain weight is constant feature.

2. Dyspnea: Prominent because of CHF. It may take form of tachypnea initially with rate increasing to 50 to 100/minute. But as condition persists with addition of CHF due to

excessive PBF lungs stiffen as compliance decreases and breathing becomes labored. However, if PBF is limited by pulmonary ostial stenosis or pulmonary vascular disease dyspnea is not seen.

3. *Cyanosis:* Extremely variable. May be minimal or absent when PBF is large. When PBF is nearly equal to systemic and CHF is absent it may be mild at rest increasing on exertion or crying. However, where PBF is low cyanosis can be extremely marked and accompanied in older children by plethora, polycyathemia and finger clubbing.

4. *General examination:* Typical infant is in CHF with hyperactive circulation and left to right shunt. Liver is enlarged and there are rales in chest. Peripheral pulses are brisk and bounding probably due to truncal valve incompetence and increased systemic run off.

5. *Heart sounds:* First HS is normal. Second HS is loud and ringing. In 50% cases it is closely split. In these cases either cusps do not close synchronously or duplicate sound is set-up by vibrations in arterial trunk.

6. *Ejection clicks:* Prominent apical systolic ejection click is heard in every case. This is characteristic of truncus.

7. *Murmurs:* Most patients have systolic murmurs. In some cases murmur is pan systolic, harsh and maximal in 3rd, 4th LICS, similar to VSD. In others murmur is ejection systolic at LSE. Rarely MDM of relative MS is heard inside apex. Continuous murmur is very rare. Early diastolic murmur is heard in 36% cases.

8. When thrill is present it is maximal at lower LSE. Occasionally also felt in upper sternum or in suprasternal notch.

RADIOLOGY

Cardiac shadow is large. Cardiac outline has no specific shape. Both left and right ventricles are enlarged and pedicle usually appears narrow. Pulmonary plethora is marked. Most characteristic feature is high origin of pulmonary arteries. This may be seen on right but more typically left. Right aortic arch occurs in 31% cases. Combination of pulmonary plethora and right aortic arch should make one suspect truncus.

ECHOCARDIOGRAPHY

Echo record shows that trunk overrides ventricular septum. There is no anterior vessel and no echo arising from pulmonary valve. Absence of pulmonary valve echo distinguishes truncus from TOF. Clinically TOF is not differential diagnosis from truncus in infancy. Cases of truncus have large LA compared to infants with TOF. 67% of truncus cases have reduplication of semilunar valve echo.

ECG

Mean QRS axis is 100°. Combined ventricular hypertrophy pattern is commonest followed by RVH and LVH.

HEMODYNAMICS

Right ventricle pressure is near systemic level. There is step up in oxygen saturation suggesting VSD. Catheter tip passes from trunk into either pulmonary artery branches or aorta. Oxygen saturation of blood in trunk is very high. This is compatible with minimal clinical cyanosis. Oxygen saturation in pulmonary arteries is same as trunk. PAP is equal to trunk pressure. Any significant gradient suggests either true or relative stenosis of ostia. Pulmonary capillary wedge, LVED and LA pressures are elevated in infants with CHF. PBF is high in such cases. 2 to 4 times of systemic. PVR is low. With time there is an inevitable development of pulmonary vascular disease with increase in PVR, PBF falls and systemic oxygen saturation lowers.

ANGIOCARDIOGRAPHY

This is cornerstone of correct diagnosis of truncus. Injection should be made in truncus and filmed in AP and lateral projections. Complete truncal anatomy can be seen.

Diagnosis

Usual presentation is of an infant in first weeks of life who has failed to thrive from birth and who has shown dyspnea. A murmur of doubtful significance is heard. Cyanosis is an inconstant feature. On examination the infant is distressed. Cyanosis is mild. Pulses are brisk. Liver and heart are enlarged. There is an ESM and marked ejection click. MDM or EDM may be heard. Second HS is single but may be split. X-ray shows enlarged heart with pulmonary plethora and right sided aortic arch. ECG shows combined, right or left ventricular hypertrophy with frontal axis of about +100.

Initial assessment is usually of a large VSD or PDA causing large left to right shunt. If cyanosis is more marked TGV with VSD may be considered. However in VSD and PDA second HS should be split. EDM are rare in TGV. Endocardial cushion defect shows LAD in ECG. Preductal coarctation of aorta may be considered since it is a common cause of CHF in this age group. Aortic atresia and hypoplastic left heart syndrome would be excluded by good pulses and presence of increased LV forces in precordial ECG. In TGV with tricuspid atresia there are usually no RV forces. Echocardiography is helpful. Definitive diagnosis is made from angiogram.

Prognosis

Poor. Median age at death 5 weeks. Only 36% children live up to 3 months of age. Only 22% children survive first year. Cause of death is CHF associated with pneumonia.

Treatment

- Initial treatment is of CHF and chest infection. However, digoxin and diuretics rarely produce significant improvement in children with large PBF. Truncal valve incompetence is cause of resistant CHF.
- Early catheterization is indicated.

Surgery

Palliative pulmonary artery banding. This reduces PBF, relieves CHF and protects lungs from progressive pulmonary vascular disease.

Corrective Surgery

Rastelli procedure. Pulmonary arteries are removed from trunk, septal defect is closed so that LV alone ejects into trunk which then becomes aorta. A conduit (valved decron tubes) is placed from anterior RV wall to pulmonary arteries. Success of operation depends upon PVR. When this is high mortality is 60%. Risk is also high in less than 5 and more than 12 years old. Preliminary pulmonary artery banding improves outlook by lowering PVR. Definitive repair with valved conduit should be done in first year of life in patients who do not have ostial stenosis and have torrential PBF. Conduit may have to be replaced by a larger one at 5 to 10 years of age.

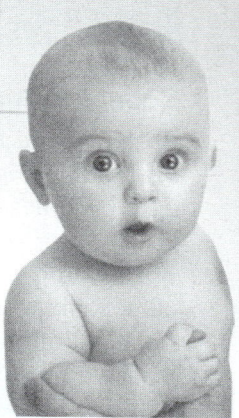

17

Complete Transposition of Great Arteries

DEFINITION

Condition in which right ventricle gives rise to aorta and left ventricle to pulmonary artery. Atria and ventricles are usually in situs solitus not inverted. Aorta is usually anteriorly situated and to right of pulmonary artery.

EMBRYOLOGY

Theories about morphogenesis of complete transposition:

1. Differential conal development theory: *Proposed by sir Arthur Keith 1909.*

   In normal different rates of growth and/or absorption of subsemilunar conuses results in subpulmonary conus bringing pulmonary artery round anteriorly and to left. While loss of subaortic conus allows aorta to sink posteriorly and to right. In transposition subaortic conus either grows or is not absorbed. Thus aorta remains high anterior and to right while subpulmonary conus is lost and pulmonary artery is low posterior and to left.

2. Straight aorticopulmonary septum theory: (*Van Meirop 1970*)

   Truncal ridges 2 and 4 rather than ridges 1 and 3 fuse to form septum. This results in nontwisting of great arteries and so an anterior aorta.

   In corrected transposition TGA is corrected by ventricular inversion.

Complete transposition occurs most commonly in situs individual with solitus atria, solitus ventricles and D transposed great arteries. Course of circulation is RA–RV aorta body systemic veins–RA as one circulation and LA–LV pulmonary artery lungs pulmonary veins–LA as other circulation. Thus two circulations systemic and pulmonary are in parallel instead of in series and obviously incompatible with life unless there is mixing which can take place at atrial, ventricular or great artery level.

Mixing at atrial level takes place through foramen ovale. Rarely there is ASD of secundum variety. This is compatible with life. Shunting at ventricular level is via VSD in membranous septum. There may be anomalies of AV valves. Shunting at great arteries level occurs via PDA or via bronchial circulation.

Pulmonary stenosis is a commonly associated congenital malformation in TGA occurring in 6% cases with intact septum and 31% of those with VSD.

Coronary arteries most commonly are of normal pattern. Left coronary artery arises from left sinus and divides into left anterior descending artery which courses down anterior interventricular sulcus down to apex and left circumflex which runs round to left. In 70% cases circumflex branch runs in front of LVOT and so could interfere with attempt at surgical relief of PS in this area. RCA arises from posterior sinus.

- Associated anomalies:
- Right aortic arch.
- Coarctation of aorta.
- Hypoplastic RV.

PHYSIOLOGY

Right to left shunt is that volume of blood which returning to right atrium crosses septum and is ejected into pulmonary artery, called as effective pulmonary blood flow. In transposition this must be balanced by and equal and opposite left to right shunt which returning to left atrium is ejected into aorta. If these two volumes are not equal over any period of time one circulation will become overfilled and other depleted of blood. Left to right shunt in TGA is also called effective systemic blood flow. In a fetus without TGA the more oxygenated blood returning via umbilical vein to inferior vena cava crosses to left atrium and perfuses upper part of body via left ventricle and ascending aorta. In TGA this blood will cross to eject through pulmonary artery and via ductus perfuse lower part of body while less oxygenated blood from superior vena cava will perfuse upper segment. This circulatory disturbance does not appear to be deleterious and most cases of TGA are born with normal or increased birth weight. After birth ductus remains patent for variable period of time. This allows some mixing between two circulations and will be associated with persistence of high pressure in pulmonary circulation when ventricular septum is intact and ductus starts to close pulmonary artery pressure drops towards normal and hypoxia and acidosis become more marked. When there is VSD, pulmonary artery pressure remains high. These patients are at risk for pulmonary vascular disease.

Classification

(Kidd and associates 1971)

Group 1: With intact ventricular septum.

Group 2: With intact ventricular septum and pulmonary stenosis.

Group 3: With VSD

Group 4: With VSD and PS.

Hemodynamically there are three groups

1. Those with inadequate communication between two circulations (group with intact ventricular septum).
2. Those with adequate communication (with VSD).
3. Those with obstruction to pulmonary blood flow (with PS).

Surgically there are two groups

1. Simple transposition (with intact ventricular septum).
2. Complex transposition (with VSD or PS or both).

Prevalence

- 9% of total congenital heart disease.
- 1 in 4500 live births.
- Male: Female ratio 1.8: 1
- There is an increased incidence of maternal diabetes. (11.4 times as frequent in TGA than in general population.
- Infants with TGA are large at birth.
- TGA is leading cause of death under 1 month of life.

Clinical Features

Presentation is in newborn period. Those with intact VS present in majority within first month of life. Those with VSD present in majority by the end of third month. There are three main clinical syndromes of presentation in newborn period:

Group 1: Hypoxia and acidosis: There is inadequate communication between two circulations. These babies are cyanosed and distressed shortly after birth. Oxygen does not help. On physical examination baby is of good size. There is cyanosis, respiratory distress, tachycardia and tachypnea. Pulses are good volume. Blood pressure normal. Apex beat not displaced. First heart sound normal. Second heart sound single or narrowly split. There is usually a faint nonspecific ejection systolic murmur. No click or other added sound. Signs of congestive heart failure develop with passage of time.

Group 2: Congestive heart failure: These patients have TGA with large VSD. There is better mixing between two circulations, so cyanosis and respiratory distress are not marked. These children present later. Rarely differential cyanosis is noted with more cyanosis in face and upper extremity than lower. This indicates that PDA is perfusing lower extremities and should always raise suspicion of coarctation of aorta or an interrupted aortic arch coexisting. On physical examination these babies appear large and well nourished. There is marked respiratory distress with tachypnea and tachycardia. Liver is enlarged. Cyanosis may be mild or marked. Pulses are usually present and forceful. Precordium is hyperactive with right ventricular lift. First heart sound is normal. Second heart sound single or closely split. There is a harsh pansystolic or long ejection systolic murmur best heard at lower left sternal edge. Diastolic murmurs are rare. Continuous murmur is uncommon to hear even though PDA may be present. CHF is severe and resistant to medical treatment. Pulmonary edema is common and chest infection supervene. Cyanosis becomes more severe.

Group 3: Pulmonary oligemia: These patients have pulmonary stenosis. They present much later. Heart failure is rare and cyanosis mild. Majority of these survive infancy. Clinical presentation is usually of a murmur and cyanosis usually in first 3 months of life. Cyanosis is variable and worse on crying. CHF is extremely rare. On physical examination baby is not distressed and may be mildly cyanosed. Pulses are good and liver is not enlarged. Precordium is quiet although there may be left ventricular or right ventricular impulses. First heart sound is normal. Second heart sound single. There is usually a harsh ejection systolic murmur at upper left sternal edge.

Occasionally pulmonary stenosis is much severe and patient presents with cyanosis marked around first week of life, severe hypoxia and acidosis with CHF. Sudden deterioration in these children is due to closure of ductus arteriosus which in face of critical pulmonary stenosis has been perfusing pulmonary circulation.

In all these clinical groups it is important to check femoral pulses because of possibility of associated problems in aortic arch, such as interruption or coarctation of aorta.

RADIOLOGICAL EXAMINATION

Fanconi in 1932 described narrow vascular pedicle at base of heart and attributed it to course of aorta in front of and parallel to pulmonary artery.

Vascular markings are either normal or increased. Heart is 'egg shaped', egg lies obliquely on its side with narrow end at cardiac apex, shoulder where pulmonary artery would be in normal and top of egg at upper right atrium.

With VSD and good mixing cardiac shadow is enlarged with both ventricles involved. Narrow superior pedicle and absence of main pulmonary artery shadow are characteristic. Pulmonary vascular markings are increased. Pulmonary edema may be present. With increasing age heart increases in size, shape becomes more characteristic and hilar vascularity becomes more increased. With PS picture may be confused with TOF. Both lung fields are oligemic, heart is small. Convex upward border to empty pulmonary artery bay rather than concave upward one typical of boot shaped heart in TOF may be helpful in differentiating.

ECHOCARDIOGRAPHY

Useful in differential diagnosis of sick cyanotic neonate. In TGA mitral and tricuspid valves are normal in excursion and are easily located. VS is normal as are LV and RV cavities. There is continuity between mitral valve apparatus and posterior border of posterior great artery and septum and its anterior border.

Relationship of great arteries can be defined.

Simultaneous visualization of both great arteries at same transducer position.

Posterior semilunar valve opens earlier and closes later than anterior one in TGA.

ECG

Sinus rhythm and normal PR interval. Normal RV dominance of newborn persists in TGA instead of regressing to left in normal heart.

Infants with group 2 (VSD) have higher incidence of combined ventricular hypertrophy.

A diminution of RV forces in TGA should alert to possibility of hypoplastic RV.

Vector provides more useful information regarding LV pressure than ECG. Because LV forces are cancelled early by increased RV forces.

Cardiac Catheterization

Diagnostic use in newborn:

1. To confirm diagnosis of TGA.
2. To determine associated lesions like VSD, PDA, PS and coarctation
3. To carry out balloon atrial septostomy.

Very desaturated blood is found in right atrium. RV pressure is at systemic level. Catheter can be passed in aorta which is also desaturated. If there is no VSD there is no step up in oxygen saturation from SVC sample to aorta sample. LA and pulmonary veins are fully saturated. LV pressure is always systemic when there is VSD.

Angiocardiography

Aorta fills on injection of RV. In VSD LV and pulmonary artery will opacify from RV injection and size and position of VSD will be seen. Hypoplastic RV can be identified.

Distribution of PBF is uneven, favoring right lung due to morphologic and hydraulic factors. Inclination of LVOT and MPA is normally to right and with time favors development of this uneven distribution.

MPA in some cases is aneurysmally dilated. Left ventriculogram will demonstrate size and nature of PS which may be valvular or subvalvular.

An aortogram should be done to exclude coarctation and other aortic arch anomaly and to define state of ductus arteriosus.

Diagnosis

Respiratory distress, cyanosis and CHF in newborn with characteristic clinical findings and negative hyperoxic test with egg shaped heart on chest X-ray, normal or rightward ECG and echocardiogram (which excludes single ventricle, truncus and hypoplastic right heart and confirms transposition).

Definitive diagnosis is by angiocardiography.

BALLOON ATRIAL SEPTOSTOMY

Introduced by Rashkind and Miller in 1966. A catheter with a latex balloon at tip is passed up IVC into RA and maneuvered across atrial septum via foramen ovale into LA. After confirmation of position of catheter tip in LA balloon is inflated with 1.5 to 3 ml of contrast material and balloon is withdrawn forcibly down into IVC. Procedure is repeated 2–3 times to ensure optimal opening. Immediate result of this procedure is an improvement in oxygen saturation. Improvement of metabolic acidosis and abolition of pressure gradient between two atria.

Rashkind balloon atrial septostomy should be carried out in all cases of TGA at time of catheterization in newborn period. Other indications of this technique are hypoplastic right or left heart syndrome and TAPVD where life depends upon circulation crossing atrial septum.

COMPLICATIONS

1. Cerebrovascular accidents:
   Incidence of thrombotic episodes varies between 17 and 24%. Venous and dural sinus thrombosis is commoner than arterial thrombosis. Pathogenesis is hypoxia and polycythemia.
2. Pulmonary vascular disease:
   Incidence is greater in TGA than in other CHD. It is universal when there is VSD and mild with intact VS.

CORRECTIVE SURGERY

Mustard procedure 1964.

It consists of removing atrial septum and replacing it with a baffle or wall made of pericardium which placed around SVC and IVC directs blood from these vessels to mitral valve and allows pulmonary venous blood to travel to tricuspid valve. If VSD is present it must be repaired.

Pulmonary artery banding prior to Mustard procedure carried out in early infancy retards development of pulmonary vascular disease.

In patients in whom pulmonary vascular disease has already arisen *palliative Mustard procedure* is done.

Correction of PS is performed by *Rastelli type procedure*. In this while VSD is being repaired pulmonary artery is detached from LV and attached to anterior aspect of RV via a decron valved conduit.

CONCLUSION

1. First a balloon atrial septostomy for all cases of TGA in early infancy.
2. *TGA with intact VS and result of atrial septostomy is good*: Total correction at 10 to 12 months.

    If result of atrial septostomy not good total correction at 4 to 6 months age.
3. *TGA with VSD*: Mustard procedure and closure of VSD at 6 months or pulmonary artery banding at 3 month with Mustard repair at 2 years age.
4. *TGA with pulmonary vascular disease*: Palliative Mustard procedure. Leave VSD alone. This improves cyanosis and symptomatology and converts a TGA with Eisenmenger reaction into straightforward Eisenmenger syndrome.
5. *TGA with VSD with PS*: Observation until 5 years age. However, if PS is severe either a systemic pulmonary Blalock Taussig shunt or complete repair by Mustard procedure and widening of LVOT or Rastelli type of operation.

These operations are not corrective and carry long-term problems of severity. Improved techniques for dealing with coronary arteries have prompted a return to great artery switching procedure.

18

Ventricular Septal Defect

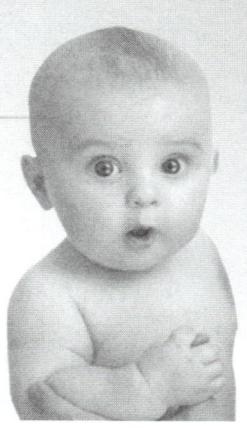

In 1879 Roger first described clinical signs of VSD. Dalrymple first described Eisenmenger complex in 1847. Eisenmenger recorded findings of similar case in 1897.

Eisenmenger complex is VSD with pulmonary hypertension and pulmonary vascular resistance sufficient to force blood from right side of heart to enter aorta.

PREVALENCE

VSD occurs in between 1.3 and 2.4 per thousand live births. It occurs with many congenital heart anomalies. In association with other anomalies VSD makes up a group that is approximately 26% of all CHD. Thus as an isolated or combined lesion VSD is present in approximately 50% of all CHD.

VSD can occur as an isolated lesion: 23% of all CHD VSD as a prime lesion with or without another defect such as PDA or MR.

Associated lesion is primary but VSD makes up the part of picture, e.g. TCF.

ASSOCIATED LESIONS WITH 100% VSD

TOF, common ventricle, persistent truncus, mitral atresia, atrioventricularis communis, aortic regurgitation, LV into RA, DORV.

- With tricuspid atresia: 90%.

- With absent aortic isthmus: 80%
- With L TGV: 65%.
- With D TGV: 56%.
- With coarctation of aorta: 16%.
- With ASD secundum: 10%.
- With PDA: 5%.

Classification

Ventricular septum develops between 5th and 7th week of fetal life and is formed by a complex union of muscular partition which is evolved between ventricles and bulbar ridges that divide great vessels. In center of heart endocardial cushions contribute to union of these structures.

VSD in outflow tract in RV are due to failure of certain muscular components to develop in fetal life. Anomalous opening is then related to particular muscle segment affected and size of defect to degree of involvement.

Muscular hypertrophy occurs in specific portions of muscle bundles of outflow tract with abnormal hyperplasia being prominent feature in certain cases particularly TOF. Either abnormal muscular hyperplasia or anomalous septal opening may be result of primordial injury and this is dependent upon timing and severity of damage to specific muscle bundles in fetal life. A variety of combined defects are due to similar episodes in other portions of heart. Endocardial cushion defects cause the lesion of atrioventricularis communis and ostium primum. Both defects and left axis deviation associated with these lesions being explained on basis of faulty fusion of bulboventricular septa producing disturbance in development of left conducting bundle branch particularly anterior branch.

Another syndrome due in part to an abnormality of junction tissue in bulbomusculature is Ebstein anomaly which leads to displacement of tricuspid valve toward apex (Grant 1961). Defect in ventricular septum may appear in variety of areas. Four areas most commonly involved in isolated form of VSD are:

1. Bulbar septal region.
2. Sinus septal region.

3. Membranous region.
4. AV canal region.

Becu and coworkers have devised a classification of VSD based on a division of RV into outflow and inflow tract. Outflow tract is defined as portion of ventricular septum that lies between pulmonary valve above and nearest part of tricuspid valve below (or papillary muscle of conus). Inflow tract is referred to as portion of septum that lies below anterior and medial leaflets of tricuspid valve.

Crista supraventricularis or ridge of septal tissue that originates from septum that lies below anterior and medial divide outflow tract into superior and inferior portions.

Lesions lying above crista are uncommon.

Greatest number of VSD lie between crista and medial leaflet of tricuspid valve. In this position they are in close proximity to aortic valve and many are directly continuous with it. A number have a small band of tissue separating them from aortic valve. While such openings are in area of membranous portion of septum Becu has demonstrated that defect is more often in muscular tissue adjoining membranous portion of septum rather than in membranous structure itself.

Defect may appear under posterior leaflet of tricuspid valve. This occurs in 15% of cases. It can be readily approached by a surgeon from RA through tricuspid valve and closed without ventriculotomy.

Defects can also pierce muscular portion of septum in various positions down to and including apex.

From embryonic and anatomic viewpoint ventricular septum in reality is a union for four septa:

1. Bulbar septum.
2. Ventricular sinus septum.
3. Retrocristal septum.
4. Atrioventricular septum.

Defects involve all four septa hence, there are four general types of VSD:

1. Bulbar septal defect.
2. Ventricular sinus septal defect.

3. Retrocristal defect.
4. AV septal defect.

BULBAR SEPTAL DEFECT

Bulbar septum is intracardiac portion of bulbotruncal septum. Bulbotruncal septum is absent in truncus arteriosus, therefore a high large anterior defect is present, limited superiorly by semilunar valves of truncus and inferiorly by crest of ventricular sinus septum anteriorly. Defects due to muscle deficiency may involve bulbar septum and may be associated with absence of moderator band. In Taussig-Bing malformation defect is large, high and anterior with same boundaries superiorly and inferiorly as defect in true truncus arteriosus, but bulbar septum is not absent. It may be well formed but it is markedly malaligned relative to ventricular sinus septum. Bulbar septum is displaced to right and lies in an anteroposterior plane whereas sinus septum is further to left and makes an angle of 40° to left relative to anteroposterior plane.

DEFECTS IN VENTRICULAR SINUS SEPTUM

This septum is common party wall that remains between excavations or evaginations of right and left ventricular sinuses. Ventricular sinus septum does not grow upward. Ventricular septum grows downwards with progressive outpouching of ventricular sinuses. Muscular defect occurs in any portion of sinus septum. It may be small or large. Single or multiple. Ventricular septum may be single or rudimentary resulting in an infrequent type of single or common ventricle. When neither ventricular sinus develops common party wall between sinuses that is ventricular septum, also is absent, this also being an infrequent type of single or common ventricle.

'Swiss cheese' ventricular septum with multiple muscular defects appears to be related to deficient septal musculature, a deficiency of stratum compactum, ventricular septum being composed of a mesh of trabeculae carneae of stratum spongiosum, hence, the numerous defects.

In case of tricuspid atresia without transposition, a muscular sinus septal defect characteristically small but occasionally large is the only communication between LV and hypoplastic RV and pulmonary artery.

JUNCTIONAL DEFECTS IN MEMBRANOUS REGION (RETROCRISTAL)

This region of membranous septum lies posterior to crista supraventricularis. This is a tripartite septum formed by its three neighbors:
1. Bulbar ridges which also forms bulbar septum.
2. Right tubercles of AV endocardial cushions which also form tricuspid valve.
3. Endocardial cushion tissue on crest of muscular ventricular septum.

Hence, retrocristal region is a functional area between ventricular septum, ventricular sinus septum and AV canal.

This junction appears vulnerable to anomalies involving any of its 3 sources. Hence, it is to be anticipated that retrocristal junctional defects are most common type.

Defects involving retrocristal membranous junction occur in following malformations:
1. As isolated retrocristal defect.
2. In TOF.
3. In origin of both great arteries from right ventricle (excluding Taussig-Bing malformation)
4. In TGV (L and D).
5. In LV–RA defect.
6. In single ventricle (left) with rudimentary (bulbar) outlet chamber.

ATRIOVENTRICULAR SEPTAL DEFECTS

AV junction is posterior relative to immediately retrocristal region. This junction normally is formed by most inferior portion of atrial septum which is septum of AV canal and by crest of ventricular sinus septum posteriorly.

Defects of AV septal junction are:

1. With patent AV canal, complete or partial (absence of AV canal septum).
2. With displacement of AV canal septum (to right, left, anterior or posterior) in association with hypoplasia or absence of either ventricular sinus.
3. With both 1 and 2.
4. With neither 1 or 2.

There is high, long posterior defect of AV canal type but without patency of AV canal and without displacement of posterior portion of ventricular sinus septum. This defect appears to represent failure of union of posterior sinus septal crest with AV canal septum without other abnormalities.

79% of VSD occur in membranous portion of septum.

ANATOMIC AND EMBRYOLOGIC CLASSIFICATION OF VSD

1. Bulbar septal defects: 8%.
   Isolated VSD.
   Taussig-Bing malformation.
   Truncus arteriosus.
   – Deficient bulbar myocardium
   – Malalignment of bulbar septum relative to ventricular sinus septum +/– bulbar septal defect.
   – Absent bulbar septum.
2. Sinus septal defects. 12%.
   Isolated muscular VSD (single, multiple, small, large).
   Tricuspid atresia.
   – Deficiency of myocardium of sinus septum.
3. Membranous region VSD. 70%.
   Isolated VSD.
   TOF
   TGA. D and L.
   LV – RA defect.
   – Deficient closure of junctional zone by bulbar ridges, right tubercles of AV endocardial cushions and by endocardial cushion tissue on crest of sinus septum.

4. AV canal region VSD. 8%.

   Isolated VSD.

   With patent AV canal, complete or partial.

   – Defective junction between atrial and ventricular sinus septa +/ – malalignment of ventricular septum relative to atrial septum +/– patent AV canal.

5. Combinations of above. 2%.

PATHOLOGY

VSD in infancy and childhood has considerable range in size, varying from 1 mm in diameter up to 25 mm. It may be circular, elliptic or eccentric. Rim may be smooth and rounded or firm and fibrotic, or ridge like. Approximately 50% of isolated VSD in childhood have diameter 75% of aortic diameter or less. When aorta is dextraposed ventricular defect is a large one and hence is associated with an augmented pulmonary blood flow and increased pressure with consequent pathology if left uncorrected over years.

Most characteristic response to increased flow and pressure is in pulmonary arteries. Prognosis both immediate and remote is intimately related to reaction in these vessels.

Pulmonary arteries have three main divisions:

1. Elastic arteries
2. Muscular arteries
3. Arterioles.

Elastic arteries are 1000 micron in diameter. Media of these vessels consist primarily of elastic fibrils with some smooth muscle cell fibers, collagen and ground substance. Elastic tissue in pulmonary trunk changes from that of fetal life and infancy as child matures. Adult pattern is established by end of second year and consist of a thinning out of media and breaking up of elastic tissue so that it becomes more regular and sparse than aorta with short fibrils branching in all directions. This is different from appearance in infancy when there are long parallel fibers with more symmetric distribution as is found in aorta. If pulmonary hypertension persists from birth elastic tissue retains its infantile appearance.

Normal muscular arteries are between 100 and 1000 micron in diameter. They are hypertrophied in newborn with a lumen to wall ratio of 1:1 or 1:2 but thin out rapidly during first year of life and then more gradually during childhood until they become thin walled structure that is characteristic of adulthood. Pulmonary arteries normally have distinct muscular media only at point of origin from parent muscular artery. Remaining course of arteriole is structured with a single elastic lamina. In presence of pulmonary hypertension there is muscular media present and hypertrophied in many small arteries down to 30 micron in diameter. There may be some relative increase in thickness of media of pulmonary muscular arteries in region of lingula. In presence of small VSD maturation of pulmonary arteries proceeds in normal fashion with normal thinning of wall. If big defect is present with large flow and increased pressure in pulmonary artery, a number of changes may occur:

1. Normal hypertrophy of small muscular arteries may persist on into infancy and childhood instead of regressing in normal fashion.
2. There are four grades of response of pulmonary arteries to increased flow and pressure:

Grade 1: Hypertrophy of medial wall of small muscular arteries (media may be 25% of diameter of external elastic lamina).

Grade 2: Hyperplasia of intima.

Grade 3: Hyperplasia and fibrosis of intima to point of obstruction in many small pulmonary arteries. At this stage pulmonary arteries tend to become tortuous.

Grade 4: Dilatation lesions. Thinning of wall beyond site of obstruction in small arteries. This may reach such proportion of sacular formation when such dilated vessels lie near air spaces that they may herniate into them and rupture causing hemoptysis. Plexiform lesions may form at site of obstruction resulting in small thin walled vessels that appear to proceed in and out of obstructed area.

Since some of obstructed vessels reach diameter of 0.2 to 0.3 mm as soon as these lesions are widespread a marked decrease in pulmonary blood flow results. In presence of VSD this may cause reversal of flow through anomalous opening of aorta and clinically may produce cyanosis on exercise or at rest.

Original dynamic responses obviously put a load on LV when pulmonary blood flow is large and resistance low. Load shifts gradually to right as resistance rises and blood flow to lungs decreases.

Changing dynamics are reflected in size and thickness of ventricular walls as well as in pulmonary arteries. VSD with a fatal outcome is classified into four groups:

1. Those with isolated VSD.
2. Those with other cardiac defects.
3. Those with noncardiac congenital defects, e.g. mongolism.
4. Those whose deaths are associated with other causes, such as pneumonia.

20% die of CHF per se. Highest mortality in first year of life. Bundle of His follows a path along posterior rim of ventricular septum and is intimately related to margin of septal defect in area of membranous portion. In its course along posterior or inferior aspect of VSD bundle gave off left ventricular branches which fan out over LV surface so that most of these fibers are not intimately related to defect itself. Right bundle continues its anteroinferior course. In some instances it is associated with margin or rim of septal defect.

Bundle pathway may present problem to surgeon when bundle is positioned in central portion of rim of heart. If defect is small one conducting tissue does not relate to defect. In TOF bundle is situated to left side of septum and below defect.

HEMODYNAMICS

Newborn Period

Most characteristic changes in child with VSD are centered on pulmonary arteries.

In normal fetus at term blood flow through lungs is thought to be 5 to 10% depending upon stage of fetal development. This flow accompanied by systemic pressure in pulmonary arteries indicates a pulmonary vascular resistance of 40000 dynes/sec/cm^{-5}. Within a few hours after birth to two to three days mean pressure in pulmonary arteries falls to less than 50% of systemic mean pressure. Flow in pulmonary artery rises to 8 ml/sec which yields a pulmonary vascular resistance of 4800 dynes/sec/cm^{-5} (one tenth of that during fetal life). During next week or two there is further drop in pulmonary vascular resistance to 2500 dynes/sec/cm^{-5}. Thereafter there is decline extending in curve during infancy and childhood that brings the mean pulmonary vascular resistance to 300 dynes/sec/cm^{-5} in 4 to 6 years and 200 dynes at 6 to 8 years of age. After that the level continues to drop slowly as long as child is growing and pulmonary artery pressure is unchanged.

Reasons for marked drop in pulmonary vascular resistance at birth when lungs expand and postnatal cardiovascular adjustment begin are:

1. Straightening of coiled distal pulmonary arteries with lungs expansion.
2. Increased blood flow through capillaries which distends them and thus tends to reduce the resistance.
3. Rise in oxygen content of arterial blood which in a reflex fashion helps to lower pulmonary vascular resistance.
4. Elasticity of pulmonary arteries which are more distensible than systemic arteries.
5. Vasomotor reflex response which may vary from hour to hour.

Opposing factors creating pulmonary vascular resistance include:

1. Thickened muscular arteries with diminished lumens.
2. Contractile response of pulmonary vasculature to increased flow and pressure.
3. Reflex effect of diminished arterial oxygen content which may occur under a variety of circumstances.

Systemic circulation also undergoes maturation process but appears to be more adapted to physiological adjustment than to anatomical changes since systemic arteries have wider range of response to sympathetic nervous system.

At birth systemic resistance based on flow of 8 ml/sec and mean pressure of 62 mm Hg is 10000 dynes. As tissue need for blood increases pressure gradually falls but rate of fall does not appear to be as precipitous as in pulmonary circulation. During first day of life systemic to pulmonary vascular resistance ratio is 2.5:1. At 2 to 3 weeks it is 2.8:1. At 1 month 3:1. At 6 month 4:1. At 1 year 5:1. After this age it varies between 5:1 and 10:1 or greater.

The anatomical changes in pulmonary arteries coincide with but do not exactly parallel physiological adjustments. In neonate there is decrease in thickness of media of small pulmonary arteries followed by further recession over period of 2 to 6 month. Maturation of pulmonary vascular tree is not complete until 4 years of age. Initial drop in pressure in the first week of life is greater than change in pulmonary vascular anatomy. When lumen of arterioles of normal lungs is related to body surface area or age of infant or child an evolutionary maturation curve similar to that comparing age and pulmonary vascular resistance is obtained.

Another parameter is elastic resistance of pulmonary artery which provides an indication of vascular distensibility of pulmonary circulation. This is 20000 dynes in neonatal period and 700 dynes at 12 to 16 years.

Thus a modest increase in pulmonary blood flow in infant is accompanied by much greater rise in pulmonary artery pressure than at later age.

PATHOPHYSIOLOGY

Pathological results of VSD are mediated through two main avenues. Both stem from effect of shunt on pulmonary arteries. First is associated with diminished PVR and CCF and second with increased vascular tone, hypertrophy of wall coupled with subsequent muscle and endothelial change that may lead to reversal of flow and inoperability.

After first month of life baby with large VSD shows a medial layer in pulmonary artery that is thicker than normal. Intimal proliferation in pulmonary arteries occur. A pulmonary blood flow 3 times normal may produce shearing forces that yield pathological changes in intima. Thinning of medial thickness occur slowly or not at all in infant with large VSD.

After birth PVR does not fall as rapidly in infant with VSD as in normal newborn. Furthermore when it does fall it may not recede to normal levels. This type of response explains delayed type of heart failure onset in VSD in interval following birth. Failure does not usually appear in healthy newborn for 4 to 12 weeks but may appear earlier in premature. Since there is a more rapid decline in PVR. Hypoxia of altitude diminishes incidence of heart failure in infant with VSD.

With an increased pulmonary blood flow in VSD normal regression of medial muscle layer in pulmonary arterioles is prevented.

There are two factors responsible for flow through a small opening in septum. Size of defect and pressure gradient between two sides. In addition to these in a small defect shunt is minimal and ceases before end of systole.

In moderate defect flow is predominantly systolic and is associated with an early but slight diastolic shunt. When defect is large one pressure is same in both ventricles and shunt depends upon differences in resistance between two circuits. When flow is large an appreciable diastolic flow is present in association with that occurring during systole.

Level of systemic arterial pressure can produce a significant effect on magnitude of shunt. Rare does one find a marked systemic hypertension with VSD but when pressure does rise in systemic circuit with this anomaly it is associated with an increased pulmonary artery blood flow and pressure. In such cases systemic pressure level may have developed in order to compensate for PVR and for more blood through lung fields. Whatever the cause there is further burden on arterial tree of lung likely to lead to development of sclerosis in pulmonary vessels.

Flow through defect may be affected by additional factors:

1. Margins of VSD may contract during systole thus reducing shunt.

2. Contraction of pulmonary infundibulum may produce some degree of narrowing of RVOT during strong ventricular systolic contractions. Occasionally narrowed outflow tract may act as resistance to further flow from RV tone pulmonary artery. Gasul in 1957 suggested that this process may proceed to anatomical infundibular stenosis over several years and thus alter dynamics of simple VSD to those of TOF.

Newborn infant makes certain adjustments and adaptations to presence of VSD. These may be described as acute or chronic. Acute element is during first few days of life. Chronic adjustments occur over several weeks or months. This includes a gradual increase in blood volume, plasma volume, total body water and pulmonary blood volume even in absence of cardiac failure. In acute stage there is an increase in heart rate and cardiac output, increased peripheral venous and arterial vasoconstriction with result that there is shift of blood volume to cardiopulmonary area. There is also increased PVR which coupled with increased blood volume tends to diminish shunt through defect. These mechanisms of compensation are brought into play by indirect action of shunt on baroreceptors of aortic arch and carotid sinus. Evidence of these compensatory mechanisms appear in neonatal period and early months of life.

Lucas in 1961 have correlated diameter of VSD with body surface area. Those with opening of less than 1 cm/m^2 surface area have only minor alteration in cardiac dynamics. When opening is more than 1 cm/m^2 of body surface area two changes are noted. Firstly in some patients there is a decrease in size of opening and thereby a reduction in blood flow to lungs. Others who have large defect show increased mortality during surgery.

During first year excessive pulmonary blood flow may manifest itself by dyspnea, frequent respiratory infections or frank heart failure.

At end of first year or in second year baby begins to improve with diminution in pulmonary congestion, increased physical activity and less dyspnea. This physiological improvement is associated with hypertrophy of media of muscular arteries of lungs with diminution in their size of lumen by hypertrophy as well as constriction and endothelial change. This improved state may last for years but it will lead to a state of persistent pulmonary hypertension, high PVR, reversal of flow through defect with clinical cyanosis and ultimately death from heart failure, pulmonary hemorrhage or infarction. This is Eisenmenger syndrome.

POSTOPERATIVE RESPONSE IN DISTAL PULMONARY ARTERIES

Once PHT with increased PVR is established for several years surgery for correction of primary cause has rarely produced any significant change in PVR. Early operation will favor postoperative decline in PVR.

Hyperreactors and hyporeactors. Pulmonary vascular obstruction. Eisenmenger complex.

Hyperreactors are patients who are likely to establish an irreversible high resistance in their pulmonary arteries. Eisenmenger first described the end stage of hyperreactors in 1897 and based on autopsy findings pointed out association of VSD with atherosclerosis of pulmonary arteries.

Woods monograph in 1958 emphasised diversity of lesions that could lead to pulmonary vascular obstruction. These included all causes of increased pulmonary flow and pressure, VSD, PDA, ASD, aorticopulmonary septal defect, L TGV with VSD, common ventricle, atrioventricularis communis, single atrium, anomalous PVD either partial or total.

Wood defined Eisenmenger syndrome as pulmonary hypertension at systemic level due to high pulmonary vascular resistance (more than 800 dynes) with reversed or bidirectional shunt through a large VSD.

Primary changes are those found in association with long standing pulmonary arterial hypertension and consist of hypertrophy of media of small muscular pulmonary arteries with fibroelastosis of intima causing thickening or occlusion. Secondary changes that help to maintain an adequate blood flow through alveolar capillaries by formation of branches of muscular pulmonary arteries that lead into thin walled structure resembling veins. These branches may arise at or proximal to site of obstruction in pulmonary arteries and may end as capillaries in alveolar walls. These collateral channels may be basis of pulmonary hemorrhage. Fully developed pathological picture is uncommon in childhood usually appears in late teens or twenties but may occur as early as 3 or 4 years of age.

Steady progression of histologic change has 5 grades:

Grade 1: Hypertrophy of media of small muscular arteries.

Grade 2: Medial hypertrophy and intimal fibroelastosis.

Grade 3: Fibrosis and vascular obstruction.

Grade 4: Evolution of plexiform collateral channels.

Grade 5: Necrotizing arteritis.

Diagnostic criteria given by Wood are present in adults with Eisenmenger complex. This is not the case in children and particularly first year of life when medial muscular hypertrophy is a normal finding. Furthermore an infant with VSD may have a PVR of 2000 dynes and yet subsequently have a drop in resistance to normal level by age 1 to 4 years. For these reasons fully developed Eisenmenger syndrome is rare in early childhood. Wood in 1958 suggested that Eisenmenger complex dates from birth with a marked reactive pulmonary hypertension from that time onwards.

Kidd in 1965 indicated that all infants have a drop in PVR in early life in presence of VSD. Some with a relatively high resistance after birth have it decline slowly others rapidly. Normal pulmonary artery pressure and pulmonary vascular resistance are likely to remain unchanged. These are invariably associated with small defects. High pressure and raised resistance lead to a slow increase in pulmonary vascular resistance and obstruction. Eisenmenger complex occurs with VSD more than 2 cm in diameter. In these cases there is large flow and moderately high pulmonary vascular resistance in childhood.

Pattern is similar in both VSD and ASD but the speed with which Eisenmenger syndrome develop is grossly different in these two lesions. High pulmonary vascular resistance of permanent nature appears early in hyperreactors with a large VSD and late in those with ASD.

Fundamental factor appears to be reaction of pulmonary arteries to flow pressure stimulus. Hyperreactivity is shown to be present in certain individuals and certain species.

The reason for difference in response of individuals has not become apparent. Pulmonary hypertension is commoner in females with ASD. Infection is commoner in severe hypertensive groups. Hypoxia is a factor in development of pulmonary hypertension.

To recognize hyper reactors catheterization should be done in each case of VSD with increased flow and resistance once in a year in first two or three years of life and large flow cases of low resistance at similar intervals. Such children may develop pulmonary vascular disease of Eisenmenger type eventually if flow is large enough. It is important to operate on hyperreactors as early as they can become clearly identified early in life before they have developed diffuse pulmonary vascular disease that is irreversible. A raised PVR in an infant or child in first two years of life is more likely to recede with normal maturation of pulmonary arteries if defect is closed during this period of physiological lability.

Cardiac Catheterization

A rise in oxygen content of one volume percent on going from RA to RV is considered as a reliable evidence of interventricular shunt. Sample taken from infundibulum are more significant and more closely resemble those of pulmonary artery.

CLINICAL FEATURES

In vast majority of children lesion is discovered in first year of life. VSD is most common cardiac anomaly identified at childhood. In classic case defect is not a large one. Loud harsh pansystolic murmur in 3rd and 4th left intercostal space is accompanied by a thrill. Cardiothoracic ratio may be normal or increased. ECG is normal. Hilar shadows may be normal or prominent. Most convincing evidence is rise in percentage oxygen saturation on going from RA to RV during cardiac catheterization or a positive angiogram into LV.

Exercise Tolerance

Usually good. Limitation of activity slight. Dyspnea occurs with vigorous effort. Babies with very large pulmonary blood flow may be dyspneic at rest.

Clinical Appearance

Color is normal as a rule. In children with advanced PVR or CCF there may be clinical cyanosis. Face, chest and body are thin. There may be prominence of precordium. Babies with large defect appear undernourished and are dyspneic at rest.

Cardiac Impulse

In mild cases with small defects heart is quiet. In large VSD with low PVR apex beat is forceful due to LVH. In PHT, RV heave is present that can be palpated over precordium on left sternal border. When both ventricles are hypertrophied, both apical thrust and RV heave are present.

Thrill

Lower precordial thrill is an important clinical sign of VSD and its confirmatory evidence.

Heart Murmurs

Pansystolic murmur is loud and harsh appearing to include both first and second heart sounds in its scope. Point of maximum intensity is between 3rd and 5th left intercostal space near sternal border. Mid-diastolic murmur may occur due to rapid inflow at beginning of diastole. Presence of this diastolic murmur is related to volume of left to right shunt and is therefore more common with large inflows and large hearts.

Heart Sounds

Pulmonary second sound is accentuated when pulmonary hypertension is present. In severe cases 3rd heart sound in mitral area occurs. It is due to rapid inflow of blood in early diastole from LA to LV. Second heart sound is normally split. Systolic click may be heard up LSE in some cases of PHT.

Radiologic Examination

To estimate size and severity of VSD and reaction of pulmonary vasculature to shunt through it.

Cardiomegaly may be due to excessive pulmonary blood flow, increased pressure in pulmonary artery and RV, CHF, Pulmonary valve insufficiency or tricuspid regurgitation.

Approximately 70% have CT ratio more than 55% in first two years of life but by age 10 years becomes 20%. This reduction in relative heart size is due to 4 factors:

1. As any child grows there may be slight reduction in CT ratio as lung volume and chest size increase in proportion to cardiac outlines.
2. There may be an absolute decrease in size of VSD.
3. There may be relative reduction in size of VSD when it is compared with increased lung volume and heart size that occurs when child develops between age of 2 and 10 years. Thus improving the ability to cope with left to right shunt.
4. In some cases there is gradual development of progressive pulmonary vascular obstruction leading to reduced pulmonary blood flow, reduced diastolic load on LV and consequent diminution in heart size (10%).

A relative or absolute decrease in size of VSD occurs in 65% cases.

Typical radiologic features are generalized enlargement of heart coupled with prominence of MPA and its major branches. LVH occurs in cases with large flow. In PHT, RVH occurs. Largest heart is found when maximum flow and pressure occur together.

LA is enlarged in cases with large shunt partly due to large flow and partly due to generalized enlargement of heart. When defect is small RA appears normal. RAH occurs when there is PHT or CHF or TR.

Hilar shadows are normal and show no pulsations on fluroscopy in cases with small shunts. When pulmonary blood flow is moderate and PAP less than systemic hilar shadows show moderate pulsations. When pressure and flow both are high hilar shadows show marked pulsations. When pressure is high and flow reduced pulsations diminish again. Pulmonary artery bulges with severe PHT.

In young children under 1 year no characteristic outline is found. Normal size to cardiomegaly are seen.

Angiocardiography

In small defects with RV contrast injection RV, pulmonary artery and left heart chambers are slightly enlarged and reopacification of pulmonary artery may be minimal or absent. Injection from RV in larger defects may show transient passage of contrast to LV and major opacification of pulmonary artery in levo phase. Position and diameter of defect can be demonstrated on LAO or left lateral views.

An aortogram is essential to exclude patent ductus or coarctation of aorta associated with VSD and to clarify whether aortic valve prolapse exists.

RV injection should be performed when there is systemic pressure in RV or in presence of pressure gradient across RVOT or pulmonary artery bifurcation in order that associated anomalies, such as DORV, pulmonary valvular or infundibular stenosis or pulmonary artery stenosis can be clearly defined.

ECG

Useful in estimating size of VSD and type of pulmonary vascular response to it, in estimating prognosis over years as well as estimating optimum size for surgery in any particular case. 1 in infant the predominant pattern is combined hypertrophy. Over 2-year-age it is predominant LVH or normal pattern.

1. In infant predominant pattern is combined hypertrophy. Over 2 year age it is predominant LVH or normal pattern. When a normal ECG pattern is present PAP is close to or

within normal range and pulmonary to systemic flow ratio is most frequently less than 2:1.

In presence of LVH pattern PAP is either normal or slightly elevated, PVR low, flow ratio between 2:1 and 3:1. When flow ratio is above 2:1 and resistance in pulmonary circuit has increased significantly combined hypertrophy is usual pattern. When flow is less than 2:1 and PVR is very high RVH pattern predominates with little or no evidence of LVH.

When a full blown Eisenmenger is clinically evident marked RVH is clearly present.

Kidd and coworkers in 1965 set forth six hemodynamic groups in VSD. When hypertrophy patterns are linked to each of hemodynamic groups a revealing relationship is indicated that is helpful in clinical assessment.

In hemodynamic group 1 with low flow and low resistance normal ECG pattern predominates in 54%. LVH occurs in 24%. Combined or pure RVH pattern in remainder. This is relatively uncommon and usually found in infancy.

In hemodynamic group 6 or Eisenmenger complex with high PVR and reversal of flow through defect pure RVH pattern is found in majority. Few show combined loading. An exceptional case presents with minimal evidence of RVH that might be considered within normal limits.

2. *QRS axis*: When mean QRS frontal axis is related to hemodynamic groups findings are as follows:

Group 1 Low flow low resistance 31°.

Group 2 Increased flow low resistance 53°.

Group 3 Increased flow slightly increased resistance 70°.

Group 4 Good flow greater resistance 84°.

Group 5 Low flow high resistance 114°.

Group 6 High resistance reversal of flow 146°.

Low flow low resistance cases have QRS axis that is within normal limits and to the left. As flow and resistance increase mean QRS axis shifts around to a point where it is deviated markedly to right. Thus direction of mean QRS axis in conjunction with other clinical data may give a clue as to state of pulmonary vasculature and height of PVR.

3. *P-wave*: PR interval is within normal limits in 95% cases. P-wave duration is prolonged in 30% cases. Notching of P-wave in lead 1 and 2 noticed in 30% cases. P-wave notching and broadening are seen in groups with either left loading or combined loading and in this group this sign is usually accompanied by tall R or deep Q. It is additional evidence of diastolic overloading of LA and LV.

When a child with VSD and high PVR also has a mitral valve anomaly with insufficiency a broad notched P-wave in ECG is seen with evidence of LV loading with increased height of R-wave in V6 or a significant Q-waves and yet have pulmonary vascular changes that are irreversible and unlikely to permit survival at the time of surgery.

4. *Counterclockwise vector*: Direction of frontal vector follows direction of axis as a rule. There are a few cases that have a counterclockwise vector with an axis of 90° or more. They have other evidences of relatively good pulmonary flow and fall into moderate or low pulmonary vascular resistance groups.

5. *Tall peaked T-wave*: Tall broad R-wave in V6 are followed by tall R-waves in same lead and is a sign of diastolic ventricular loading. Tall broad QRS complexes over right precordium with tall R-waves following them are indicative of marked RV overloading. In such cases prognosis is poor and associated with increased pulmonary vascular resistance.

6. Q-waves: 25% of VSD show Q-waves of 4 mm or more in V6. This is associated with other evidence of LV diastolic overloading such as tall R in V6, deep S in V1 or notching of P-wave. There is left axis deviation and a pulmonary to systemic blood flow ratio of 2:1.

VECTOR CARDIOGRAPHY

Horizontal vector gives more accurate complete picture of electrical impulse from heart since ordinary precordial leads do not go all the way round the chest as a rule and may not as accurately reflect maximal positions of electrical activity. A comparison of vectorcardiograms over a period of several months or years may more accurately reflect changes occurring in relationship of one ventricle to the other and therefore further reflect changes in pulmonary vasculature.

Horizontal plane vector in normal heart or in presence of small VSD reveals a counterclockwise loop and a voltage pattern that is within normal limits for the age. Axis of this vector is usually between 0° and + 60°. In RVH or loading pattern horizontal vector is clockwise and its dominant portion is anterior and to the right. Axis is between +70° and +150° and direction of vector is clockwise. In LV overloading or hypertrophy vector is counterclockwise in direction and to the left, somewhat similar to normal pattern but with increased voltage and axis of vector may be within normal range or veer round beyond 0° to a negative axis.

Combined loading or hypertrophy pattern in horizontal vector shows a wide variety of loops since many combinations of both right and left loading may be present. Thus there may be a clockwise or counterclockwise loop or it may be a figure of 8 loop with terminal portion clockwise. Maximum septal vector increases with rising pulmonary vascular resistance.

ECHOCARDIOGRAPHY

Left to right shunting at ventricular level produces volume overloading of LA and LV. This is shown echocardiographically as increased LA and LV dimensions. Degree of LAE is related to measured left to right shunt. This enables one to separate large (more than 2:1) from small (less than 2:1) shunts. These findings are similar to those seen in PDA.

Aneurysmal transformation of VSD may be recognized by abnormal echoes appearing on right septal surface. Association of PHT may be recognized by an enlarged thick walled RV and abnormal systolic time intervals as determined by pulmonary valve leaflet motion.

Echocardiogram thus provides the clinician with left to right degree of shunting and PVR by noninvasive technique. As such it is of value in patient's initial assessment and long time follow-up.

Diagnosis

VSD is usually present when there is a loud harsh systolic murmur maximum in 3rd and 4th intercostal space with or without a thrill in a child who has no obvious cyanosis. Presence of increased hilar shadowing is of value in confirming diagnosis. ECG may show LVH, RVH, BVH or a normal tracing. Heart is enlarged to some degree. Cardiac catheterization shows a rise in oxygen content on entering RV. There may be insignificant rise even in presence of definit VSD. Hydrogen electrode in RV or LV angiogram locates such minimal shunts.

Even with this technique a shunt may not be recognized and it may be necessary to augment it by norepinephrine or angiotensin. These drugs force a sufficient shunt through a small defect by raising LV pressure.

Differential Diagnosis

1. *Pulmonary stenosis*: Difficulty arises in first 6 months of life when point of maxim intensity of murmur is difficult to define and may be misleading. In pulmonary stenosis cyanosis is present. Murmur is maximum in pulmonary area. Poststenotic dilatation of pulmonary artery on X-ray. RVH on ECG. In doubtful cases cardiac catheterization is required.

2. *Aortic stenosis*: Murmur is characteristically located over aortic area, shorter with systolic click or split first heart sound. ECG shows a deep S in V1 when LVH is present. In doubtful cases left heart catheterization is required.

3. *Infundibular stenosis*: Murmur low in precordium and accompanied by a thrill. RVH in ECG is characteristic. There is lack of pulsations in hilar shadows. Second heart sound is fainter in pulmonary area.

4. *VSD with ASD*: An unusually large heart with bulging pulmonary artery and pulsating hilar shadows associated with VSD murmur but with signs more severe than in majority of cases when defect is isolated. ECG evidence of marked RVH pattern with strain. Deeply inverted T-waves over precordium and depressed ST segment in same leads

with RAD in standard leads. Large RA. CCF with large heart. In presence of any of these signs one should do cardiac catheterization.

5. *PDA with VSD*: Continuous murmur over pulmonary area coupled with characteristic murmur over lower precordium.

6. *Coarctation of aorta with VSD*: This is a common association. Femoral arteries should be felt and BP taken. Raised LV pressure produces intense murmur.

7. *TOF*: 15% cases have no history of cyanosis during first year of life while at rest. Cyanosis appears on crying or breath holding. RVH is fairly marked in ECG that suggests true diagnosis. Presence of right aortic arch is helpful in making diagnosis.

8. *Endocardial fibroelastosis*: These cases may have murmur over lower precordium simulating VSD. Such murmurs are due to aortic or mitral valvular disease. Marked LVH pattern with strain occurs in ECG.

9. *TGV*: When associated with tricuspid atresia there may be only slight cyanosis with pulsating hilar shadows. LVH and failure are seen.

10. *Common ventricle*: Murmur is similar to VSD since there is narrowing at entrance of outflow tract to aorta. Majority of cases show cyanosis at rest which increases with activity. 80% of them have evidence of TGV. Many L TGV X-ray is characteristic. Cardiac catheterization is required.

VSD WITH CHF

Heart is more likely to fail in first year of life. Some infants are premature. Prematurity leads to either a weaker myocardium or lower pulmonary vascular resistance or premature may have a high incidence of VSD.

Therapy consists of digitalization, oxygen, diuretics and antibiotic.

Most children who have myocardial inadequacy will eventually need surgical closure. Infant can be managed medically to control CHF till optimum time for surgery arrives.

Failure precipitated by respiratory infection requires antibiotic and decongestive therapy.

Surgical intervention may be urgent in VSD with failure due to associated cardiac anomalies.

SPONTANEOUS CLOSURE OF VSD

Closure can occur naturally by an adherent medial leaflet of tricuspid valve which is rare. Small defects close in first 7 years of life in majority. However, the process continues in adult life. If a baby is born with small VSD, chances of its closure by adult life are 60 to 70%. Muscular septal defect closure is more than membranous ones.

Mechanisms for spontaneous closure:

1. Fibrosis of margins of defect.
2. Adherent tricuspid valve cusp that seals off the defect.
3. Fistulus tracks surrounded by reactive fibrosis.
4. Low defects in muscular portion of septum that close when muscles hypertrophy.

ANEURYSMS OF MEMBRANOUS SEPTUM

First described by Laennec in 1826. It may be an isolated phenomenon or associated with other cardiac anomalies particularly VSD. It is also described with a variety of Arrhythmias and conduction defects.

Mall's theory concerning origin of this malformation: Congenitally weakened state arising from a mildly dextraposed aorta.

More likely explanation is adherence of some portion of tricuspid valve to the area of ventricular defect.

Majority have a small left to right shunt when associated with VSD. Presence of aneurysm may facilitate spontaneous closure of VSD. An early systolic sound preceding the pansystolic murmur with a clicky quality is recognized between LSE and apex and is best heard in expiration. Systolic murmur has late systolic accentuation.

Incidence of aneurysm of membranous septum in isolated VSD is 70% (Freedom 1974).

DECREASE IN SIZE OF DEFECT WITHOUT COMPLETE CLOSURE

1. PAP and shunt through defect both decrease.
2. Cardiothoracic ratio decreases. ECG changes in similar direction suggest a decrease in pressure and flow due to decrease in size of defect.

Reduction in size may be absolute in some cases. In others it is due to an increase in muscular development of septum. During ventricular systole the defect may itself contract significantly.

Decrease in size of defect occurs in defects less than 5 mm in size in infants and less than 10 mm diameter in older children.

DEVELOPMENT OF INFUNDIBULAR PULMONARY STENOSIS

Gasul and associates in 1957 first described development of infundibular pulmonary stenosis in a child who previously had an isolated VSD.

Incidence of this complication varies with hemodynamic group concerned. It does not occur in group 1, 5 or 6. It occurs in 5 to 10% cases of group 2, 3 and 4. All of these groups have flow ratio of more than 2:1 initially.

Specific angiographic measurements appear useful in detecting early or those cases who have certain anatomical features of TOF but without coronal gradient across RVOT. In these cases as a result of underdevelopment of distal pulmonary infundibulum a deviation of crista supraventricularis in outflow tract and pulmonary valve give rise to an increased RVOT angle. This angle is useful in recognizing those cases who will ultimately develop TOF picture over a period of time. Normal RVOT angle is 40°. (range 20 to 46°).

In TOF outflow tract is more horizontal in relation to ventricle and makes an angle of 65°.

Right aortic arch is associated with VSD and is help in recognizing those that are likely to have progressive infundibular stenosis.

CLINICAL SYNDROME OF EISENMENGER REACTION

It is a phase of VSD spectrum that is more characteristic of second and third decade of life, since vascular changes occur at a slow pace.

Incidence of Eisenmenger complex with VSD is 10 to 20%. In children 10%. In adults 16 to 20%.

Clinical Features

Fully developed clinical picture of Eisenmenger syndrome is slow in appearing in childhood. Clinical signs and symptoms begin to appear with diminished exercise tolerance, cyanosis first with exercise and later at rest, failure to thrive, retarded growth, clubbing of fingers and polycythemia. Obvious cyanosis during childhood is rare before 10 years of age. Those who develop cyanosis early are more likely to run a stable course and therefore have slightly improved prognosis. Pulmonary diastolic murmur of valve insufficiency begins to develop particularly in those with dilated pulmonary artery and slowly progressive pulmonary vascular disease.

Radiologic Examination

There will be a decrease in CT ratio from that seen in first and second year of life. Pulmonary artery bulges more prominently. Central hilar shadows pulsate but lung fields beyond hilar areas is clear in majority of cases. In advanced cases heart failure, pulmonary valve insufficiency and tricuspid valve insufficiency may cause some enlargement of heart. Progressive cardiomegaly is characteristic of relatively small group of cases that continue to have pulmonary vascular disease after VSD has been closed. Complications:

- Congestive heart failure.
- Pulmonary thrombosis.
- Hemoptysis.
- Bacterial endocarditis.
- Brain abscess.
- Paroxysmal tachycardia.

Treatment

In children with VSD whose pulmonary arteries are hyperreactive management should be preventive. Cardiac catheterization should be carried out in first few months of life in VSD infant with cardiomegaly, CHF and ECG changes. Catheterization should be repeated if CHF continues, large shunt persists and QRS axis shifts to right in ECG with RVH, indicating rise of resistance in which case surgery is indicated. Surgery may be done at 6 months to one year of age with advent of new techniques of hypothermia and approach to closure of defect through RA. If surgery is successful then progressive pulmonary vascular disease is prevented. If operation is delayed until after the child is 2-year-old pulmonary vascular disease may progress even if VSD has been completely closed.

Surgical closure of VSD in classic Eisenmenger syndrome carries surgical mortality that is prohibitive. Even if patient survives there may be no benefits and vascular disease is not impeded. It may at times be speeded up.

Eisenmenger syndrome is strong contraindication to pregnancy.

PROGNOSIS IN VSD

There are a number of factors that shapes clinical course of a child with VSD:

1. Size of defect.
2. Response of pulmonary vascular system to increased flow and pressure.
3. Presence of associated cardiac and noncardiac defects.
4. Patient's response to pneumonia, CHF and endocarditis. Natural history of VSD is frequently a dynamic process that is improving at various rates in infancy and childhood. Prognosis in isolated VSD appears to be good on the whole.

Possible courses that may be followed by a child with VSD are:

1. Defect may get smaller.
2. Defect may close entirely.

3. Defect may remain same size as child grows. In fact this is a reduction in size of anomaly provided it is less than diameter of aorta or less than 1 cm per meter body surface area.

4. Defect may get larger as child grows.

5. Progressive pulmonary vascular obstruction may occur rapidly over a period of 2 to 4 years in severe cases otherwise slowly over a period of 10 to 60 years. Response is likely to be more rapid if defect is large one.

6. Patient may develop CHF and has either favorable or unfavorable response to decongestive therapy. Patient may particularly susceptible to pneumonia or highly resistant to it.

7. Course may be unfavorable if there are associated non-cardiac anomalies of a serious nature particularly in neonatal period.

8. Bacterial endocarditis may occur (one in thousand patient years).

9. Infundibular narrowing of a minor degree may be present at birth which will progressively narrow RVOT and thus protect pulmonary vasculature.

10. Child with isolated VSD may be operated upon successfully.

11. A few patients with moderately elevated PVR may go onto develop progressive pulmonary vascular disease with fatal termination after they have been operated upon successfully and septal defect closed.

12. Once a child with VSD has reached teen age prognosis is good. 4% close spontaneously after they have reached adolescence or adult life. Only 1% develop endocarditis.

SURGERY FOR VSD

Modern technique for closure of VSD involves cardio-pulmonary bypass with aid of pump oxygenator. Successful results are also reported with hypothermia.

Median sternotomy incision is preferred. It provides an easier quicker approach and is better for pulmonary function postoperatively. Defect is repaired by teflon or decron patch. Pulmonary artery banding:

Modest degree of pulmonary stenosis has protective effect on pulmonary vasculature and yet may permit a relatively good exercise tolerance with minimum of cyanosis. Shunt through VSD is controlled by pulmonary artery banding.

Surgery for VSD in the first year of life:

Subramanian prefers to use transatrial approach in which tricuspid valve is pulled aside and does not need to be incised or detached. Under hypothermia heart is relaxed and defect is closed with decron velour patch with continuous suture.

If a child with VSD is going to require surgery it is usually evident in first year of life either because of CHF or cardiomegaly with progressively increasing pulmonary vascular resistance. Approximately 5% of babies in first year of life with isolated VSD should have operation in first year unless there is evidence of pulmonary valve stenosis or infundibular stenosis that protects lung fields and diminishes or eliminates possibility of failure. There may be certain circumstances when banding operation is required, e.g. multiple large swiss cheese holes in septum or when there is a complicated defect present, such as coarctation of aorta with VSD and a double operation to completely correct both anomalies would require excessive time and excessive risk. Management of child with large VSD requires first of all observation and catheterization to outline pathology and anatomy present. Child should be adequately treated medically and if response is good operation can be delayed till later part of first year. If defect shows marked diminution in size surgery may become unnecessary. If medical treatment is inadequate to contain failure complete correction operation is indicated within a few days or a few weeks depending upon infant's progress. Child should be recatheterized during second half of first year in those who have had heart failure whether heart remains large or becomes smaller in order to be certain about pulmonary vascular resistance. If PVR is increasing surgery is required even though baby looks improved and failure is absent. After 2 years of age successful closure of VSD may cause a drop in PAP but rarely in PVR. Data are thus in favor of early surgery when complicating effects of flow, pressure can be controlled or prevented or reversed.

Selection of VSD cases for surgery:

1. Optimum age for closure of uncomplicated VSD is 1 to 3 years but many will require surgical correction in first year of life. All cases with pulmonary to systemic flow ratio of 2.5:1 or more at 2 year age may be considered for closure at optimum time. Direct closure of defect is indicated in early life when infant is in CHF that will not respond to medical management especially in first six months of life.

2. Children with pulmonary to systemic flow ratio of under 2.5:1 with normal PAP can wait.

3. Children with CHF in first year of life require surgery. Many will respond to medical therapy. 20% are intractable and require surgical correction.

4. Each infant with VSD with CHF, cardiomegaly and ECG changes should be catheterized in first year of life and if there is evidence that PVR is rising catheterization should be repeated yearly until the course is clarified.

5. Children with high PVR and low pulmonary blood flow with obstructive pulmonary vascular disease over age-2-year are poor risk for surgical correction and have an excessively high rate of mortality at operation.

6. Children with high PVR whose vasoconstriction is relaxed by use of oxygen or relaxant drugs are suitable for surgical correction.

COARCTATION OF AORTA WITH VSD WITH OR WITHOUT PDA

If an infant survives first six months of life with this combination he is likely to live on for several years. In neonatal period a loud systolic murmur is heard over precordium, pansystolic accompanied by a thrill. Acyanotic at rest but cyanosis appears on crying. Majority are dyspneic. 60% have features of failure. CT ratio varies between 50 and 80% with prominent hilar shadows on X-ray chest. Aortic systolic pressure ranges 70–140 mm Hg. Femoral arteries rarely palpable. Pulse feeble. ECG shows combined hypertrophy pattern, RV loading pattern and LV loading pattern. Mortality is over 50% in first 6 months of life. 50% of these patients do not respond to digitalis.

VSD WITH AR

Incidence: 2% of VSD cases (Keith)

5% (Nadas 1964)

Importance of this syndrome is that it invariably leads to decreased exercise tolerance and heart failure after a latent period varying from 2 to 50 years. After onset of significant symptoms associated with progressive dyspnea a fatal outcome is likely to occur. Anatomy: Syndrome is characterized by high VSD with a little or no tissue separating defect from aortic valve. Right aortic cusp is the one most frequently defective. It has a dilated pouch appearance and sags into LVOT over area occupied by VSD. Its margin is usually thickened. Content of aorta may spill into LV or through VSD into RV during each diastolic pause. Occasionally deformed aortic cusp prolapses into RV sufficiently to partly obstruct the ventricular shunt. Posterior cusp may be involved either alone or in association with a deformed right coronary cusp. Occasionally the anomalous cusp is pulled down by a fibrous band attached to it from below. LV and RV are enlarged and hypertrophied. RVOT obstruction occurs in 25 to 50% cases. Usual cause of aortic insufficiency is an elongation and inversion of margin of one cusp. Other defects, such as fenestration of aortic valve or diffuse involvement of all 3 valvular cusps may occur. Occasionally syndrome is accompanied by calcification of aortic valve. Small muscular pulmonary arteries have medial hypertrophy.

Classification: Type I subcristal type associated with protruding right or noncoronary cusp of aortic valve.

– Without pulmonary infundibular stenosis.

– With infundibular stenosis.

Either adjacent to pulmonary valve or few mm away from pulmonary valve.

Type 2 supracristal type occurring below pulmonary valve but through which prolapsed right coronary cusp of aortic valve has appeared.

Infracristal type is divided into three categories:

1. Adjacent to right coronary cusp.
2. Adjacent to noncoronary cusp.
3. Midway between the two.

Infundibular stenosis can occur with subpulmonary as well as infracristal type of VSD.

Clinical Features

Murmur may be noted in early infancy. Baby is asymptomatic. CHF is unlikely to occur until second decade but reported as early as 4 years of age.

There is a loud harsh systolic murmur accompanied by thrill maximum in 2nd 4th left intercostal spaces. It is accompanied by a blowing diastolic murmur down the LSE. There may be a continuous murmur heard over left precordium. Heart is enlarged to left with forceful apical impulse. An inflow diastolic murmur may be heard inside apex.

Early diastolic murmur of AR down the left sternal border is rarely heard before 2 years of age. It is invariably present by 14 years of age.

A systolic murmur well heard in first and second LICS and accompanied by thrill is indicative of additional lesion of infundibular stenosis.

Peripheral signs of AR are present with a Corrigan pulse, increased systemic systolic pressure and decreased diastolic pressure. Pressure in LV always exceeds that of RV and pulmonary artery. So there is no cyanosis or clubbing. Exercise tolerance is good in majority. CHF occurs infrequently in pediatric age group.

ECG

LVH loading pattern is characteristic with deep S in V1 and tall R in V6 and increased depth of Q in V6. Occasionally T-wave in V6 is depressed.

Axis varies from 0 to +150°. 80% have less than 90°.

Radiology

Generalized cardiomegaly with LV configuration. RV slightly to moderately enlarged. Pulmonary artery is prominent on left border. Peripheral pulmonary vessels are increased. In a few patients major vessels are pulsatile. Ascending aorta is prominent and pulsates more vigorously owing to high systolic and low diastolic pressure.

Cardiac Catheterization

Left heart catheter should also be inserted. Oxygen rise in entering RV of 15 to 20% is found. Pulmonary to systemic flow ratio is low 2.5:1. RV pressure is moderately elevated. Pulmonary systolic pressure does not increase more than 35 mm. Resistance in pulmonary circuit is within normal range. A gradient between RV and PA of more than 15 mm Hg suggests infundibular stenosis.

Treatment

Children with large heart and CHF should be operated upon promptly. Prolonged medical management of such cases may not be satisfactory.

Hartmann and Weldon in 1972 recommended reconstruction of aortic valve by shortening free edge of cusp so that all distances from corpora arantii to commisural attachments are equal. Homograft replacement of aortic valve is preferred to repair. For severe defect closure of VSD with aortic valvuloplasty is advised. A number of subcristal defects are associated with commissural malformations or bicuspid valves. In such cases aortic valve replacement is recommended.

VSD WITH VENTRICULOATRIAL COMMUNICATION

This consists of a VSD with an anomalous opening in tricuspid valve which permits a communication between LV and RA. It is oval in shape and is associated with fusion of tricuspid valve to margins of VSD so that neither LV nor RA communicates with RV through the anomaly. With each ventricular systole blood is forced in a jet like stream into RA.

Classification

1. Defect between LVOT and RA above the annulus of tricuspid valve.
2. Defect as in 1 and defect in ventricular septum below the anomalous valve.
3. Defect just below annulus of tricuspid valve so that LV communicates with RA through a segment of septal leaflet of tricuspid valve fused to margins of septal defect.
4. Defects in both tricuspid valve and ventricular septum but not fused together.

Physical Examination

Apex beat increased in force slightly. There is a harsh systolic murmur best heard in 3rd and 4th LICS accompanied by thrill. Moderate cardiomegaly with LAE and RA dilatation is characteristic. This creates a cardiac silhouette that is ball like.

Cardiac Catheterization

There is rise in oxygen content on passing from vena cava to RA between 5 and 40%. Further rise on proceeding into RV. RAP is normal or slightly elevated. Pulmonary to systemic blood flow is 2:1.

ECG

LV loading. RBBB. Combined hypertrophy. Enlarged P-wave of RAH is noted in 75% cases.

Angiography

With tip of catheter in LV a characteristic shadow with immediate filling of RA from LV before RV shows opacification. It may also reveal enlarged heart chambers and dilatation of central and peripheral branches of pulmonary artery. Dye dilution curve demonstrates a tracing characteristic of left to right shunt. An injection into left ventricle with hydrogen sensitive catheter in RA will show an immediate response in a typical curve.

Diagnosis

Several diagnostic possibilities present when arterialization of RA blood is found during cardiac catheterization, such as ASD, intraventricular septal defect with tricuspid insufficiency, LV to RA defect with or without tricuspid valve involvement and aneurysm of sinus of Valsalva with an opening into RA. A long harsh systolic murmur with thrill is rarely found in ostium secundum but may occur in atrioventricularis communis. However, AVC has a characteristic ECG pattern and one can easily pass the catheter from RA to LA without difficulty as well as demonstrate evidence of mitral insufficiency.

Aneurysm of sinus of Valsalva is accompanied by rapid onset of failure when a sudden opening occurs between the sinus and RA. A diastolic murmur of AR is also heard.

Tricuspid insufficiency with VSD is likely to occur when failure is present and this is an uncommon event in LV to RA anomalies. LAD occurs.

Treatment

Indications for operation are similar to those in simple ostium secundum. In more severe cases indications are those similar to combined ventricular and atrial septal defects. VSD should be closed and operative closure of anomalous opening of tricuspid valve should be carried out.

All of these patients should be operated upon in early childhood. Optimum age of surgery being after 2 years of age unless CHF or cardiomegaly is present.

At operation atrial defect is repaired. Tricuspid leak is repaired. RV should be explored to exclude a second defect.

19

Single Ventricle

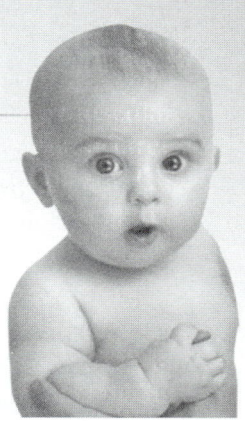

A condition where one ventricular chamber receives both mitral and tricuspid valves or a common atrioventricular valve. This definition excludes mitral and tricuspid atresia.

In its commonest form single ventricle is a single left ventricle with small outflow chamber. Both D and L transpositions are common.

Holmes heart is a single ventricle with normally related great vessels and pulmonary stenosis.

ANATOMY AND EMBRYOLOGY

Basic problem is a large VSD. There are four types:

Type A is most frequent 78%. It is single left ventricle. RV sinus or inflow tract is absent. A small rudimentary RVOT which represents RV infundibulum communicating with single left ventricle through bulboventricular foramen. This chamber lies anteriorly and either to right or left and so ventricular inversion. The diminutive outflow chamber usually gives rise to aorta since transposition is nearly 6 times more common than normal relationship of great arteries in single ventricle. In these cases pulmonary artery arises from large left ventricle.

Type B is single RV with complete absence of LV sinus 5%.

Type C has equal amount of right and left ventricular sinus myocardium 7%. This group is nearest to "Huge Ventricular Septal Defect" concept.

Type D 10% development of neither ventricular sinus.

In Van Praagh's series 83% were in visceroatrial situs solitus, i.e. in usual position with RA on right along with liver and LA on left along with stomach.

Only 3% had visceroatrial situs inversus.

In 13% cases visceroatrial situs was indeterminate (Heterotaxy). All these cases had asplenia.

Direction of ventricular looping determines relative position of right and left ventricles. D loop is seen in situs solitus normal and in D transposition with RV on right and L loop is seen in situs inversus individual and in L transposition with RV on left. The great vessels are transposed and aorta arises above RVOT. In cases without an outflow chamber the same relationship between great arteries is called malposition.

Concept of single ventricle as faulty development of ventricular septum has been challenged by de La Cruz and Miller who introduced the concept of "Double Inlet LV". They proposed that the terms single and common ventricle be confined to the entity in which ventricular septum is absent or represented by only a small muscular ridge and in which both atria empty into and both great arteries arise from same chamber. This fits in with type C of Van Praagh classification. These cases are rare. Most frequent form of this anomaly (type A) is a double inlet left ventricle. Anderson and his colleagues in 1977 have posed a question. Is the single ventricle type A a morphological left ventricle or is it a morphologically primitive ventricle? The distinctive feature of primitive ventricle is absence of the posterior ventricular septum, i.e. that portion which interposes between AV valves. Thus type A single ventricle of Van Praagh is not a morphologic left ventricle but is a primitive ventricle with an outlet chamber.

The embryologic basis of this group of anomalies is faulty alignment of AV canal in relationship to two developing ventricles. On completion of formation of bulboventricular loop both atria relate only to primitive ventricle part of cardiac tube. The part which is going to form the LV. In order for AV canal to relate to RV which is going to form from bulbus cordis part of tube the atria must expand to the right and ventricular part of tube move to left. As the RA makes more complete functional contact with RV this ventricle develops normally. However, if this movement is incomplete the tricuspid valve may straddle ventricular septum and RV is hypoplastic. If this does not take place at all both AV valves relate solely to LV and RV will be solely represented by infundibulum.

Double inlet RV, single RV, straddling mitral valve are examples of excessive displacement of AV canal towards bulbus cordis.

Commonest type of single ventricle is a large LV with small RVOT.

Associated anomalies: Both venous returns pass into a common chamber from which mixed blood is ejected into great arteries. These great arteries are transposed. Obstruction to ventricular outflow is frequent. Incidence of obstruction to both pulmonary and systemic flow is equal. All cases of D transposition have some degree of subaortic stenosis at site of bulboventricular foramen together with preductal coarctation or atresia of aortic isthmus. With L transposition 73% cases have subaortic stenosis and 50% have pulmonary outflow tract obstruction (pulmonary stenosis and pulmonary atresia).

Other lesions are ASD (Both primum and secundum), single atrium, TAPVD. These last two conditions occur with asplenia.

Clinical Features

Because of major circulatory changes in these children they commonly present in early childhood.

In first major clinical group pulmonary blood flow is small in fetus because of collapsed lungs and high PVR.

After birth when there is no pulmonary stenosis pulmonary blood flow will start to increase markedly as PVR falls. This circulatory overload will give rise to rapid breathing, fatigue, poor feeding, failure to gain weight, respiratory distress and congestive heart failure. cyanosis is not prominent in these children. Chest shows a hyperactive precordium with diffuse cardiac impulse. First heart sound loud. Second heart sound single or narrowly split. Murmur is pansystolic or long ejection in type. Mid-diastolic flow murmur of rapid ventricular filling or a third heart sound may be noted.

In second clinical group those with limited pulmonary blood flow cyanosis will be prominent presenting feature and heart failure rare. Children resemble TOF and have cyanosis at birth or may become cyanosed with time. Cyanosis increases with crying or exertion. In children with small pulmonary blood flow precordium is quiet with a localized cardiac impulse. There may be a systolic thrill. First heart sound normal. Second heart sound single. There may be a harsh grade 3 to 4 systolic murmur best heard at base of heart and frequently as well in second RICS and second LICS due to often more medial portion of pulmonary artery.

Radiology

In those cases with increased pulmonary blood flow heart is enlarged with pulmonary plethora. A narrow pedicle may suggest D transposition. L transposition is suggested by a prominence on upper left border with a sloping shoulder formed by ascending aorta.

In majority of cases with PS pulmonary vascularity appears normal and heart is only mildly enlarged or may be normal. Only when obstruction to pulmonary blood flow is very severe or there is pulmonary atresia is there pulmonary oligemia. In later stages obliterative changes take place in pulmonary vasculature. With increase in PVR pulmonary blood flow falls hence heart decreases in size and peripheral lung fields will clear. Hilar pulmonary artery prominent.

Echocardiography

There is no ventricular septum in usual position. In some cases, however, a small septum may be located high and anterior in outflow area and probably represents bulbar septum demarcating outer chamber. Great arteries can be seen and recognized as transposed or not. Demonstration of two distinct atrioventricular valves simultaneously without an intervening ventricular septum is diagnostic.

ECG

Initial forces in QRS axis are generated by septal depolarization. A pattern with Q-waves in right chest leads is suspicious. Additionally however Q-waves may either be absent completely or present in all leads. LAD occurs in children with single ventricle and normally related arteries. Large R- and S-waves from V1 through V6 is usual pattern. However, both RVH and LVH patterns can be seen separately. Abnormal AV conduction may also occur with first and second degree heart block.

Hemodynamics

Diagnosis of single ventricle is made by cardiac catheterization and angiocardiography. Catheter passing up IVC enters a large ventricular cavity through tricuspid valve. There is a step up in oxygen saturation which may vary from location to location in ventricular chamber and which is at systemic pressure. Entry into great arteries may be easy or may necessitate use of Swan Ganz catheter. If atrial septum is crossed the catheter enters the same ventricular chamber through left AV valve. A catheter passed retrogradely into heart via aorta will lie either in anterior outflow chamber or passing through bulboventricular foramen enter common ventricular chamber. Aortic oxygen saturation may be reduced depending upon pulmonary blood flow. Complete mixing in common chamber is rare and favorable streaming, i.e. streaming of pulmonary venous blood to aorta and systemic venous blood to lungs is more likely to occur when there is L transposition. More complete mixing occurs in pulmonary stenosis. It is of major importance to assess the pulmonary outflow tract, to measure pressure there and to determine whether there is pulmonary stenosis or whether a low pulmonary blood flow is due to progressive pulmonary vascular disease.

ANGIOCARDIOGRAPHY

1. Type of single ventricle, i.e. with or without an outflow chamber can be identified. Cine angiocardiography may

demonstrate in LAO projection the presence or absence of ventricular septum.

2. Outflow chamber can be defined. It is medial and anteriorly situated in D transposition and lateral and anterior in L transposition.

3. Relationship of great arteries can be recognized. With D transposition aorta arising anteriorly from outlet chamber will be on right and pulmonary artery posteriorly on left. With L transposition aorta will be anterior and on left. Ascending aorta will form upper left cardiac border and pulmonary artery arises posteriorly and to the right.

4. Obstruction to pulmonary outflow can be seen. Pulmonary stenosis can be valvular or subvalvular. When there is no transposition the obstruction can be at bulboventricular foramen.

5. Obstruction to systemic outflow can be defined. Commonly the obstruction is at bulboventricular foramen or in restrictive outflow chamber.

6. State of atrioventricular valves can be assessed. From point of view of reconstructive surgery, AV valve may be normal, inverted in L transposition or common as seen in AV canal type of defect. One or other can be absent. Finally the valve may straddle the bulboventricular septum.

7. Associated lesions can be diagnosed, e.g. PDA and coarctation of aorta.

Diagnosis

This is most commonly made in newborn or young infant who is mildly cyanosed and in respiratory distress if not in frank CHF. In the group with large pulmonary blood flow differential diagnosis is from complete TGV with VSD, DORV, persistent truncus arteriosus or from a large left to right shunt, e.g. VSD, PDA with PHT.

In second group with pulmonary stenosis and diminished pulmonary blood flow differential diagnosis is from TOF, TGV with PS and DORV with PS.

Treatment

Initial problem is in newborn period. Here prognosis is worse if there is pulmonary atresia as pulmonary blood flow is dependent upon continued persistence of ductus arteriosus. Early and successful systemic pulmonary anastomosis possibly preceded by prostaglandins infusion may be life-saving.

In newborn digitalis and diuretics should be administered if heart failure is present. Chest infection should be treated with appropriate antibiotics.

If heart failure persists pulmonary artery banding should be carried out to limit pulmonary blood flow, relieve heart failure and to protect pulmonary vasculature from development of progressive pulmonary vascular disease.

Separation of ventricular cavity is feasible now in both common variety with an outlet chamber and where there is no outlet chamber.

Main features of successful repair are mapping of conduction system intraoperatively, stable fixation of prosthetic septum and relief of pulmonary outflow obstruction, whether natural as in PS or iatrogenic as in pulmonary artery banding.

Complete transposition can be dealt with by Mustard procedure.

In conclusion there is a possibility that the child who has survived infancy (either by fortunate anatomy or by successful palliation) may be a candidate for successful repair of single ventricle.

20

Aortopulmonary Septal Defect

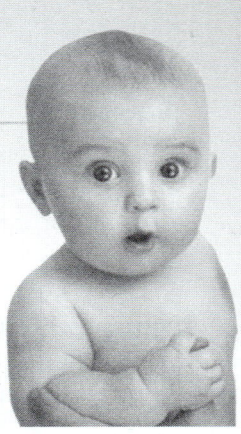

When embryo has crown rump length of between 9 and 13 mm spiral aortopulmonary septum should fuse and finally separate aorta from pulmonary artery. A failure of this process leaves a localized gap between two great arteries just above their valve origin.

Pathology

Defect consists of round or oval communication of variable but often large size. Defect lies between left side of ascending aorta and right wall of MPA just anterior to origin of right MPA branch. Condition is isolated in 50% cases but associated CVS anomalies are common, e.g. PDA, VSD, ASD secundum, interrupted aortic arch, coarctation of aorta, subaortic stenosis, anomalous origin of coronary artery, pulmonary arteriovenous fistula, TOF, origin of right pulmonary artery from aorta and right aortic arch. Ventricular hypertrophy is present its degree and distribution being related to size of defect and status of lung vascular field.

CARDIAC CATHETERIZATION

Dynamics are similar to large VSD or PDA. Systemic pressure levels are seen in RV and pulmonary artery and large left to right shunt in pulmonary arterial level. Aortic pulse pressure will be wide. By end of infancy there will be evidence of high PVR.

Angiography

This permits separation of patients with aortopulmonary septal defect from those with true truncus arteriosus or PDA. Other associated CVS anomalies can be defined likewise by angiocardiography.

Clinical Features

In usual case with large defect tachypnea is an early sign during infancy. Baby is acyanotic at this age. CHF is common. Pulses are bounding. Murmur appears within a few weeks which is non-specific, short, ejection in type along LSE. Occasionally pansystolic or loud. There is often an MDM and occasionally pulmonary valve incompetence may be evident. Second heart sound is narrowly split and pulmonary valve closure is accentuated. In patients with high PVR mild cyanosis may be seen. Pulses are more likely to be normal and frequently a short murmur, loud pulmonary ejection sound and loud single heart sound. In 10% cases there is no symptom. These patients with small defect are detected by murmur during routine examination. Murmur is continuous and localized to 2nd LICS. Second heart sound is normal. Near normal PAP. Additional CVS malformations may be masked by aortopulmonary septal defect, e.g. in PS of TOF or anomalous coronary artery.

RADIOLOGY

Heart is slightly, moderately or grossly enlarged depending upon size of defect and state of PVR. With large defect there is cardiomegaly with left atrial enlargement and prominent lung vascularity. Aortic knuckle is not enlarged. Right aorta is common especially in patients with associated VSD.

ECG

May be normal or show slight LVH in small defects. In large usual defects varying degree of frontal plane QRS axis, RVH, CVH or LVH will reflect status of pulmonary vascular bed.

Diagnosis

For large defect features are of left to right shunt. Bounding pulse might suggest diagnosis of PDA. Alternative of truncus arteriosus is unlikely because of clear cut splitting of second heart sound in aortopulmonary septal defect.

Echocardiography may detect two separate great vessels roots. VSD with ductus or AR can be simulated by aorto-pulmonary septal defect.

In majority with small defect patient may be considered to have an isolated PDA and referred for surgery without confirmatory catheterization and angiocardiography. Any patient with apparent PDA who shows even slightest departure from classic diagnostic features, e.g. atypical nature, duration or position of murmur, discordant features in ECG or chest X-ray should be submitted for catheterization study.

Treatment

Operative closure of defect. Patients with small defect can be repaired electively after infancy. In those with large defect with complicating anomalies repair may be necessary during infancy. Reasonably effective medical control of CHF allows deferral of operation to later part of first year of life. Failure to maintain good control argues for early surgery.

Earlier techniques employed ligation or division of defect as is used in PDA. After introduction of cardiopulmonary by-pass for repair of this malformation an approach through pulmonary artery was suggested by Schumaker and later by Putamen and Gross. After which Wright and colleagues devised transaortic closure method now in vogue.

As diagnostic and management decisions are confined to first or second year of life the operation in patients with high PVR in aortopulmonary septal defect will not be required.

21

Cardiac Arrhythmias

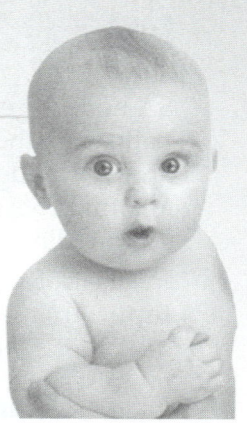

Normal heart rate in infants and children:
- 0–24 hours 88–166/min.
- 1 day–1 week 100–188/min
- 1 week–1 month 125–188/min.
- 1–3 month 115–215/min.
- 3–6 month 125–215/min.
- 6 month–1year 115–188/min.
- 1–3 year 100–188/min.
- 3–5 year 68–150/min.
- 5–8 year 75–150/min.
- 8–12 year 51–125/min.
- 12–16 year 38–125/min.

Normal rhythmic cardiac contraction is initiated by spontaneous depolarization of sinoatrial node. This depolarization generates an impulse that spreads sequentially through atrial wall and specialized internodal tracts to atrioventricular node and then to His bundle and its branches to reach Purkinje network and to excite ventricular muscle. SA node lies in RA wall adjacent to SVC. Measuring 5 mm into 20 mm it consists of muscle cells surrounding a central artery. Close to its center primitive 'P' cells are identifiable. Peripherally both purkinje like fibers and undifferentiated cells are found. These 'P' or pale cells are probably pacemaker cells of sinus node and similar cells can be found in AV node. Central artery is derived from RCA in 60% and LCA in 40% of hearts.

SA node is generously innervated with both sympathetic and parasympathetic fibers. Three internodal pathways connect SA and AV node and a further tract connects SA node to left atrium. These tracts conduct impulses more rapidly than surrounding atrial myocardium.

Fibers of all three internodal tracts intermingle near AV node. Input area of AV node may be considered in two main divisions. Most fibers enter the crest of node delivering impulses that must traverse the entire node. Some fibers enter much more distally bypassing most of central nodal fibers and connecting almost directly with His bundle. Impulses carried in this later pathway may avoid normal delay inherent in conduction through AV node. These are potential pathways for abnormal conduction and reentry mechanism.

AV node lies subendocardially just inferior to coronary sinus ostium and medial leaflet of tricuspid valve connected above with internodal tracts and below with His bundle which penetrates fibrous skeleton of heart. True AV nodal fibers do not show spontaneous depolarization and are therefore nonautomatic and cannot normally assume pacemaker function. Automaticity can develop in coronary sinus portion of node and adjacent junctional tissue between node and bundle. His bundle and Purkinje cells can also assume pacing function. Nodal and junctional region is supplied by specific artery derived from RCA in 92% and left circumflex in 8% hearts. AV node is less well innervated than SA node and its supply is largely parasympathetic from left vagus. His bundle and its branches are also supplied by vagus. His bundle penetrates cardiac skeleton to reach crest of muscular portion of interventricular septum. From the point where it emerges it gives off fasciculi of left bundle which divides into two major branches and discrete branches. Anterior branch runs anterosuperiorly to ramify over anterior half of left septal surface and endocardium of anterior LV. Posterior branch is directed posteroinferior over posterior half of septum and posteroinferior surface of LV. These two branches run to their respective papillary muscles merging peripherally with

Purkinje network which facilitates rapid spread of excitation. From Purkinje subendocardiac plexus an extensive intramyocardial network carries impulse through septum and free ventricular wall.

Right bundle branch forms distinct tract along lower margin of crista supraventricularis to moderator band. Close to anterolateral papillary muscle it divides into three terminal rami continuous with Purkinje networks of inferior, anterior and lower septal surfaces of RV.

RBB and anterior division of left bundle derive their blood supply from LAD coronary artery while posterior division of left bundle is usually supplied by posterior descending coronary artery.

James in 1970 has shown that AV node and His bundle arise as separate structures in embryo and normally fuse in first gestational month. In patients with congenital complete heart block there appears to be a failure of fusion although both structures may be present.

Lev in 1971 has described absence of communication between atrial musculature and AV node or His bundle in congenital AV block. This may be due to a malformation of central fibrous body during absorption of bulbus.

Conducting system in congenital heart malformations may have an abnormal course, its continuity may be interrupted or there may be accessory communications in addition to or in place of usual pathways. Complete or partial AV block, RBBB, left hemiblock and WPW syndrome relate to these conditions. Both persistent atrioventricularis communis and tricuspid atresia are associated with characteristic early excitation of posterior parts of LV. In atrioventricularis communis posterior LBB fascicles have a relatively early origin from common bundle and anterior fascicles appear deficient. RBB appears to have an abnormally prolonged course. Similar abnormalities are found in patients with tricuspid atresia.

In congenitally corrected transposition connecting AV node is situated anteriorly in RA at lateral junction of pulmonary and mitral valves.

An anteriorly situated bundle descends into morphologic LV and encircles anterolateral quadrant of pulmonary outflow tract before descending onto anterior septum and bifurcating. Bundle branches are inverted. In cases with VSD bundle is related to anterior quadrant of defect. In single ventricle normal posterior AV node is rudimentary while an accessory anterior AV node is found at roof of RA. This later node gives rise to an AV bundle descending in outflow tract of posterior vessel to lay in right margin of foramen between main and outlet chambers. Bundle bifurcates astride septum between chambers to give a typical left bundle to main ventricular chamber and right bundle tissue to outlet chamber. In contrast in true common ventricle in which AV orifices enter separate sinuses slightly subdivided by remnant of posterior ventricular septum conducting tissue usually lies on a posterior muscular ridge.

PHYSIOLOGY

Arrhythmias may result from disorder of impulse formation or impulse conduction or both. Under normal physiological conditions most cardiac fibers are nonautomatic and a steady potential difference of 90 mv can be recorded across cell membrane, interior being negative with respect to exterior. This resting membrane potential is abolished by excitation being momentarily reversed. RMP is then restored in three different phases of repolarisation. This whole sequence of electrical events is termed action potential. An external electrical stimulus provokes an action potential only if the stimulus is sufficient to lower the RMP to a critical threshold potential approximately 65 mv in normal cardiac fibers. Automatic cardiac fibers are self-excitatory and their action potential are characterized by slow spontaneous depolarization during resting phase probably due to a time dependent decrease in potassium efflux. This diastolic depolarization is unique to pacemaker fibers. When threshold potential is reached an action potential is generated and a wave of excitation spreads to adjacent nonautomatic fibers. Such automatic cells are found in SA node, interatrial tract, coronary sinus portion of AV node, junctional region and in His Purkinje system. Under appropriate conditions many of these automatic cells assume pacemaker capacity but this function normally resides in SA node and all other latent pacemaker cells are suppressed by wave of excitation originating from SA region. Traditional view is that SA activity is enhanced by sympathetic stimulation and suppressed by vagal stimulation. Increased vagal activity slows spontaneous diastolic depolarization and increases RMP of sinus node. Excessive vagal activity may arrest both SA and atrial activity. Pacemakers are subject to a frequency dependent suppression. Pacemaker tissue stimulated at a frequency in excess of its intrinsic rate exhibits a temporary inhibition of its pacemaker ability when stimulation ceases. This overdrive suppression accounts for temporary ventricular standstill occurring during excessive vagal stimulation or following the sudden onset of complete heart block.

Many arrhythmias result from changes in automaticity that may be influenced by alterations in rate of diastolic depolarization, maximum diastolic potential and threshold potential. Catecholamines increase rate of spontaneous depolarization in His Purkinje system therefore, enhancing their pacemaker potential. A rise in temperature, hypoxia, elevated PCO_2 and stretching of myocardium all tend to augment the automaticity and increase the risk of latent pacemaker usurping the sinus node. Other dysrrhythmias especially premature beats and ectopic tachycardia may result from reentry pathways secondary to areas of abnormal refractoriness coupled with entry and exit block. Finally defects of conduction may result in temporary or permanent forms of heart block of varying degree.

DISORDERS OF IMPULSE FORMATION
SINUS TACHYCARDIA

Persistently elevated heart rate above expected for age. It usually shows slight variation in rate over a period of hours and usually slows slightly during carotid sinus massage returning to original rate when pressure is released. Sinus tachycardia is often a compensatory response and has numerous causes including exercise, emotion, anemia, fever, infection, heart failure, hemorrhage, shock, thyrotoxicosis, adrenaline, atropine, etc. ECG shows normal P-waves. Each followed by a normal QRS complex. P-wave duration, PR and QT interval are shortened. ST depression and flattening or inversion of T-wave may develop if tachycardia is prolonged and may persist for for 12 to 24 hours after tachycardia ceases. Treatment of sinus tachycardia is directed towards the cause. Attempts to reduce heart rate by digoxin in absence of heart failure are misguided.

Sinus Bradycardia

A persistent heart rate less than 90 in infants and less than 60 in children. This may occur in healthy individual, athletes, infectious fever, such as scarlet fever during convalescence, acute nephritis reflexly due to hypertension, raised intracranial tension and jaundice. It also occurs in 20% cases of acute rheumatic fever. Presence of heart block should be excluded by ECG.

Sinus Arrhythmia

Irregular impulse formation by sinus node is present in most children. There are two varieties. In one heart rate increases toward end inspiration and slows again during expiration. This variation is related to diminished vagal tone during inspiration. In other less common type the arrhythmia bears no relationship to respiration and most often occurs during administration of digoxin or morphine.

Premature Beats (Extrasystole)

May be atrial, junctional or ventricular in origin. Most are due to reentry pathways. A small area of myocardium remains refractory and consequently unresponsive to next normal impulse which bypasses the area. Later retrograde conduction returns to the area which is now responsive forming focus for premature systole. Less commonly a true ectopic focus due to heightened automaticity or existence of a parasystolic focus may account for premature beat. Incidence 1 to 2% in normal children and 4 to 6% in those with heart disease.

Premature beats may occur in acute rheumatic fever and other forms of myocarditis. They are less often a feature of digoxin toxicity than adults. Most children with premature beats are asymptomatic but some may be conscious of missing a beat. ECG is diagnostic. Atrial premature beats are typified by a distorted or inverted P-wave and normal QRS complexes except when they are very premature and fail to be conducted. Premature junctional beats are recognized by inversion of P-wave which just precedes, coincides with or just follows the QRS. Ventricular premature beats may originate anywhere in ventricles and cause sequential activation of ventricles resulting in slurred, wide QRS complexes and T-waves of opposite polarity. No preceding P-wave is observed. Ventricular premature beats are followed by full compensatory pause. Exercise tends to abolish the premature beat in normal heart while in diseased heart they become more frequent. Symptomatic and frequent premature beats respond to propranolol. Mild sedation may help to relieve anxiety.

PAROXYSMAL SUPRAVENTRICULAR TACHYCARDIA

Sudden rapid supraventricular (atrial or atrioventricular junctional) regular rhythm with a ventricular rate of between 140 and 240 beats per minute. This may be paroxysmal, repetitive or occasionally sustained. PSVT may be regarded as a series of rapidly repeated premature beats. Paroxysms start suddenly, lasts seconds, hours or days and end abruptly. PSVT occurs in one out of every 25000 children.

ETIOLOGY

PSVT may occur in association with cardiac catheterization, cardiac surgery when hypoxia, electrolyte disturbance and pH changes contribute.

Digoxin toxicity may produce PSVT with AV block. 70% cases of WPW syndrome experience one or more episode of PSVT.

Other factors are emotional stress:
- Hyperthyroidism
- Hemochromatosis
- Cardiac tumors
- Childhood infections
- CHD especially Ebstein anomaly
- Skull fracture
- Blow on chest
- Rheumatic heart disease.

There is slightly higher incidence of neurosis, peptic ulcer and syncope in one or other parent than is found in general population. There is association of PSVT with infections.

Mechanism

1. Circus movement or gross reentry theory: His bundle recordings taken during onset of PVST have helped to document its initiation following atrial premature beats. PSVT due to reentry has following features:
   - It is initiated or terminated by an atrial premature beat.
   - During its establishment there is a regular sequence of cycle length.
   - Once established the paroxysm has fixed cycle length.
2. Unifocal or run of atrial ectopics theory: Consisting of a run of supraventricular ectopic beats from a single ectopic focus of enhanced automaticity.

Clinical Features

Some children are totally unaware of a fast rate. HR in them is usually less than 200/minute.

Majority of children over 5 year are aware of sudden onset of tachycardia and usually stop whatever activity they have undertaken and sit or lie down. They may appear pale. Occasionally tachycardia may proceed for days and weeks without showing any more sign or symptoms.

The children are usually aware of a need for keeping quiet. They do not wish to move about. They show anxiety.

Cases arising in infancy show most dramatic features. They are quite ill with ashen complexion, cyanosis of lips, cold clammy skin, subnormal temperature, irritable movement of head and arms and enlargement of liver, rales in chest and evidence of edema. Fever may occur as illness progresses especially when it is associated with infections.

In atrial tachycardia heart sounds are extremely constant in intensity. A short faint systolic murmur is heard in a number of cases but this disappears when rate decreases. Chest pain is not common.

Leukocyte count is markedly elevated, up to 25000/cu mm. CHF is related to duration of attack in infancy. If duration is less than 24 hours, failure rarely occurs. It rarely occurs with HR less than 200/minute.

CHF occurs in 36% cases in first year of life but only rarely in those over that age.

Prolonged PSVT may produce a fall in stroke output and BP. In presence of cardiac disease collapse may occur. Chest X-ray may show cardiomegaly with or without pulmonary edema.

ECG

Ventricular rate ranges from 140 to 240/minute. Ventricular complexes are normal in configuration but occasionally aberrant ventricular conduction may widen QRS complex and make differentiation from ventricular tachycardia difficult. P-wave is buried in preceding T-wave and is impossible to distinguish. Secondary ST depression and T-wave inversion may occur. Once normal sinus rhythm is restored ECG may show atrial premature beats coupled to preceding normal beat.

Lown-Ganong-Levine syndrome is short PR interval with normal width QRS.

Diagnosis

PSVT must be differentiated from sinus tachycardia, atrial flutter and when aberrant QRS complexes are present from ventricular tachycardia. Carotid sinus massage may assist in differential diagnosis. In cases where, there are P-waves difficult to detect an ECG recorded with an esophageal or intra-atrial electrode will often reveal atrial mechanism and permit distinction between atrial tachycardia with aberrancy and ventricular tachycardia.

Treatment

Many attacks terminate spontaneously. It is worth attempting conversion by reflex stimulation of vagus nerve. This can be achieved by unilateral carotid sinus massage. The patient should be recumbent with head tilted back and to one side. The artery is compressed against vertebral column as high up in neck as possible. Heart beat is monitored with a stethoscope on precordium. As soon as the arrhythmia stops pressure should be released. If massage on one side is unsuccessful the opposite side should be tried but never both together.

Steady eyeball pressure applied just below supraorbital ridges also produce vagal stimulation and may terminate tachycardia. However, detachment of retina has occured as complication. Induction of vomiting or Valsalva maneuver is occasionally effective in terminating attack.

In infant and young children digoxin is drug of choice. 80% of attacks are terminated within one to two days after use of this drug and commonly after first dose. Dose 0.06 mg/kg. Give half of this dose immediately intramuscular. One fourth in 4 to 6 hours and another one fourth in 8 to 12 hours. One-tenth of total digitalizing dose is then given every 12 hours as maintenance dose.

A few patients in first year of life do not respond to digoxin especially those associated with WPW syndrome or congenital heart anomalies. In these patients propranolol 0.1 mg/kg given as slow intravenous injection is effective and second drug of choice unless failure is severe.

In desperately ill patients or those who fail to respond to digoxin and propranolol electrical DC countershock should be tried. An initial shock of 10 watt/second is effective in infancy. Parasympathomimetics like edrophonium or neostigmine may be effective either alone or combined with carotid sinus massage. Edrophonium can only be given IV and is a specific inhibitor of cholinesterase. In infancy 0.5 mg is given over a period of 30 seconds while patient's cardiac rhythm is monitored. In older children 2 mg is given initially and if this is ineffective a further 5 mg can be tried after 10 minutes interval. Toxic effects include excessive vagal stimulation, nausea, diarrhea, salivation, muscle twitching, hypotension. Both atrial and ventricular asystole may be observed. Should AV block be produced it may be reversed by 0.5 to 1 mg of atropine IV.

Quinidine and procainamide have also been used successfully. Both have serious side effects and should be reserved for resistant cases.

In older children many attacks terminate spontaneously.

Prevention of Recurrences

Digoxin maintenance is continued for six months. If paroxysms are occuring every once or twice a year no preventive therapy is necessary.

Precipitating causes should be identified and removed. If maintenance digoxin fails to prevent recurrences propranolol 5 to 10 mg TDS alone or in combination with digoxin may help. In more resistant cases quinidine 60 to 200 mg daily or procainamide 30 to 50 mg/kg/day in divided doses may be tried. Conversion of supraventricular tachycardia to sinus rhythm by an appropriately timed atrial or ventricular premature beat induced by implanted pacemaker and control of frequent PSVT in WPW syndrome by a permanently implanted pacemaker with electrodes attached to left atrium is being done. The pacemaker is set to pace at 108 beats/minute and is turned on during a paroxysm by holding a magnet over implanted unit. This converts each paroxysm back to sinus rhythm.

Prognosis

Good in vast majority of cases. Mortality is less than 2%. Presence of CHD especially cyanotic increase risk.

74% cases have recurrence in follow-up.

Most significant prognostic feature is related to age of onset. If onset occurred in first 4 months of life recurrence rate is 22%. If onset is after 4 months of age recurrence rate is 83%.

PAROXYSMAL VENTRICULAR TACHYCARDIA

Rare in childhood. Apart from cardiac catheterization is associated with serious heart disease.

Bellet's criteria in ECG

1. Paroxysmal beats must be ectopic in origin and conform to those observed as isolated ventricular premature beats before onset of paroxysm.
2. QRS complexes should be widened and notched (more than 0.12 second).
3. First step of paroxysm should bear same relationship to preceding normal beat as a ventricular premature beat bears to previous beat.
4. Ventricles beat regularly or slightly irregularly at rate 130 to 180/minute while atria beat more slowly regularly and independently.
5. Occasional ventricular captures are observed (conducted beats from atria with narrow QRS).
6. Ventricular fusion beats (from combined ectopic and sinus beats).

If all above are present diagnosis of ventricular origin is highly likely.

In difficult cases His bundle ECG showing His potentials relating to atrial activity only, will be diagnostic.

The arrhythmia is seldom tolerated for long without developing cardiac decompensation, i.e. substernal pain, dyspnea, shock, syncope and CHF especially if there is underlying heart disease. Treatment depends upon underlying cause and patient's general condition. Lidocain is specially effective in ventricular arrhythmias. IV bolus 1 to 2 mg/kg is effective within 1 to 2 minutes and suppresses ventricular activity up to 20 minutes. If arrhythmia recurs a continuous IV infusion at rate of 15 microgram per kg is usually effective in suppressing ventricular ectopic activity and may be continued for many hours. IV Quinidine or procainamide may also revert ventricular tachycardia to sinus rhythm. Electric countershock with DC converter is treatment of choice for drug resistant episodes of PVT not due to digoxin.

REPETITIVE PAROXYSMAL TACHYCARDIA

Continuously recurrent runs of paroxysmal tachycardia with intermittent return to NSR for a few beats. Atrial form is most common. This tachycardia may persist for many months or years. Average rate including burst of tachycardia and NSR is between 120 and 180/minute. Most children withstand this rate well. Digitalis is needed when there is excessive rate and heart is enlarged or if failure appears cardioversion or electric shock can be tried. Prognosis is good. Most cases return to NSR. Tachycardia does not interfere with normal life.

Persistent Paroxysmal Atrial Tachycardia

These cases are refractory to all forms of therapy.

Cardiomegaly, cardiac failure, hepatomegaly occur.

Palpitation and awareness of heart beat are most common symptoms usually accompanied by slight shortness of breath on exertion. No associated disease, such as myocarditis or hyperthyroidism is found in these cases. Electrical countershock should be tried in these arrhythmias. Tachycardia at times be a contributory cause of death.

Atrial Flutter

Rare. May develop anytime from fetal life up through childhood. Majority appear in infancy most commonly in newborn.

Two types:

Type 1: Congenital atrial flutter is recognized prenatally or within first week of life. More common. Has an equal sex distribution and responds to digitalis in 50% cases.

Type 2: Paroxysmal atrial flutter. First recognized after age 3 weeks. Predominantly in males and infrequently responds to digoxin. Atrial rate varies between 200 and 450. Ventricular rate being half to one-third or one-fourth depending upon block degree. Ventricles beat at a rate that does not produce cardiac failure.

Diagnosis is established by finding typical F-waves in ECG giving a regular saw tooth appearance to the tracing. Ventricular rate may be regular with a degree of block or may vary if degree of block changes. Electrical DC countershock is the preferred treatment. Prognosis is good in type 1. It is poor in type 2 when associated cardiac malformation is present or periods of atrial fibrillation occur.

ATRIAL FIBRILLATION

Uncommon in childhood. May occur in older children with advanced RHD or as a result of digoxin intoxication especially if serum potassium is lowered. Tumors of heart involving atria, e.g. Hemartoma may also precipitate this AF. ASD as cause of AF is uncommon in childhood.

Heart beat is rapid and continuously irregular with varying intensity of heart sound and a marked variability of cardiac impulse. Heart failure may or may not accompany it. Pulse may be so weak that only a few beats are felt.

ECG defines irregularity of ventricular beats and reveals small f-waves occurring at 300 to 500 per minute representing abnormal atrial contractions. Ventricles beat at rate of 150 per minute. Both rapid ventricular rate and loss of atrial contribution to ventricular filling impair cardiac output especially during exercise. Digoxin 0.06 mg per kg in divided doses as rapidly as required slows ventricular rate. One-fourth of digitalising dose should be given IV and repeated in 15 to 30 minutes until digitalization is complete. Then digitalization may be carried on with one-fifth of digitalising dose as long as it is necessary to control ventricular rate. Some cases revert to normal rhythm others will need such therapy continuously. Electrical countershock may be effective in converting AF to sinus rhythm although recurrences are common.

WPW SYNDROME

An entity characterized by paroxysmal tachycardia and between attacks ECG abnormalities including short PR interval, widening of QRS interval and delta wave. Delta wave is a slurring of initial portion of QRS complex and represents premature ventricular excitation. QRS duration 0.1 second is criterion of this condition. Importance of syndrome lies in susceptibility of patient to tachyarrhythmias and because ECG may simulate serious heart disease.

WPW syndrome results from premature excitation of one or other ventricle occurring when sinus impulse partially or completely bypasses normal AV junctional pathway. Several potential anomalous pathways have been described. Kent first described anomalous AV pathways. James has described bypass fibers around AV node. Maheim and Clerc have reported fibers connecting conducting bundles to ventricular system. Existence of these pathways which may be involved alone or in combination allows rational explanations to be made of ECG features of classic WPW and its variants.

These variants include a normal PR with prolonged QRS and prominent delta wave or a short PR with delta wave but normal QRS duration.

Lown described association of short PR interval with normal QRS duration and configuration.

All these variants may be associated with paroxysmal tachycardia. Unlike classic WPW syndrome the Lown-Ganong-Levine syndrome is common in females.

True incidence of WPW syndrome is 0.1% of unselected children and 0.5% with suspected heart disease. 40% children with WPW syndrome have associated CHD, commonest is Ebstein anomaly, L transposition of great arteries and familial or primary myocardial disease. 70% are males. Several reports of familial occurrences are there. No pattern of inheritance is established. Classic WPW has been divided into type A and B.

Type A is characterized by large R-wave in right precordial leads. Type B shows large S-wave in same leads.

Findings suggest that anomalous pathways involve left bundle and left ventricle in type A and right ventricle and right bundle in type B. Combination of bundle branch block with WPW is uncommon but may occur. In such cases vectorcardiogram may be helpful. In both conditions there is a relative delay in activation of one ventricle which is manifested in VCG by increased proximity of dots in vector loop. In WPW this delay always involves initial portion of loop while in LBBB or RBBB delay is seen in mid section of loop.

Premature beats and tachyarrhythmias occur in 70% cases of WPW syndrome. PAT is commonest but atrial fibrillation and flutter also occur. Occasionally ventricular fibrillation may cause sudden death. Retrograde conduction via anomalous pathways with reactivation of atria is basic mechanism underlying arrhythmia.

Prognosis depends upon frequency and severity of paroxysmal tachycardia episodes and on presence or absence of associated cardiac defects. Infants with otherwise normal heart who first develop PAT under 6 months have best prognosis although WPW pattern may persist bouts of tachycardia usually cease. Patients presenting for first time at older age are most likely to suffer recurrences. When an associated heart lesion is present prognosis is that of basic defect.

Digoxin is preferred for treatment. Propranolol also may terminate tachycardia. Atropine by enhancing normal conduction and quinidine or procainamide by increasing refractoriness of accessory pathways may all tend to normalize ECG between attacks. Propranolol is most valuable in preventing attacks of recurrences.

Amiodarone can be used in controlling tachyarrhythmias. In drug resistant episodes cardioversion is successful. Intracardiac electrode catheter used to provoke premature atrial depolarization or retrograde atrial depolarization by ventricular stimulation may terminate supraventricular tachycardia by interrupting re-entry pathways.

For recurrent WPW tachycardia a high frequency radio pace maker is implanted. During attacks pacemaker is switched on by magnet held near generator. Fixed rate competitive pacing terminates attacks.

Technique of epicardial mapping has resulted in successful surgical interruption of anomalous conducting pathways.

AV JUNCTIONAL RHYTHMS

Uncommon and transient in children. If sinus node fails to pace heart or if its intrinsic rate falls below that of AV junctional region, AV junction may assume pacemaker function usually with a rate between 40 and 60/minute. Occasionally AV junctional automaticity may be enhanced so that its rate exceeds that of sinus node resulting in junctional tachycardia. Finally should AV node fail to conduct atrial impulses, AV junction may again assume pacemaking. Automatic fibers also lie close to coronary sinus ostium and are capable of assuming pacemaker function producing coronary sinus rhythm.

Junctional rhythm is often a transient feature in rheumatic and other myocarditis, during cardiac catheterization and surgery or during therapy with digoxin and parasympathomimetic drugs. They may follow Mustard operation for transposition when they may be permanent. Bacos in 1960 has described a familial association of junctional rhythm.

In CHD presence of junctional rhythm indicates partial anomalous venous return to right atrium or a persistent left superior vena cava associated with ASD (coronary sinus rhythm). ECG is diagnostic. P-wave may precede, coincide or follow QRS and is inverted or abnormal in shape. Occasionally it may be absent. QRS is of normal width and configuration but occasionally shows aberrant conduction. In coronary sinus rhythm PR is normal or slightly short (0.1 to 0.07 second). P-wave is negative in lead 2 and 3 and often peaked. Its axis is deviated to left. Junctional and coronary sinus rhythms are usually transient and treatment is directed toward underlying cause. AV junctional tachycardia is sometimes paroxysmal when causative factors, clinical features and treatment are similar to PAT.

AV HEART BLOCK

Partial or complete.

Partial may be first or second degree.

All may be temporary, intermittent or permanent.

PR interval represents total conduction time of cardiac impulse from SA node through atria, AV node, His bundle and its branches to the onset of ventricular activation. His bundle ECG demonstrates four components of conduction:

1. Intra-atrial
2. AV nodal
3. His bundle
4. Bundle branches and Purkinje network.

All degrees of block may develop at any of these sites.

First degree heart block:

Abnormal delay in AV nodal region and manifest as a prolongation of PR interval. First degree heart block may be defined as PR interval prolongation greater than maximum PR interval for heart rate and age.

PR interval may be abnormally prolonged during rheumatic fever. There is no difference between patients with carditis and those without cardiac involvement.

Viral infection, diphtheria, vagal stimulation, digoxin, propranolol may all be associated with first degree heart block which may also follow cardiac surgery or may occur during cardiac catheterization.

PR interval more than 0.18 second in congenital cardiac anomalies:

- L or corrected transposition of great arteries 57%.
- Ebstein disease 50%.
- ASD 43%.
- Coarctation of aorta 12%.
- Complete anomalous PVD 8%.
- PDA 3.4%.
- PS 3%.

- TOF 2%.
- PR prolongation is not seen in tricuspid atresia. First degree heart block may be suspected clinically by softening of first heart sound. It does not cause symptoms and does not require treatment.

Second degree heart block

Progressive lengthening of PR interval in succeeding cycles until the impulse fails to be conducted to ventricles and a ventricular beat is dropped. Cycle then repeats. Usually PR interval increments get smaller until beat is dropped. This phenomenon was first described by Wenkebach in 1914, also called Mobitz type 1 block. It occurs in association with same conditions that cause heart block. In less common second type of second degree heart block ventricular beats are dropped without previous PR prolongation and PR interval is constant for conducted beats. Dropped beats may occur periodically or constantly when ventricular complexes occur only after every second, third or fourth atrial beat resulting in 2:1, 3:1, 4:1 AV block. This form of second degree heart block is due to bilateral bundle branch problems. This is called Mobitz type 2 block and indicates a more serious prognosis often progressing to complete heart block. On auscultation first heart sound may progressively diminish in intensity. Exercise or atropine may double ventricular rate in 2:1 heart block. If they do not do so and ventricular rate is below 60 complete heart block is present.

Complete AV block

Absolute failure of atrial impulse to be transmitted to ventricles. Atria and ventricles beat independently. Atria in response to SA node and ventricles at a slower rate responding to a pacemaker situated in lower AV junctional region, His bundle or more distally. In general the lower the pacemaker lies in conduction system the slower the idioventricular rate. Complete AV block may result from lesions proximal to, within or distal to His bundle and may involve a single lesion within the bundle or multiple lesions in each of the three fascicles.

COMPLETE HEART BLOCK

Two types:
1. Congenital:
   Isolated 67%.
   Associated with heart disease 23%.
2. Acquired:
   Postoperative 40%.
   Acute rheumatic fever 2%.
   Acute streptococcal infection 1%.
   Pathogenesis:

Origin of congenital AV block due to:

1. Discontinuity between atrial musculature and more peripheral conducting system.
2. Interruption of His bundle.
3. Pathologic change in an aberrant conduction system. Complete heart block may occur in association with L transposition of great arteries, atrioventricularis communis, endocardial fibroelastosis, and VSD.

   Temporary complete heart block has been attributed to mumps, diphtheria and rheumatic fever, digoxin and quinidine.

Clinical Features

Congenital complete heart block may be detected *in utero* suggesting fetal distress, it is more often not discovered until child is few years old.

Congenital complete heart block rarely causes symptoms and is usually compatible with normal growth and development. In isolated form problems are most likely to occur during infancy. There is an association between syncopal attack and heart rate. If rate falls less than 40/minute, syncopy is likely. Systolic ejection murmurs are common probably as result of increased stroke volume. First heart sound varies in intensity. Faint atrial sounds may be heard during long diastolic pauses. A rapid inflow type of diastolic mitral murmur may be present. Venous pressure is elevated and venous cannon waves may be seen whenever right atrium contracts against a closed tricuspid valve. Slow ventricular rate results in increased stroke volume and end diastolic volume of heart. Consequentely CT ratio on chest X-ray is greater than 55%.

ECG shows complete heart block and in 50% of patients LVH is present.

Prognosis

Sokes Adams attacks can cause death. A wide QRS complex with LBBB pattern suggests a poor prognosis. Ventricular rate at birth under 30 beats per minute with multifocal QRS complexes carry an unfavorable significance and suggest prenatal toxic or inflammatory etiology rather than developmental defect. Acquired complete heart block is almost always a surgical problem and follow closure of VSD or *intracardiac* repair of Fallot tetralogy. It may also complicate ASD closure, Mustard operation and procedures on mitral valve. It may occur temporarily in immediate postoperative period. Some patients develop complete heart block months or even years after their surgical procedures. Pattern of left anterior hemiblock associated with RBB and prolonged PR interval may give a clue to those patients at risk of developing late complete heart block.

Acquired heart block is usually associated with slower idioventricular rate, wider QRS complexes often of abnormal contour, less response to exercise, congestive heart failure and syncope. Prognosis is grave and treatment is always required.

Treatment

Congenital complete heart block requires no treatment unless syncope or unremitting heart failure develops.

Temporary acquired heart block due to drugs, acute rheumatic fever or renal failure can be managed with temporary transvenous pacing catheter lodged in RV.

Permanent complete heart block or acquired heart block causing symptoms should be managed by insertion of permanent pacing unit. In older children most satisfactory combination is a demand unit buried in axilla and attached to transvenous pacing catheter in RV apex. In small children unit is best attached to epicardial electrode because of possible displacement by growth. Chief advantage of demand unit is that it avoids competition with patient's own rhythm, whenever patient's heart accelerates above present pacemaker rate an inhibitory circuit is activated that prevents further stimulus discharge until ventricular rate falls once more below critical level.

Although isoproterenol given IV or sublingually increase heart rate in complete heart block its use is limited therapeutically. Its effect is too unpredictable, risk of ventricular tachyarrhythmia too great, to permit its use except under emergency situation where temporary pacing is not possible.

Artificial Pacemaker

Attempts to control heart beat by direct electric stimulation were described in early 1800. In 1952. Zoll restored effective cardiac action in patients with Adams Stokes attacks by transthoracic pacing. This successful demonstration stimulated further research culminating in Chardaek's completely implantable system powered by mercury cell battery. Furman showed that permanently implanted transvenous catheter could be used to stimulate RV. Direct transvenous endocardial pacing is preferred method but in children, growth may displace transvenous pacing catheter from RV apex. At present epicardial electrodes placed during thoracotomy are preferred.

There are two types of pacemaker units. One is fixed rate unit in which pacing is independent of electrical activity of heart. Although these pacemakers are relatively simple and less prone to premature failure they carry risk of competition with patient's intrinsic rhythm especially if sinus rhythm is restored. If pacemaker stimulus falls during vulnerable period of ventricular depolarization, ventricular fibrillation may be induced. Ventricular inhibited demand pacemakers stimulate only when patient's rate falls below present pacemaker's rate, otherwise patient's own QRS complex is fed back to unit and generator suppressed.

Ventricular triggered stand by pacemakers sense normally occurring QRS complexes and immediately discharge into absolute refractory period of these beats. If there is no spontaneous beat pacer will discharge at its preset escape interval.

Atrial synchronous pacing requires two electrodes. An atrial electrode senses P-wave and heart is paced after suitable delay by a ventricular electrode. A long refractory period prevents rapid ventricular pacing in event of ventricular tachycardia, fibrillation or flutter.

Early models of demand pacemaker could be inhibited by external electrical equipment, such as electrical shavers, radar sources, cautery and microwave grills. Improved generator screening has reduced risk in later models. Functional life of all types of generators is 24 to 36 months. Lithium based cells and nuclear power source based designs may last for 8 to 10 years.

CARDIOAUDITORY SYNDROMES

Association of congenital deafness with prolongation of QT interval in ECG, episodes of syncope and risk of sudden death is Jervell and Lange Nielsen syndrome (1957).

QT prolongation, syncope and sudden death in absence of deafness is Ward syndrome (1964).

Both syndromes may occur on familial basis.

Incidence of QT prolongation in congenitally deaf children varies between 0.1 to 1%. Syncopal attacks begin after 1 year of life and are due to paroxysmal ventricular fibrillation or short periods of asystole. Attacks are precipitated by fear or other emotional stimuli and may be fatal.

This syndrome represents an abnormal response to adrenergic stimulation. Alternative hypothesis are abnormality in vascularization of SA node and in myocardial metabolism. Beta blockers are effective in majority of patients, otherwise left sympathectomy is completely effective and also shortens QT interval.

This condition should be suspected in any deaf child who suffers from convulsions.

ECG is diagnostic.

Sick Sinus Syndrome

Disease of SA node or injury secondary to suturing of cannulation of SVC during cardiac bypass may result in SSS.

Failure of impulse formation at SA node or failure of transmission of sinus impulse to depolarize atrial myocardium causes bradycardia, but symptoms are unlikely unless there is also failure or delay in onset of escape rhythm originating in junctional region. Symptomatic sinus node disease usually implies additional conduction tissue disease beyond sinus node. Periods of sinus arrest, bradycardia, slow or rapid junctional rhythm, supraventricular ectopic beats and supraventricular tachycardia including atrial flutter and fibrillation may all occur in same Patients though ventricular ectopic activity is uncommon. Occurrence of both bradycardia and tachycardia in same patient gives rise to alternative name of brady tachy arrhythmic syndrome.

Classification

Type 1: Sinus bradycardia or sinus arrest predominates.

Type 2: paroxysmal tachycardia predominates.

Preceding cardiac surgery most commonly a Mustard correction of transposition, patch closure of ASD, repair of TAPVD and correction of TOF and viral myocarditis are associated. Symptoms include palpitation, nonanginal pain, dyspnea and pallid spells.

Treatment is indicted when symptoms are significant or CHF is present. Drug therapy with digoxin or propranolol may supress paroxysmal tachycardia but may cause profound bradycardia between such episodes. Cardioversion carries an increased risk in these patients but it is often necessary to terminate persistent tachycardia. Patients with syncope or intractable heart failure due to bradycardia may require insertion of permanent cardiac pacemaker.

HIS BUNDLE ECG

Pioneered by Scherlag in 1969. Coupled with simultaneous recording of surface ECG, HBE can provide more precise localization of site of block or delay in patients with conduction defect, analyzing arrhythmia and studying WPW syndrome. Several ECG patterns may be associated with a risk of developing subsequent complete heart block, e.g. RBBB with LAD, LBBB with RAD.

HBE recorded from these patients may eventually prove predictive in indicating which patients are at higher risk by unmasking conduction problems in apparent in surface ECG. HBE has been used to study effect of various drugs on conducting system.

DIGOXIN

In addition to its positive ionotropic action digoxin has several effects on heart muscle.

High doses of digoxin produce slowing of conduction velocity especially through AV node and His bundle. This action being partly direct and partly vagal.

PR prolongation seen in ECG reflects this action which also explains AV dissociation and complete heart block in digoxin toxicity.

Digoxin in therapeutic doses shortens refractory period of atrial and ventricular muscle while prolonging functional refractory period of AV node. These combined effect underlie slowing of heart rate in atrial fibrillation. Shortened ventricular refractory period is seen in ECG as reduced QT interval.

Automaticity is induced in Purkinje fibers and in toxic doses is increased in all areas of heart except SA node. Occasional ventricular premature beat may occur with moderate doses. With increased doses ventricular bigeminy are seen eventually leading to ventricular tachycardia and ventricular fibrillation. Digoxin is indicated for supraventricular ectopic rhythm associated with rapid ventricular rate which often convert to sinus rhythm after digitalization.

Atrial fibrillation responds to digoxin by slowing of ventricular rate. Degree of block is increased by digoxin in atrial flutter, thereby reducing ventricular rate. Digoxin is effective in preventing recurrence of paroxysmal supraventricular tachycardia in infants. Almost any known arrhythmia can be caused by digoxin toxicity. However, in children ventricular premature beats are less common than conduction disturbances, such as SA block, AV dissociation and AV junctional ectopic rhythm. When digoxin toxicity is suspected the drug should be discontinued. Blood pH, electrolytes should be determined. Hypokalemia and metabolic acidosis should be corrected. In patients with advanced degree of AV block due to digoxin, potassium salt is contraindicated because of their action of prolonging AV node refractory period. Both lidocain and phenytoin are effective in treatment of ventricular tachycardia due to digoxin. Phenytoin is more useful as it reverses digoxin induced prolongation of AV conduction. Phenytoin is also most effective drug for suppressing supraventricular tachyarrhythmia due to digoxin.

Junctional or His bundle conduction disturbances respond to atropin.

LIDOCAINE

Indicted in treatment of cardiac arrhythmias complicating cardiac surgery, myocardial infarction and digitalis intoxication. It has little effect on atrial arrhythmias.

It acts by reducing ectopic rhythm formation in ventricles, e.g. paroxysmal ventricular tachycardia, paroxysmal ventricular fibrillation, ventricular ectopics. Metabolized in liver quickly when given IV its action is rapid in onset and lasts for short duration. Myocardial depression may occur with large doses. Drowsiness, muscle twitching, hallucination and seizures may occur. Hypotension and rhythm disturbance, such as sinus tachycardia, sinus bradycardia and sinus arrest are rare.

Dose IV bolus 1 to 2 mg per kg given over 30 to 60 seconds. IV continuous infusion 15 to 25 microgram per kg per minute.

Quinidine

Naturally occurring alkaloid in cinchona bark. Quinidine depresses myocardial contractility, reduces excitability and slows conduction velocity. Quinidine is used to convert atrial fibrillation into sinus rhythm and to prevent its recurrence and to suppress paroxysmal tachyarrhythmias of both supraventricular and ventricular origin. Although premature beats normally do not require treatment quinidine will often effectively suppress them. Nausea, vomiting and diarrhea are common. Tinnitus, vertigo and other features of cinchonism may develop. Thrombocytopenia is reported. Sudden death due to ventricular fibrillation may occur. Hypotension complicates IV use. Quinidine should not be given to patients receiving digoxin.

ECG of patients on quinidine shows wide QRS complexes with QT prolongation and sinus bradycardia with PR prolongation. Dose 3 mg per kg.

Propranolol

Beta adrenergic blocking drug with direct myocardial action which is responsible for its antiarrhythmic action. Direct action is independent of circulating catecholamine and sympathetic activity.

Dose IV 0.1 mg per kg slowly and 1 mg per kg per day. Drug of choice in recurrent supraventricular tachycardia associated with WPW syndrome.

Propranolol should be tried in patients with supraventricular tachycardia who are refractory to digoxin. Also effective in treating arrhythmias due to digoxin toxicity except those associated with AV conduction disturbance in which it may increase degree of block. Propranolol may cause hypotension and bradycardia, myocardial depression which may precipitate CHF. It should not be used in asthmatics as it causes bronchial constriction.

Phenytoin

Decreases SA node automaticity and increases AV node conduction velocity. It reverses prolongation of AV conduction produced by digoxin. Depresses automaticity in His Purkinje system. It has a little effect against supraventricular arrhythmias. IV route should be used in emergency and under ECG control. Dose 1 to 3 mg per kg. Oral dose 1 to 3 mg per kg 8 hourly. Maximum plasma levels are reached in about 12 hours of oral administration. Metabolized in liver the drug should be given in reduced doses in liver disease.

Side effects: Sleepiness, nystagmus, ataxia, confusion, disorientation, hypotension, bradycardia, cardiac arrest and myocardial depression.

Defibrillation

Lown in 1962 used it first for treatment of ventricular fibrillation. It is effective in defibrillating hypoxic heart. High energy unsynchronized discharge between 50 and 400 watts per second combined with correction of acidosis and hypoxia. Precipitating causes should be corrected. A continuous infusion of lidocaine 1 to 3 mg per kg may prevent further fibrillation.

ELECTRICAL COUNTERSHOCK

DC converter delivers a synchronized shock to heart usually coinciding with peak of R-wave thereby avoiding the vulnerable period of ventricle in which ventricular fibrillation may be induced. The shock simultaneously discharges all fibers excitable at that instance, abolishes all re-entry pathway and provided the sinus node is healthy restores normal sinus rhythm. While depolarizing the heart, countershock stimulates both parasympathetic and sympathetic cardiac nerves and causes catecholamine release. This autonomic stimulation may be responsible for postconversion tachy brady arrhythmias which can be minimized by keeping stimulus strength low and can be blocked with atropine or propranolol. Attempted cardioversion of arrhythmias due to digoxin toxicity is often followed by serious postconversion arrhythmias especially ventricular tachycardia or fibrillation. DC countershock is contraindicated in arrhythmias due to digoxin toxicity.

DC countershock is indicated in children with paroxysmal supraventricular tachycardia which are resistant to carotid sinus massage and digoxin. Other indications are atrial fibrillation and flutter and paroxysmal ventricular tachycardia.

Contraindications

- Recent onset of arrhythmia.
- Repetitive arrhythmia.
- Recent systemic or pulmonary embolus.

Cardioversion in children is performed under light general anesthesia. Digoxin is withheld for 24 hours prior to conversion and there is no need for anticoagulation. The patient issue connected to a cardioverter which is provided with an oscilloscope so that ECG can be viewed simultaneously. Patient is well oxygenated. An initial low energy discharge of 10 watt per second is applied which if ineffective is followed by 50 watt per second shock.

Defibrillator and IV lidocaine should be available in case ventricular tachycardia or fibrillation supervenes. Pulmonary edema, elevated serum enzymes and transient ST elevation are rare complications.

DIAGNOSTIC APPROACH TO CARDIAC ARRHYTHMIAS

Arrhythmias may be benign, asymptomatic, life-threatening or non life-threatening.

Asymptomatic arrhythmias are detected because of an irregular pulse or by an ECG taken for other indications.

Benign arrhythmias usually disappear after exercise and regular sinus tachycardia is seen.

Carotid sinus massage can be used to differentiate tachyarrhythmias as follows:

Sinus tachycardia—slight slowing. Rapid rate on release. Paroxysmal supraventricular tachycardia—abrupt termination or no effect.

Paroxysmal supraventricular tachycardia with AV block— slows. Rapid rate on release.

Atrial flutter—ventricular rate halved due to increase in AV block.

Ventricular tachycardia—atrial slowing. Ventricular rate unchanged.

Patient with symptoms suggestive of arrhythmia but in whom ECG is normal pose a problem.

Sometimes arrhythmias may be provoked by graded exercise test. Introduction of portable systems allowing continuous recording of a single lead ECG for periods often up to 24 hours has facilitated investigation of elusive intermittent arrhythmias. His bundle electrocardiogram permits precise localization of conduction defects.

Atrial pacing may unmask an unsuspected impairment of AV conduction.

Measurement of sinus node recovery time can confirm presence of impaired SA node function.

Once an arrhythmia has been identified its significance must be determined.

Whether they require treatment will depend upon frequency and severity of symptoms.

22

Heart in Anemia

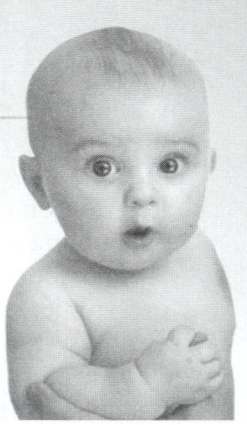

When hemoglobin level drops below 7 gm%, an increase in cardiac output occurs. Below 3.5 gm% cardiac enlargement is found with or without CHF.

Increased cardiac output is associated with reduction in total peripheral resistance. Blood volume is reduced and venous pressure is increased.

In severe anemia cardiac enlargement is the rule. Heart is increased in size and weight particularly left ventricle. Fatty degeneration and microscopic foci of myocardial necrosis have been described. Dilatation of heart and hypertrophy are both found. An increase in cardiac output gives more workload to myocardium. The blood supplying heart has diminished oxygen carrying capacity producing some degree of hypoxemia in tissues. These two factors lead to cardiac hypertrophy.

Clinical Features

Pallor, lassitude, hyporexia, dizziness, dyspnea on effort due to anemia alone or at times associated with CHF.

Part of clinical picture of heart disease in anemia may be due to underlying cause, such as hemorrhage, leukemia, hemolytic anemia or severe iron deficiency. In presence of such etiological factors careful examination of heart should be made. Heart rate is increased 10 to 30 beats per minute over usual rate for the age.

Blood pressure is lower than normal with wide pulse pressure. Hands are warm and moist. There may be capillary pulsations. Apical beat is more forceful than usual. Pulse is fuller and more readily palpable. First heart sound is normal or booming and distinctly increased, simulating mitral stenosis. Second sound is finely split. Third heart sound is frequently present. Heart murmurs are the rule but may be occasionally absent. Atypical systolic murmur transmitted to axilla or systolic murmur down left sternal edge. At times a rapid inflow type of diastolic murmur follows third heart sound just inside apex. Aortic diastolic murmur may be recognized down left sternal edge and is due to dilatation of aortic valve ring. Murmur is not closely related to heart size. Murmur appears to be due to accelerated blood flow and reduced viscosity. It usually persists after cardiac enlargement has disappeared and is more intimately related to hemoglobin level of blood. It disappears when hemoglobin level returns to normal. Heart failure may occur in severe cases. Heart failure is high output type. There will be dyspnea, edema, hepatomegaly, cardiomegaly, murmurs, third heart sound followed by inflow diastolic murmur proceeding at times to gallop rhythm.

ECG Changes

Flattening or inversion of T-wave, low amplitude of T, prolongation of PR interval, depression of ST segment, increased voltage over left precordium indicative of left ventricular hypertrophy.

Treatment

For infant and children with heart involvement in anemia transfusion is the treatment of choice but blood must be given cautiously to avoid overloading circulation and precipitating acute CHF. Packed cells may be used if many transfusions are indicated. Iron medication or specific therapy may be indicated.

23

Heart in Blood Diseases

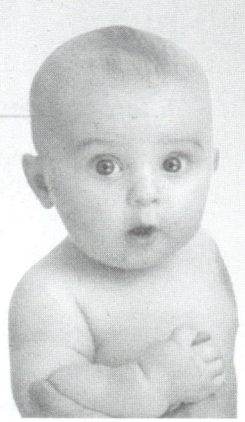

POLYCYTHEMIA

This is present in cyanosed patients with right to left shunt. Rise in hematocrit is due to an increased red cell mass with plasma volume remaining in normal range. Blood viscosity rises exponentially once hematocrit exceeds 50%. This leads to sluggish circulation, excessive deoxygenation, aggravation of peripheral cyanosis and tissue hypoxia. In extreme cases there may be headache, dizziness and general malaise. Thrombosis is a distinct danger in patients with hematocrit over 70% who become dehydrated or are subject to excessive temperature. Iron deficiency aggravates tendency to thrombosis. Selective removal of red cells with their replacement by plasma or albumin decreases viscosity, increases peripheral blood flow, improves oxygen availability to tissues and reduces bleeding at surgery.

Hemostatic Defects

Deficiency of vitamin K dependent factors (prothrombin, 7, 9, 10) and consumable factors (fibrinogen, 5, 8). Disseminated intravascular coagulation may occur. Liver hypoxia secondary to vascular stasis in CHF causes deficiency of vitamin K dependent factors. Coagulation defects are more common in cyanotic rather than acyanotic heart disease. Postoperatively defects are more severe.

Thrombocytopenia

Common in cyanotic patients. Its severity is related to degree of hypoxia and polycyathemia. Platelet survival is diminished while production is normal or increased. These changes are associated with increased platelet stickiness and aggregation to ADP.

There are two mechanisms:

1. Tissue hypoxia results in lactic acidosis which causes increased platelet adhesiveness.
2. Platelet adhesiveness increases in direct proportion to red cell volume. Increased red cell breakdown causes an increased release of ADP into circulation with resultant increased platelet aggregation and reduced survival. Thrombocytopenia is further aggravated by destruction or loss of platelets during extracorporeal circulation. This state may persist for 1 to 2 days postoperatively. When platelet count drops below 50000/cu mm a platelet transfusion should be considered. In severely thrombocytopenic patients preoperative reduction of red cell mass may help.

Fibrinolysis

Before and during surgery EACA reduces bleeding in cyanotic patients on prolonged extracorporeal circulation.

Blood Changes Secondary to Cardiac Surgery

Hemolytic anemia due to traumatic damage to red cells following surgery in which prosthetic valve or teflon patches have been inserted. Damage is due to high shear forces and abnormal hemodyanamics caused by cardiac surgery. Schistocytes and spherocytes are seen in peripheral blood. High reticulocyte count, polychromasia, elevated indirect bilirubin and reduced serum haptoglobin are evidence of hemolysis. Large quantity of iron may be lost in urine resulting in iron deficiency. Some improvement may occur with time as abnormal surfaces may get covered with endothelium. Long-term iron therapy may be required to compensate for urinary losses.

Platelet survival is reduced in patients with heart prosthetic valve. Platelet consumption is not active enough to prevent thrombopoiesis from maintaining a normal platelet count. However, it may be related to high incidence of thromboembolic complications. Administration of dipyridamol or aspirin returns platelet survival to normal and may be useful to prevent embolization.

Thalassemia

Recurrent pericarditis probably viral, without effusion. Arrhythmias, atrial and ventricular premature contractions, incomplete bundle branch block, first degree heart block, shifting pacemaker and sinus arrhythmia occur in young patients. Prolonged conduction atrial flutter and fibrillation, paroxysmal atrial tachycardia and AV dissociation are typical of advanced disease.

CHF is preceded by cardiomegaly. Initial episode occurs at 14 years of age.

24

Heart in Glycogen Storage Disease

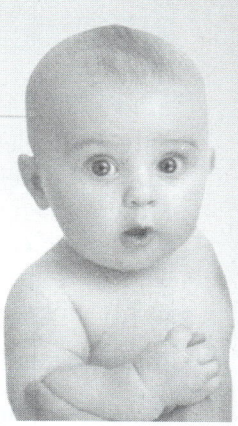

Clinically characterized by enlargement of heart, muscular weakness and macroglossia. In majority heart is severely affected and death may occur in infancy.

First described in 1932 by Pompe.

Cardiac type is a separate entity from hepatic type of glycogen storage disease.

In 1964 Hers demonstrated that tissues from normal individuals contain an acid alpha-1, 4-glucosidase. This enzyme activity is absent in type 2 glycogen storage disease. Enzyme lack occurs throughout body but cardiac involvement plays major part in early onset of symptoms.

Classification

Van Hoof 1972.

- Type 1 Glucose-6-phosphatase deficiency. Liver and kidney are involved. 26% prevalence.
- Type 2 Acid alpha-glucosidase deficiency. Generalized disease. Prevalence 15.6%.
- Type 3 Amylo-1, 6-glucosidase deficiency. Liver, muscle, RBC. Prevalence 20%.
- Type 4 Branching enzyme deficiency. Liver. 0.3%.
- Type 5 Phosphorylase deficiency. Muscle principally involved.
- Type 6 Hepatic phosphorylase deficiency. Liver. 39%.
Type 7 Phosphofructokinase deficiency. Muscle.

Pathogenesis

Deficiency of acid alpha-1, 4-glucosidase causes accumulation of glycogen in many organs throughout body, mainly heart, liver and skeletal muscle. Glycogen increase is also found in leucocyte, kidney, mucous secreting cells of GIT, muscle fibers of urinary bladder, blood vessels and pyramidal cells of cerebral cortex. There is no hypoglycemia. No ketonuria. GIT, lactose and adrenaline tolerance tests are normal.

Clinical Features

Onset is between 2 and 6 months of age. There is anorexia and failure to thrive. Rapid or labored respiration is evident due to

CHF: Infection may be precipitating event. Vomiting and intermittent cyanosis may occur.

Signs: Baby is poorly nourished and acutely ill in 50% cases. Liver is enlarged due to heart failure and increased glycogen deposition. Macroglossia is seen in 25%. Skeletal muscle weakness may be demonstrated.

Heart: Enlarged. Generalized enlargement is characteristic, involving ventricles chiefly. Cardiac murmur is usually at apex and not widely propagated. Gallop rhythm may be noted.

Radiology: Generalized cardiomegaly. Left atrial enlargement. Hilar congestion.

ECG: Heart rate is over 140/minute. Conduction time is less than 0.12 second in 85% cases. QRS interval is wide. T-wave is inverted in lead 1 in 70% cases. Precordial leads show LVH in 80% cases.

Diagnosis

Family history is helpful. Baby has cardiomegaly in first year of life with poor appetite and failure to thrive with large tongue and muscle weakness. There is absence of specific heart murmur occurring in noncyanotic baby who has LVH, normal axis and short PR interval in ECG. Muscle biopsy shows an increased glycogen content (over 1% of net muscle weight). Definitive diagnosis depends upon demonstration of deficiency of acid alpha-1, 4-glucosidase enzyme in tissues coupled with increase in glycogen, e.g. in WBC. Early diagnosis is achieved by amniocentesis. Cultured amniocytes reveal deficiency of critical enzyme.

Differential Diagnosis

Left ventricle hypertrophy in early life:

- Endocardial fibroelastosis.
- Coronary calcinosis.
- Anomalous left coronary artery from pulmonary artery.
- Aortic stenosis.
- Coarctation of aorta.
- Coarctation of aorta does not present much difficulty when blood pressure is taken.
- Anomalous left coronary artery from pulmonary artery has a suggestive ECG picture.
- Aortic stenosis has typical murmur and angiocardiogram. Coronary calcinosis has associated calcification of vessels of many organs of body seen in X-ray.
- Endocardial fibroelastosis is commonest cause of CHF with LVH in first year of life. It shows more marked picture of LVH, normal PR interval and QRS interval.
- Muscle biopsy revelation of excess glycogen is most important differentiating feature.
- Any baby who presents with floppiness suggestive of amyotonia congenital or Werdnig-Hoffmann syndrome must be considered as possibly suffering from glycogen storage disease of heart.

Prognosis

Condition is uniformly fatal. Death occurs in first year of life. Increasing deposits of glycogen in heart muscle interferes with its function causing progressive weakness and enlargement of heart leading to CHF. Failure is precipitated when baby contracts an infection.

Weakness of musculature throughout body may lead to difficulty in swallowing and respiration.

TREATMENT

Trial of digitalis first until diagnosis is established. Second to see if life can be prolonged by that means. Specific enzyme replacement is treatment of choice.

25

Heart in Mucopolysaccharidosis

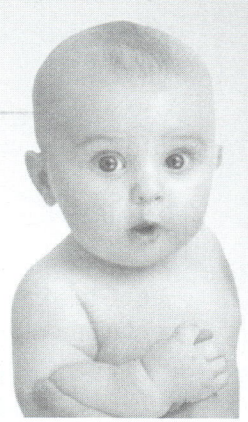

MPS are a group of inherited metabolic disorders in which there is impaired degradation of various glycosaminoglycans due to defective or absent activity of specific lysosomal enzymes. Disorders are characterized by deposition of MPS in various organs of body and by mucopolysacchariduria.

First examples of MPS were noted by John Thompson between 1900 and 1913.

First case report appeared in literature in 1917 (Hunter) and 1919 (Hurler).

Ellis in 1936 introduced term gargoylism to describe ugly faces and dwarfism characteristic of some types of MPS.

In 1952 Brante isolated dermatan sulfate from liver of two patients of Hurler syndrome.

Clinical Features

MPS are characterized by abnormal storage and excretion in urine of excess quantities of mucopolysaccharides. Various syndromes are differentiated on basis of clinical signs, substance in urine and by measurement of activity of specific mucopolysaccharide catabolizing enzymes.

All MPS except Hunter syndrome are transmitted as autosomal recessive. Hunter syndrome is X-linked disorder. There are no signs of disease in heterozygotes.

Classification

By Mc Kusick in 1972 on basis of specific enzymology and use of corrective factors.

1. *MPS Type 1 H (Hurler syndrome)*: Some children are recognized in first few months while others may be 8 to 12 months old before diagnosis is made. Infants have chronic nasal discharge, frequent upper respiratory infections and occasional episodes of pneumonia. Classic gargoyle facies develop slowly during first year and continue to progress throughout life. Hepatosplenomegaly, inguinal and umbilical hernias, deafness, clouding of cornea, lumber gibbus, claw hands and deformity of chest are seen. Growth slows in second year and ceases in 4th year. Mental deterioration is severe to moderate. Mitral regurgitation and aortic regurgitation are most common cardiac involvement. Death due to cardiopulmonary complications at 7 to 10 years occurs.

2. *MPS Type 1 S (Scheie syndrome)*: Intelligence is normal. Other features of type 1 H are present but to a minor degree. Clouding of cornea and aortic valve disease is common.

3. *MPS Type 1 HS Compound*: Features of both type 1 H and S are present. These children have severe boney changes, short stature, gargoyle facies, hernias and hepatosplenomegaly but mild mental retardation. These are probably offsprings of a Hurler carrier and a Scheie carrier.

4. *MPS Type 2 (Hunter syndrome)*: Clouding of cornea is not seen clinically and development of lumber gibbus is rare. Signs resemble type 1 H closely although they are less marked. Deafness is prominent. Mitral regurgitation and aortic regurgitation are present.

5. *MPS Type 3 (sanfilippo syndrome)*: These children present with mild to moderate mental retardation at 2 to 4 years age. Growth slows at 7 to 8 years. They have severe aggressive behavior problems. Heart disease is described.

6. *MPS Type 4 (Morquio syndrome)*: Spondyloepiphyseal dysplasia is hallmark of this condition with clouding of cornea and deformities of teeth. Intelligence is normal but

odontoid hypoplasia and other spinal deformities may cause spastic paraplegia or other neurological symptoms. Death may occur due to acute atlantoaxial subluxation. Aortic regurgitation appears during adolescence.

7. *MPS Type 6 (Maroteaux-Lamy syndrome)*: Dwarfism is primary feature of this disease. Intelligence is normal. Other features of type 1 H are present. Skeletal changes are so marked as to cause death from cardiorespiratory complications at an early age. Specific descriptions of cardiac abnormalities have been made.

8. *MPS Type 7 (Sly syndrome)*: Beta glucuronidase deficiency.

MUCOLIPIDOSIS

Several conditions have clinical features that resemble those of MPS. Affected children do not excrete increased quantities of mucopolysaccharides in their urine but have similar radiological findings and usually have cardiac involvement. Commonest cardiac defects are mitral regurgitation and aortic regurgitation.

Mucolipidosis include:

1. *Type 1 (GM 1 Gangliosidosis)*: Multisystem disorder due to defect in beta galactosidase activity. These children fail to thrive, have hepatosplenomegaly, cloudy cornea, cherry red spots and abnormal facies. Chest X-ray shows infiltration of lungs. Histologically lung alveoli are filled with foamy histiocytes which are also found in bone marrow. Mitral insufficiency is often severe causing CHF in first 6 months of life.

2. *Type 2 (I cell disease)*: Syndrome with growth failure, boney changes, mental retardation and gargoyle features but with little hepatosplenomegaly and usually clear corneas. Cardiac involvement develops at end of first or second year of life.

3. *Type 3 (Pseudo Hurler dystrophy)*: Milder form. Presents with restriction of joint movements in second year of life. Children are short, have scoliosis, hip dysplasia and mild mental retardation. Fine corneal opacities are found on slit lamp examination. Cardiac involvement is rare.

CARDIOVASCULAR FEATURES

Over half of cases of MPS show evidence of heart disease. Aortic regurgitation is most frequent clinically, although at autopsy mitral valve is most frequently involved. Grade 1 to 2 typically decrescendo systolic murmur which starts after first heart sound lasts for about half systole is heard. This is due to mitral regurgitation or tricuspid regurgitation. Occasionally suggestive of mild pulmonary artery stenosis. Murmurs increase in amplitude with passage of time as the disease process causes ever increasing damage to heart valves. First heart sound may be diminished. Second heart sound in pulmonary area is greatly accentuated. Third heart sound is frequently heard at apex.

Cardiomegaly or CHF may be presenting feature of cardiac involvement. In others sudden death.

29% cases have systemic hypertension.

Cardiovascular disease is associated with every form of MPS except type 7. Its clinical expression has been evident as aortic valvular disease (almost all aortic regurgitation) and terminal CHF. Hypoxia from respiratory obstruction together with compromise of left ventricle function from combination of accumulation of mucopolysaccharides in myocardium, presence of systemic hypertension, valvular regurgitation and coronary artery disease accounts for cardiorespiratory demise.

Presence of heart murmur in MPS leads to diagnosis of congenital heart disease particularly VSD, PS, AS, MR, corpulmonale and anemic heart disease.

Echocardiography will be useful in diagnosis by identifying abnormal left ventricle dimensions and by showing mitral and aortic valve abnormalities.

ECG

Prolongation of QT interval, RVH, LAE, combined ventricle hypertrophy and first degree heart block.

Cardiac Catheterization

Mild pulmonary hypertension, MR, AR, PR are seen. Indices of left ventricle function obtained by LVEDP and response to angiotensin infusion are abnormal.

Pathology

Dawson in 1954 demonstrated abnormal storage of mucopoly-saccharides in parenchymal cells and fibroelastic tissues throughout body. Patients excrete mucopolysaccharides in urine: chondroitin sulfate B (dermatan sulfate) Heparan sulfate and keratan sulfate.

Dermatan sulfate is stored in spleen, bone, brain and kidneys. Heparan sulfate is stored in liver.

Symptoms are produced by effect on organ structure and function and by interference with growth.

Stored mucopolysaccharide produces a diffuse disease that varies in both its clinical and pathological picture depending upon speed, degree and site of accumulation of abnormal substance as well as on nature of affected material itself. Most commonly eyes, heart, bones, brain, liver, spleen and skin are affected. In 80% cases hypertrophy of heart is reported. Left ventricle is more affected than right ventricle. Endocardium in either ventricle may be thickened. Heart valves are affected in over 60% of cases. Regurgitation is commonest clinical sequelae but if process is extreme then stenosis may occur. Mitral valve is most commonly involved on autopsy. Chordae tendineae may be thickened and shortened. Characteristic microscopic picture is swollen and vacuolated appearance of cells in connective tissue of all layers of heart particularly of valves and intima of main vessels and coronary arteries. Electron microscopy has revealed two types of abnormal cells. One a glycolipid cell and the other containing an acid mucopoly-saccharide.

Over 30% of autopsies in children show marked narrowing of coronary arteries. Pancreatic, renal, cerebral and splenic arteries show minimal intimal involvement. Narrowing of these arteries is due to plaque formation and it is probable that these contain mucopolysaccharides and thus are different from true atheromatous plaques. Gross changes in myocardial fibers are less common although chronic myocarditis is described.

BIOCHEMISTRY

Mucopolysaccharides are macromolecules composed of disaccharide units of hexosamine and either hexuronic acid or hexose. They are O sulfated in either sugar and may be N sulfated (heparan sulfate). They are covalently bound to peptide or small protein.

- Children with MPS excrete 3 to 20 times the normal quantity of MPS in their urine.
- Type 1 H. Hurler syndrome. Urinary MPS Dermatan sulfate and heparan sulfate. Enzyme defect: alpha iduronidase.
- Type 1 S. Scheie syndrome. Dermatan sulfate and heparan sulfate. Alpha iduronidase.
- Type 2. Hunter syndrome. Dermatan sulfate. Sulfoiduronate Sulfatase.
- Type 3 A. Sanfilippo syndrome. Heparan sulfate. Heparan sulfate Sulfatase.
- Type 3 B. Sanfilippo syndrome. Heparan sulfate. N-acetyl alpha-D-glucosaminidase.
- Type 4 Morquio syndrome. Keratan sulfate. N-acetyl hexosamine sulfate sulfatase.
- Type 6 Maroteaux-Lamy syndrome. Dermatan sulfate. Aryl sulfatase B.
- Type 7 Atypical. Beta-glucuronidase.

MPS are lysosomal defects due to inactive lysosomal hydroxylase. Increased incorporation is due to block in degradation of mucopolysaccharides that these cells formed at normal rates. Mucopolysaccharide storage results from defect in factor that is present in genotypically different cells. For complete degradation of macromolecules each of specific glycosidases and sulfatases must be active. Defect in activity of any one results in failure of catabolism and thus storage.

Radiology

There is abnormality of bone texture with loss of trabeculations and thinning of cortex. Long bones, ribs and metacarpals become wider and misshapen. Lumber vertebrae are notched. Skull has prominent frontal bones and shallow sella turcica. There is decrease in mastoid and ethmoid air spaces. Cardiac enlargement is generalized. Pulmonary artery segment prominent.

Diagnosis

MPS may be diagnosed by specific clinical appearance, genetic history, X-ray of spine, ribs, long bones and hands and combination of laboratory tests.

Mucopolysaccharide excretion in urine of 24 hours is quantitated as mg of hexuronic acid excreted per 24 hours. Normal excretion is less than 20 mg per 24 hours. Patients with type 1, 2 and 6 excrete 5 to 10 times the normal. Patients with type 3 excrete 2 to 4 times the normal. Patients with type 4 excrete keratan sulfate which contains no hexuronic acid. For quantitation of different species mucopolysaccharides are isolated on different DEAE cellulose columns and separated by cellulose acetate electrophoresis. Electrophoretogram can be quantitated by densitometery. Using Sulfate 35 incorporation mucopolysaccharide storage can be demonstrated by cultured fibroblasts.

Enzymological diagnosis is not generally available for all MPS because of the substrates that must be synthesized in laboratory. Sulfatase defect can only be demonstrated with S 35 labelled substrate which have limited shelf life because of radioactive decay.

N-acetyl-alpha-D-glucosaminide as 4-methyl-umbiliferryl derivative is commercially available for diagnosis of Sanfilippo B syndrome. Sulfate 35 heparan sulfate for diagnosis of Sanfilippo A syndrome.

In families with previously affected infant antenatal diagnosis of MPS can be considered.

Treatment

Supportive therapy for orthropedic problems, respiratory infections and CHF may postpone the end and is indicated especially in those with normal mental development.

Valve replacement for severe mitral regurgitation may be performed. Corneal grafting particularly lamellar grafting is tried successfully.

Major problem is inactivity of specific enzymes.

Hurler in 1919 and Ernould 1949 tried thyroid and pituitary extract without effect.

Vitamin A, prednisolone and diet low in vitamin C stimulate synthesis and release of lysosomal hydrolases.

Infusion of normal plasma and leucocytes produces clinical improvement in MPS 1 H and MPS Type 2.

Specific enzyme replacement therapy is now available at select centers.

26

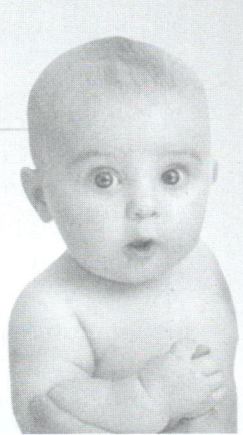

Heart in Marfan Syndrome

In 1896 Marfan described five and a half year old girl who had long limbs, hyperextensible joints, atrophied musculature and an abnormally long head (dolichocephaly). Her feet and hands were particularly slender (spider legs).

Marfan labelled the condition "Dolicho steno melie". Achard in 1902 reporting on 18-year-old girl with this disorder used term "Arachnodactyly".

Association of heart disease with Marfan syndrome was first reported by Salle in 1912 in two and a half month old infant with obvious features of this syndrome at birth and evidence of aortic and tricuspid valve disease at autopsy.

ETIOLOGY

Marfan syndrome is heritable disorder of connective tissue, transmitted as autosomal dominant. About 50% of offsprings are affected.

De novo mutations occur in not more than 15% of cases. There is relationship between this presentation and advanced paternal age.

There may be abnormal serum seromucoid levels (Bacchus). Increased urinary excretion of hydroxyproline has been demonstrated in patients under 20 years age. This may be reflection of their increased growth.

Primary defect may be in elastic tissue. Deposition of metachromatic material may precede elastic tissue changes.

Fundamental lesion may be overaccumulation of chondroitin sulfate C.

Collagen produced by fibroblasts from patients with Marfan syndrome is abnormally soluble.

Pathology

CVS abnormalities are found in over 90% cases of Marfan syndrome at autopsy. Main lesions are aortic and pulmonary arterial aneurysms, aortic and pulmonary valvular incompetence. Mitral regurgitation and true congenital malformations of heart.

Aorta: Fusiform aneurysm of ascending aorta is most common. Dilatation extends from aortic valve to innominate artery, portion of aorta that normally undergoes maximum hemodynamic stress. This change creates typical 'waterflask' appearance of aorta on aortogram.

Aneurysm of sinus of Valsalva. Process starts at aortic ring and may cause so much sacculation of aortic cusps and dilatation of ring that aortic regurgitation may be present without true aneurysmal formation of ascending aorta. This finding is common in children.

Dissection of aorta with or without previous dilatation may occur. This may cause death due to cardiac temponade by hemopericardium.

Dissection of innominate and carotid arteries.

Fusiform aneurysm of descending aorta.

Microscopically there is total destruction of aortic architecture. Elastic fibers are interrupted and scarce. Smooth muscle tissue is hyperplastic and irregular. Vasa vasorum invade media. Cystic spaces are filled with metachromatically staining material.

Pulmonary artery: Aneurysmal dilatation and dissection of aneurysms may occur.

Valves: Significant mitral regurgitation is the commonest CVS problem in Marfan syndrome. CHF due to MR is reported as early as 4-month of age. Mitral valve in Marfan syndrome is described as redundant, folded and thickened with almost cartilaginous translucency. Chordae are thickened and elongated. Valve bulges into left atrium. Rupture of chordae and avulsion of posterior leaflet is reported. Microscopically there is myxomatous degeneration in valves.

Apart from hemodynamic upset these lesions may cause, they may predispose to infective endocarditis.

CLINICAL FEATURES

Congenital heart malformations are common:
- Patent foramen ovale.
- ASD primum and secundum.
- Ventricular septal defect
- Tetralogy of Fallot
- Patent ductus arteriosus
- Coarctation of aorta
- Pulmonary artery stenosis
- Partial anomalous pulmonary venous drainage

Severely affected cases of Marfan syndrome will be recognized at birth. Many are thin during first year. Where relatives have been tall and thin the physical picture in an affected infant is usually accepted by parents. Sporadic cases are more likely to seek medical treatment for failure to thrive. As the child grows, excessive height, wasted appearance, deformed chest or scoliosis may make family consult a doctor. Visual difficulty may be emphasized on entry to school. Symptoms of early fatigue, limb pains and failure to gain weight appear. Heart murmur and minor ECG changes may confuse the picture with rheumatic fever. In adolescent girls psychologic difficulties become prominent. In childhood some cases present with dyspnea due to CHF. Physical appearance of a severe case is characteristic: wasted look is due to combination of excessive length of bones of extremities, poor musculature and lack of subcutaneous fat. Inadequate musculature results in scoliosis and kyphosis. Excessive overgrowth of length of ribs results in chest deformities or pectus excavatum. Nose, ear and teeth are misshapen. Skull is dolichocephalic. Palate is narrow and high arched. Ocular abnormalities occur in 75% cases. They include dislocation of lenses, tremulous irides, deformed anterior chamber or cornea and myopia. Respiratory symptoms may be related to infection in abnormal lungs or to spontaneous pneumothorax.

Symptoms due to CVS lesions may appear in childhood, related to MR and AR. Chest pain due to aortic dissection is rarely seen. MR is commonest finding. Classic pansystolic apical murmur may be heard but often the murmur is mid to late systolic. Mid systolic clicks or multiple non ejection clicks near the apex are commonly a clue to presence of prolapsed mitral valve leaflet. Mitral murmur varies with position of patient and is maximal with patient upright so that from being late systolic in recumbent position it may become pansystolic when patient sits upright. AR or PR is suspected when an early diastolic decrescendo murmur is heard along LSE. Ejection click may also be audible in patients who have dilatation of great vessels. Severe AR is more common in males. Musical, vibratory or buzzing systolic murmur in aortic area indicates dissection of aorta. Murmur is believed to be generated on fibrous cords in lumen of aorta or on lips of an endothelial tear.

Radiology

Heart may be normal appearance. Two characteristic radiologic pointers to vessel involvement in childhood are dilatation of ascending aorta and peculier bulge in usual position of RVOT due to sacculated descent of pulmonary valve cusps. The later is often mistaken or left atrial enlargement. In severe cases there may be moderate to gross cardiac enlargement.

ECG

Cases with MR and AR develop LVH. Changes of subendocardial ischemia may be present. Conduction abnormalities and arrhythmias have been described. They include RBBB, LBBB, junctional rhythm, atrial flutter and fibrillation, WPW syndrome and complete heart block. Incomplete RBBB, PR and QT prolongation may be due to changes in small coronary arteries and general as well as specific cystic degeneration of nodal arteries.

ECHOCARDIOGRAPHY

91% cases have evidence of MVP. 60% show increased aortic root dimensions. Females have more frequent mitral valve abnormalities and males aortic root abnormalities.

Cardiac Catheterization

Right and left heart catheterization will confirm hemodynamically significant valvular lesion and congenital malformations.

Angiocardiography

Aneurysmal dilatation of aortic sinuses is demonstrated, is a very early sign and may be seen in infants without frank CVS disease. Dilatation of root of MPA is demonstrated by selective angiocardiography from right ventricle. MR with or without aortic root alterations can be demonstrated following LV contrast injection.

DIAGNOSIS

Classic case of a tall thin child with long fingers and toes, chest deformity and poor eyesight is unlikely to be missed. Diagnosis is certain if dislocation of lens and positive family history is present. In patients with negative family history late paternal age can provide supportive evidence for mutation.

Most important differential diagnosis is from homocystinuria. This metabolic disorder results from one of several possible enzyme deficiencies inherited as autosomal recessive traits. Physical appearance of homocystinuria closely resembles that of Marfan syndrome. Affected individuals are tall and thin. Scoliosis and pectus deformities are common. Joint action is tight as compared to Marfan. Osteoporosis and bone fractures are common. Lens dislocation is common after age of 10 years, occurs downwards and usually of more marked degree than Marfan syndrome. Mental retardation is present in 50% cases. Psychiatric disturbances and seizures are common. Light complexion and premature grey hair is usual. There is malar flushing on exercise or exertion and an increased incidence of thrombosis in medium size arteries and veins after adolescence. Death may occur from coronary thrombosis in young. Infarction of brain, heart, kidney, lungs eventually occurs. Such patients are at increased risk of contraceptive pills. Valvular lesions and vascular rupture do not occur in homocystinuria. A positive cyanide—nitroprusside test on urine is suggestive of homocystinuria and urine chromatography establishes the diagnosis. Patients of homocystinuria are treatable by dietary restriction and specific vitamin therapy. Incomplete forms of Marfan syndrome are called 'Formes frustes'. Families with unequivocal examples of the disorder may contain some members with only one manifestation. A tall slender physique, dislocated lens or heart involvement may be the solitary evidence of Marfan syndrome. Formes frustes pose a problem when family history is negative. Similar physique may occur in some black population and eunuchoidism. Severe wasting from a variety of disorders may superficially resemble Marfan syndrome. Cardiovascular formes frustes involve mitral valve only or aortic valve only. Some familial cases of MVP may be CFF. Similarly idiopathic pulmonary artery dilatation, aortic aneurysm and aortic or mitral insufficiency as isolated findings warrant a closer inspection for other features of Marfan syndrome. However, diagnosis of Marfan syndrome can usually not be made with complete confidence when ectopia lentis or a positive family history are not found.

Prognosis

Life expectancy is greatly reduced in Marfan syndrome. Mean age at death is 32 years. Cause of death almost always is cardiovascular. Aortic lesion taking the highest toll (rupture of aortic aneurysm and aortic dissection). Mitral regurgitation may cause death from CHF or during cardiac surgery. Infective endocarditis is also a cause of death.

Treatment

There is no treatment for underlying disorder. Assistance for ocular defects is necessary. Correction of associated malformations, such as cleft palate, scoliosis, chest deformity is indicated. Attempts to curb excessive growth by inducing precocious puberty have been made. A trial of medical treatment with propranolol 120 to 160 mg per day may be conducted to prevent aortic dissection. Since aortic dissection and rupture are result of medial degeneration plus hemodynamic stress reducing this stress may delay rupture. Propranolol reduces myocardial contractility and decreases pulsatile force in aorta.

Cardiac surgical procedures include excision of aortic aneurysm with bicuspidation of aortic valve (excision of noncoronary aortic leaflet to decrease valve surface), graft replacement of ascending aorta and prosthesis and replacement of mitral valve.

27

Diseases of Coronary Arteries

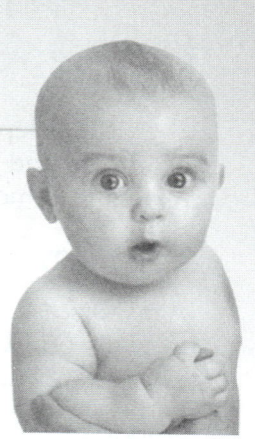

Various forms of involvement of coronary arteries in infants and children include:

- Specific infection.
- Hyperplastic changes.
- Sclerosis.
- Calcification.
- Arteritis.
- Thrombosis.
- Aneurysms.
- Fistuli.
- Congenital defects of coronary arterial system.
- Various syndromes.
- Hypertension.
- Atherosclerosis.

The rubella syndrome may involve coronary arteries with intimal proliferation and at times changes in internal elastic lamina and media. Such changes occur in rubella at the time of birth or in few weeks following it.

Calcification may occur in infants who have widespread necrosis of an artery. Newborns may have necrosis of media in septic states such may be site of development of subsequent calcific deposits.

Histological changes are seen in coronary arteries in various infections in childhood.

Calcium deposits in internal elastic lamina of iliac arteries of infants and young children is described. This finding is related to hemodynamic load on iliacs early in life.

CORONARY CALCINOSIS

A rare disease in infancy characterized by deposition of calcium in walls of a variety of vessels throughout body. Coronary arteries are affected as part of this pathological picture.

Pathology

Coronary vessels are raised, tortuous, calcareous, showing prominently on surface of heart. Myocardium is hypertrophied. Left ventricle more than right ventricle. Myocardial infarction may occur.

Earliest change is seen in internal elastic lamina of various sized arteries throughout body. Calcium deposition may assume appearance of ring or segment of a circle. Intimal proliferation and thickening may occur.

Since lesions are widespread many organs are affected.

Clinical Features

These babies are affected in first 2 to 8 months of life. The infant appears well in neonatal period. Later presents a sudden onset of signs and symptoms which last from 1 to 5 days.

Dyspnea is noted first coupled with an ashen grey color of face suggesting shock. Respiratory rate increases. Signs of CHF appear. Gallop rhythm is heard. Normal axis and LVH with strain pattern are seen in precordial leads.

Diagnosis is based on sudden onset dyspnea, CHF, shock and LVH in ECG.

Differential diagnosis includes aortic stenosis and coarctation of aorta. Differentiation is by angiocardiogram, catheterization and phonocardiography.

Biochemical or adrenal insufficiency may lead to a similar cardiovascular collapse.

In Endocardial fibroelastosis ECG will show more LVH than in coronary calcinosis.

Anomalous left coronary artery from pulmonary artery has a characteristic ECG pattern.

Glycogen storage disease may be associated with family history. Radiological evidence of calcification in vessels over surface of heart is diagnostic.

Treatment

These babies should receive oxygen and digitalis since it may not be initially possible to exclude endocardial fibroelastosis or coarctation of aorta, conditions that will respond to therapy.

ANOMALOUS LEFT CORONARY ARTERY FROM PULMONARY ARTERY

Originally described by Abrikosoff in 1911.

Bland in 1932 recorded an ECG in an infant with this condition.

Incidence

0.24% of all CHD. Once in 300,000 children.

Most babies die in first year of life. Survival into adulthood is possible due to large right coronary artery which supplies collaterals to left ventricle.

Pathology: Left coronary artery arises from base of pulmonary artery somewhat posteriorly. Left ventricle is enlarged to aneurysmal proportions with dilated chamber. Right ventricle wall is small and compressed.

Patchy fibrosis is apparent in left ventricle at apex and anterior myocardium.

There is an increase in elastic tissue and disintegration of muscle fibers. In advanced cases calcareous infiltration may be apparent in anterior portion of left ventricle.

Many infants have evidence of endocardial fibroelastosis. More common in females.

Focal atelectasis may be seen in lung tissue adjacent to enlarged heart. Alveoli may show chronic passive congestion of CHF.

Hemodynamics

Before birth oxygen content of blood in right ventricle and left ventricle are same. Pressure is similar. Thus anomalous LCA from pulmonary artery has no deleterious effect on heart.

Cardiovascular adjustments after birth include fall in pressure in right ventricle and pulmonary artery as compared to that in left side of heart. Coronary artery arising from pulmonary artery will thus be receiving blood under low pressure or the flow may be reversed. Collaterals from right coronary artery supplying left ventricle. Left coronary artery merely acting as a vein. Some of coronary blood supply to left ventricle must come during diastole. Since in infants diastole may be shortened than systole a further inadequacy of blood flow to left ventricle results. Pathological changes occur over a period of week to months and lead to a failure of left ventricle. Tachycardia and circulatory inadequacy of CHF further increase the ischemia of left ventricle.

Clinical Features

Infants with this anomaly appear normal at birth. Symptoms appear in second or third month of life. These are of discomfort, CHF and respiratory infections.

Irritability and discomfort occur intermittently during day. A look of anxiety or pain may be suggested on baby's face. Episodes of pain and distress may occur after feeding and are anginal in origin. Also due to angina paroxysms of distress with pallor, sweating and dyspnea have been reported. Symptoms due to CHF are dyspnea, tachycardia, wheeze, cough and secondary cyanosis.

Physical Examination

Baby is usually well developed but may at times appear underweight.

Tachypnea is the rule and baby appears uncomfortable and irritable.

Minor degree of pallor is common. Intermittent cyanosis may be noted with crying. Crying is likely to occur in paroxysms and may be associated with pallor, profuse sweating and shock. Respiratory rate is between 50 and 100/minute. There is evidence of respiratory distress. Fine rales may be heard in lungs. Liver is enlarged. Definite edema is uncommon. Evidence of respiratory infection is present with fever, cough, nasal discharge and rales in lungs. Heart murmurs are usually not heard.

Radiology

Heart size and shape vary. There is marked enlargement with blunt apex protruding down and out into left axilla. Left cardiac border is full and convex. Right atrial shadow appears small in comparison to left cardiac enlargement. Lungs fields are congested. In LAO view LV protrudes back overlapping the vertebral column markedly.

Under fluroscope cardiac borders appear quiet. LV is greatly enlarged. Hilar shadows are congested but not pulsating. Barium swallow shows a normal left aortic arch. LA may be enlarged. RV is not enlarged but its border appears more active than LV in LAO view.

Angiocardiography

Demonstrates small RV giving rise to normal pulmonary artery and branches, greatly enlarged LV with round symmetrical shape.

Usually the flow is from left coronary into pulmonary artery. So LCA is not demonstrable.

Aortogram shows absence of LCA at base of aorta and reveals RCA clearly. Collaterals then fill the LCA branches and make visible the LCA and its attachment to pulmonary artery.

ECG

The pattern is of anterior myocardial infarction. There is a QR pattern and inverted T-waves in lead 1 and avL accompanied by deep Q in V5 and V6 with inverted T in V5V6. ST segment is raised over left precordium followed by T-wave that is cove shaped and symmetric in outline.

Diagnosis

In infancy it is based on following criteria:
- Features appear in first year of life.
- Irritability and pain on feeding.
- CHF in second to fifth month of life.
- Pneumonia is common.
- Little or no cyanosis.
- Gross cardiomegaly on X-ray.
- ECG evidence of anterior myocardial infarction.

Thalium 201 myocardial perfusion scan gives direct confirmation of infarction by showing wedge shaped defect in image of LV wall.

Selective angiogram with tip of catheter at base of aorta will demonstrate the RCA only and no evidence of LCA arising in its usual place.

Differential diagnosis: Of LVH, e.g. EF, tricuspid atresia, AS, PDA, coarctation of aorta, VSD, myocarditis, coronary calcinosis. A marked Q-waves followed by an inverted T-wave is present in avL in anomalous LCA. This pattern is rarely found in EF.

Prognosis: In infants with symptoms and signs it is uniformly poor. A few cases reach adult life. The infant who dies early has no communication between RCA and LCA branches.

Treatment

Group 1: Those who have survived infancy because of sufficient collateral circulation from RCA to LCA. Such cases can be helped by saphenous vein bypass graft between aorta and anomalous coronary. This aorticocoronary bypass graft technique is limited to children over 2 to 3 years age.

Group 2: Those cases that present in infancy. 85%. Oxygen, digitalis, diuretics are initiated early while surgery is being considered.

Several surgical techniques are in use:
1. Ligation of anomalous coronary at its origin. Sudden death may occur on clamping.

2. Use of a systemic artery to anastomose to anomalous coronary.

3. Aorticopulmonary window can be tunneled to LCA. An orifice of 5 mm diameter is made in adjacent walls of aorta and pulmonary artery at the same level as anomalous coronary orifice. The vessels are then anastomosed in side to side fashion.

MYOCARDIAL INFARCTION IN CHILDHOOD

Causes

4% of autopsies in pediatric age group have some evidence of myocardial infarction.

1. Congenital anomalies of coronary circulation: Anomalous origin of left coronary artery from pulmonary artery.

2. Occlusion of a main coronary vessel may take place during difficult delivery or at newborn period. Newborn will present with signs of low systemic perfusion, e.g. low volume pulse, acidosis, pulmonary venous congestion. ECG shows anterolateral myocardial infarction pattern. LDH level over 1500 units. Significant rise in SGOT and CPK are reported.

3. Atherosclerosis in childhood may occur due to progeria, diabetes and homozygous type 2 hyperlipoproteinemia.

4. Miscellaneous causes:
   - Embolism.
   - Inflammatory diseases.
   - SLE.
   - Syphilis.
   - PAN.
   - Interstitial myocarditis.
   - Degenerative diseases.
   - Hypertension.
   - Thrombocytosis.
   - Trauma.
   - Aneurysms.
   - Fibroelastosis.

- Tumors.
- Congenital aortic stenosis.

Atherosclerosis

Histological investigations of arteries from infants and children dying accidentally suggest that a significant number are developing early atherosclerosis.

Lobstein in 1829 introduced term arteriosclerosis. Moon in 1957 associated degeneration, regeneration and deposition of mucopolysaccharides and of intimal fibrosis as characteristic of early nonlipid phase of atherosclerosis. Fatty streaks appear in endothelium of aorta in first year of life universally. They may develop into atheroma, remain unchanged or regress. When such streaks are associated with disintegrating cells of lipid debris they appear more likely to develop into atherosclerotic plaques.

All children have some evidence of aortic fatty streaking by 5 years of age but such streaking appears late in coronary arteries and does not occur until age 20 years. Advanced atherosclerotic lesions develop by progression and transformation appear to vary from one artery to another and among racial groups. To prevent fatty streaking or progression of fatty streaks to more advanced lesions a program to control dietary habits, blood lipid levels, hypertension should be directed towards first two decades of life.

At birth aorta is clear of fatty streaks. During first two years all infants deposit lipid in some portions of aorta until by age 5 it is present in all aorta. There is characteristic localization of lipid deposit in aortic valve rings, in region of ductus scar and just below orifices of intercostal arteries.

In young persons the process of atherosclerosis of coronary arteries may proceed independently and is not necessarily part of generalized atherosclerosis.

Coronary atherosclerosis is common in those having hypertension.

Factors of stress and turbulence are related to pathology of bicuspid aortic valve. Evident lipid streaking in such cases is due to altered hemodynamics. This leads to atherosclerotic changes. Congenital bicuspid aortic valve occurs in 1% of normal population, 7% of children with CHD particularly coarctation of aorta, VSD and EF (19% of VSD).

Type 2 hyperlipoproteinemia is characterized by distal disease of coronary circulation (92%) and involvement of left coronary artery (42%).

Type 4 hyperlipoproteinemia is characterized by localized lesions in proximal part of coronary arteries (65%) with infrequent occurrence of coronary artery stenosis (15%).

Kaplan in 1976 mentioned that there is a latent ischemic heart disease in many children with familial hypercholesterolemia as proved by exercise ECG changes of ST depression of 1 mm or more in V5.

Newborn: Musculoelastic intimal thickenings are found forming pads at branch sites. Lipid is present extracellularly or intracellularly in smooth muscle cells.

Age 2 to 9 years: Intimal thickening continued to increase. Age 15 to 19 years: There is presence of focal deposits of debris from disintegrating lipid cells. Foci of lipid necrosis occur where there is thickening of intima near bifurcation of vessels.

Progeria

A condition that is characteristically associated with generalized atherosclerosis and coronary thrombosis in childhood. Out of total 32 cases reported the youngest patient is 7-year-old. Lipid levels are moderately raised and are not comparable to those seen in most cases of type 2 hyperlipoproteinemia.

- Risk factors for atherosclerosis:
- Family history of atherosclerotic pathology.
- Hyperlipidemia.
- Hypertension.
- Diabetes mellitus.
- Obesity.
- Diet rich in saturated fat, cholesterol, sucrose.

- Cigarette smoking.
- Habitual physical inactivity.
- Males are more susceptible than females.

Genetic traits of arterial wall of structure, function, metabolism, permeability and nutrition or deterioration of vessel wall with age.

Effect of testosterone, hypothyroidism, obstructive liver disease.

- Specific drugs.
- Psychic stress.
- Occupation.
- Culture.
- Trauma.

HYPERLIPIDEMIA

This as a cause of atherosclerosis may be acting in early infancy. Primary hyperprebetalipoproteinemia is a frequent finding in young adults with occlusive vascular disease. Familial hyperlipoproteinemias especially type 2 which are associated with premature coronary artery disease might be helped with a suitable diet.

Familial hyperlipoproteinemia has been divided by Frederickson and Lees in 1965 into 5 groups on basis of ultracentrifuge and electrophoretic findings:

Type 1: Hyperchylomicronemia, Hypertriglyceridemia is characterized by eruptive skin xanthoma, abdominal pain, lipemia retinalis, marked increase in serum triglycerides and typical electrophoretic pattern. It is brought about by delayed clearance of exogenous lipid use to a lipoprotein lipase deficiency and may be treated by low fat diet. It is rare autosomal recessive condition. It does not appear to be associated with premature atherosclerosis.

Type 2: Hyperbetalipoproteinemia due to excessive production or inadequate clearance of low density lipoproteins. It may have its onset in childhood with arcus cornea, tendon and tuberous xanthomata, accelerated atherosclerosis and an increase in serum cholesterol. Serum triglycerides are normal or slightly increased. Plasma is clear. Electrophoretic pattern is characteristic. Such cases can be treated with low cholesterol diet, use of polyunsaturated fatty acids and drug therapy. This group is inherited as autosomal dominant with incomplete penetrance. Heterozygotes show only arcus senilis.

Type 3: Onset is in adult life with atherosclerosis of coronary and peripheral vessels and tuberous eruptive lesions. Cholesterol and triglycerides are increased. There is abnormal glucose tolerance and characteristic broad beta electrophoretic pattern. It is treated with drugs, low carbohydrate diet and weight control. Inherited as autosomal recessive.

Type 4: Onset in adult life with obesity, abdominal pain and CVS disease. Cholesterol is normal or slightly increased and triglycerides are markedly increased. Glucose tolerance is abnormal. Characteristic prebeta band in electrophoretic pattern. There may be eruptive tuberosities in skin. It can be treated with weight control, carbohydrates restriction and drug therapy.

Type 5: Onset in early adult life with obesity, abdominal pain, hepatosplenomegaly and lipemia retinalis. Cholesterol is normal or increased. Triglycerides are increased. Glucose tolerance is abnormal. There is combined chylomicron and prebeta electrophoretic pattern. Treatment with weight control, low fat and carbohydrates and addition of drugs or hormones. In children most cases are type 2 with cholesterol over 94th percentile level. Borderline cases may be due to dietary excess. Severe forms are related to genetic abnormalities and are referred to as familial type 2. Inheritance is via single mutant allelic gene causing elevation of cholesterol and increase of LDL.

Serum cholesterol level in infants and children:

At birth: 55–120 mg/100 ml.

At 2 weeks: 96–99 mg %.

At 4–6 weeks 120–190 mg%.

Concentration of LDL in cord blood permits identification of children of parents with type 2 hyperlipoproteinemia. When cord blood LDL exceeds 41 mg% this is confirmation of lipid abnormality.

Prevention

1. Early control of diabetes. Poor control of hyperglycemia is associated with hyperlipidemia which accelerates arterial changes.
2. Control of obesity. Low sucrose diet with carbohydrates regulation and 25% fat.
3. Avoidance of smoking.
4. Physical activity. Endurance exercises enhance cardiovascular fitness. Exercise increases coronary collateral vascularization, vessel size, myocardial efficiency, efficiency of peripheral blood distribution and return, electron transport capacity, fibrinolytic capability, arterial oxygen content, RBC mass and blood volume, thyroid function, growth hormone production, tolerance to stress, prudent living habits and joie de vivre (Fox 1972).

   It may decrease serum triglycerides, cholesterol, glucose intolerance, obesity, platelet stickiness, heart rate, vulnerability to dysrrhythmias, neurohormonal overreaction and strain associated with psychic stress.
5. Dietary management of hyperlipoproteinemia:

   Diet 1. Strictly controlled diets specifying exact quantities of foods to be taken, involves more work in menu planning, more likely to achieve greater reduction in blood lipids.

   Diet 2. Less rigid diet arrived at by listing foods to be avoided. Suitable for babies with mildly elevated serum lipids.

28

Cardiac Tumors

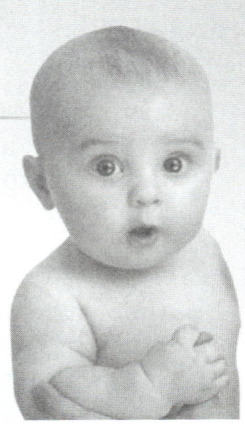

CLASSIFICATION

A. Clinically unimportant tumors:
1. Congenital blood cysts found on heart valves.
2. Focal myxoma are small lesions on valves.
3. Lambes excrescences are villous projections on valves.
B. Rhabdomyoma are associated with tuberous sclerosis.
C. Intramural fibroma of myocardium of left ventricle or interventricular septum.
D. Myxoma of atrial wall in region of fossa ovalis.
E. Sarcoma mural and polypoidal.
F. Pericardial tumors include teratoma, fibroma, lipoma, angioma, leiomyofibroma.
G. Miscellaneous tumors:
1. Lipoma.
2. Hemangioma.
3. Lymphangioma.
4. Congenital cysts.

Clinical Features

Intramural Tumors

Mostly asymptomatic. Presenting feature is usually an abnormal cardiac contour on X-ray chest. Calcification of tumors may be seen. Cardiac murmur is heard if tumor encroaches cavities. Association of rhabdomyoma and tuberous sclerosis presents with convulsions and mental retardation. Severe CHF may occur sometimes. ECG shows hypertrophy pattern, arrhythmias, intermittent WPW syndrome and complete AV blocks and pattern of myocardial infarction.

Pericardial Cysts and Tumors

Abnormal contour of heart on X-ray or rapid pericardial effusion. CHF and tamponade are common. Persistent pericardial effusion is suggestive in infants.

Intracavitary Tumors

Often bizarre picture includes sudden onset of dyspnea, loss of consciousness, CHF, cyanosis, shock and death. Some of these features are precipitated by change of posture. Murmur of mitral stenosis is found which changes with posture. Embolic episodes are frequent due to fragmentation of tumor mass or thrombus formed on tumor surface. Intractable CHF is described. Echocardiography is useful diagnostic tool.

Treatment

Successful removal is reported. It depends upon early diagnosis involving angiocardiography.

Cardiac tumor should be suspected in child if any of following are present:

1. Unusual heart shape particularly with protrusion from left ventricle.
2. ECG with abnormal wide deep Q-waves and ST deviation or abnormal T-waves. (infarct pattern)
3. Underlying disease: Leukemia, tuberous sclerosis or primary malignant tumor in some other organ.
4. Organic murmur that varies with body posture.
5. Persistent pericardial effusion in infant.

29

Aortic Stenosis

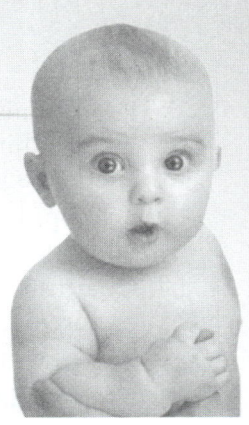

INCIDENCE

7% of heart diseases.

6th most frequent malformation.

Types

1. Valvular aortic and discrete subaortic stenosis.

2. Muscular subaortic stenosis.

3. Supravalvular aortic stenosis.

Valvular aortic and discrete subaortic stenosis is commonest cause of left ventricular obstruction in children. Stenosis may be present at birth or may be acquired by fibrosis and calcification of a congenitally malformed but originally unobstructive valve.

Rheumatic aortic stenosis is exceedingly uncommon in children.

Pathology

Types of congenitally abnormal valve:

1. Unicuspid aortic valve have either a central orifice without lateral attachment to aortic wall or an eccentric orifice with one lateral attachment to aortic wall at level of orifice.

2. Bicuspid aortic valve in which cusps are arranged either to left and right with anterior and posterior commissure or cusps are positioned anterior and posterior with right and

left commisures. Such bicuspid valves open less completely when a third raphe or false commissure is present and they coapt less well in diastole.

3. Tricuspid aortic valve with marked disparity in cusp size which may lead to fibrosis and calcification.

4. Quadricuspid aortic valve usually functions normally but on rare occasions develops stenosis.

Valves with fewer cusps are more likely to be stenotic.

Unicuspid valves are stenotic from birth.

Bicuspid and abnormal tricuspid valves are nonobstructive at birth but thicken and calcify in response to hemodynamic stress.

Discrete subaortic stenosis accounts for 1/10th of all cases of aortic stenosis in childhood.

Acquired lesions of aortic valve are common in patients with subaortic stenosis due to jet lesions causing thickening and fibrosis of valve leaflets. Consequentely aortic valve often becomes incompetent in these patients. Subaortic stenosis may be due to incomplete atrophy of bulbus cordis. It may result from maldevelopment of endocardial cushion tissue of AV canal that usually forms anterior leaflet of mitral valve.

Subaortic stenosis may also occur in lesions of mitral valve, such as accessory valvular tissue or abnormal insertion of normal or cleft mitral valve leaflet to interventricular septum.

Finally subaortic stenosis may occur as part of an endocardial cushion defect or be caused by an obstructive bulboventricular canal septal defect in single ventricle complexes.

Types of subaortic stenosis:

Type 1: Consists of a thin discrete membrane lying immediately beneath aortic valve.

Type 2 is situated 1 cm below aortic valve and embodies a fibromuscular ring that narrows outflow tract and may encroach on anterior leaflet of mitral valve. Occasionally a fibromuscular tunnel narrows left ventricle outflow tract for several centimeters. Significant obstruction to left ventricle ejection leads to concenteric hypertrophy of left ventricle with little dilatation. Thickened ventricle offers more resistance to filling. Left ventricle end diastolic pressure rises. Corresponding elevation in left atrial, pulmonary artery and right ventricle pressure occur and both left atrium and right ventricle enlarge and hypertrophy. Occasionally marked left ventricle myocardial fibrosis develops. Poststenotic dilatation of ascending aorta occurs due to localized increase in aortic wall distensibility. Turbulent blood flow creates vibrations that damage elastic fibers and breakdown links between collagen fibers in aortic wall.

In infants aortic stenosis may be associated with left ventricle hypoplasia and endocardial fibroelastosis. Abnormal left ventricle offers inflow obstruction from left atrium which may enlarge, stretching foramen ovale leading to left to right shunting at atrial level. Hypoplasia of aorta is rare.

Cook in 1947 described a rare form of acquired aortic stenosis complicating xanthoma tuberosum hypercholesterolemia in which stenosis is due to xanthomatous infiltration of aortic valve. Aortic valve calcification is rare before 15 year age.

CLINICAL FEATURES

Most children with AS are asymptomatic and grow and develop normally. Heart murmur is discovered on routine examination. 70% of cases are asymptomatic.

Dyspnea and CHF are common in first year of life. Between 1 and 5 years signs and symptoms are rare. Between 5 and 15 years dyspnea and syncope are common. Angina is a rare finding in childhood.

Growth curve shows normal height and weight for age. CHF is likely to occur when AS is associated with some other heart lesion, such as endocardial fibroelastosis or PDA.

First heart sound is normal. ESM begins shortly after S1. It is diamond shaped with crescendo—decrescendo quality and ends before aortic valve closure. The murmur is best heard over aortic area and is well conducted to neck especially right side. In infants murmur may be maximum at LSE and apex. Intensity of murmur is useful in predicting aortic valve gradient. ESM is always preceded by ejection click that coincides with sudden arrest of ascent of domed stenotic valve when its elastic limits are met. This abrupt deceleration of oncoming column of blood causes high frequency vibration recognized as ejection click. This sound is best heard near apex and down LSE and does not vary with respiration. Absence of click in congenital AS is rare but implies an immobile valve due to extensive thickening of valve cusps. Audible ejection clicks are absent in SAS therefore absence of ejection click favors localization of obstruction to below the valve.

LV ejection is prolonged resulting in delayed aortic valve closure with consequent alteration in second heart sound which may become narrowly split or single or may exhibit reversed splitting with P2 preceding A2. A thrill is palpable in aortic area. Early diastolic murmur due to associated regurgitation is common. Unlike valvular and supravalvular stenosis, subvalvular stenosis may be associated with an apical middiastolic rumble due to obstruction to left ventricular filling by encroachment of anterior mitral valve cusp on mitral valve orifice as well as on LVOT. An audible S4 may be heard in any form of severe LVOT. LVH may be appreciated on palpation but heart is not significantly enlarged unless there is associated AR or LVF. In event of failure the murmur becomes softer or disappears especially in infants. Arterial pulse may be normal. Carotids may be week.

NONINVASIVE ASSESSMENT OF AORTIC STENOSIS

Radiology

Infants with AS and CHF have cardiomegaly and pulmonary edema. Older children without failure may show some LV and LA enlargement when narrowing is severe. Dilatation of ascending aorta occurs seen as a double shadow on upper right border of heart in large percentage of cases of valvular stenosis but is rarely seen in association with subvalvular stenosis. Calcification of aortic valve is rare.

ECG and Vectorcardiography

Pattern of LV strain with ST depression and T-wave inversion in leads V5,V6.

Increased LV voltages with widened angle between mean QRS and T-vectors to greater than 100° in frontal plane often occurs in severe stenosis.

Flattened or inverted T-waves in V6 are consistent with severe AS assessed clinically.

Attempts to correlate ECG with other signs of AS have been made with objective of improving clinical estimates of severity from ECG alone, hoping to avoid cardiac catheterization, for patients with small pressure gradients. Final criterion based on multivariate analysis involved only the intensity of systolic murmur, presence or absence of early diastolic murmur and voltage of Q and R-waves in lead V6.

Left ventricle aortic systolic gradient could be predicted from 13 (murmur score on 0 to 6 scale reduced by 1 in presence of EDM) + RV6 − 6 (QV6) − 9.

LVH in vectorcardiogram results in an abnormal shift of mean spatial QRS posteriorly, superiorly and to left with an increase in maximal QRS forces and a widened QRST angle.

Following features indicate severe stenosis with a peak systolic gradient of over 50 mm Hg:

1. Frontal axis of T-wave + 10, zero or − 10.
2. Sum of frontal and horizontal QRST angles more than 100°.
3. R/T ratio in V5 or V6 greater than 10.

If anyone of these criteria are positive there is 80 to 90% chance that peak systolic gradient between LV and aorta is over 50 mm Hg.

Exercise ECG

With pressure gradient exceeding 50 mm Hg, ST depression exceeding 2 mm occurs on exercise.

With pressure gradient less than 50 mm Hg there is no ST depression on exercise.

Echocardiography

In bicuspid aortic valve eccentricity of aortic valve closure and multilayered diastolic echoes can be seen in aortic root. This sign becomes unreliable in presence of VSD or TOF.

In patients with good LV function peak systolic pressure in LV is estimated from ratio of end systolic wall thickness over end systolic cavity dimension multiplied by 237. By subtracting measured systolic pressure (taken by sphygmomanometer) an aortic valve gradient is obtained. This method is suitable for coexistent mitral or aortic regurgitation.

In discrete subaortic stenosis echo features are aortic valve closure in early systole with persistent valve closure throughout remainder of systole, coarse fluttering of leaflets and absence of asymmetric septal hypertrophy.

SAS produced by long muscular narrowing of LVOT may be appreciated by narrowing of LVOT seen on echo sweep from LV to aortic root. Premature aortic valve leaflet closure occurs. Cross sectional echocardiography improves accuracy of localizing LVOT obstruction.

PULSE WAVE ANALYSIS AND SYSTOLIC TIME INTERVALS

Correlation of arterial pulse with aortic valve gradient or calculated orifice size has been studied. Results show that ejection time index, maximum rate of rise of carotid pulse and timing of peak of systolic murmur best correlated with severity of obstruction in adults. In children the pulse wave form is modified by compliant arteries and therefore valueless in assessing severity of aortic stenosis.

DIAGNOSIS

Cardiac Catheterization

Even in severe AS it is possible to pass a catheter retrogradely across aortic valve to LV. In infants this procedure may be carried out by passing a catheter through foramen ovale to left atrium and left ventricle.

Angiography delineates level and anatomy of obstruction. LV chamber can be outlined. Wall thickness and presence of mitral regurgitation can be seen. Mobility of aortic valve, orifice position and size, size of valve ring and presence of poststenotic dilatation can be confirmed.

Differentiation of valvular from subvalvular ring stenosis

Male: female ratio

- 5.8:1 in valvular AS
- 1.9:1 in subvalvular AS
- EDM more common in subvalvular AS.
- Ejection click is heard in 90 to 100% cases of valvular AS.
- X-ray shows much dilatation of ascending aorta in valvular AS. Not much in subaortic stenosis.
- MDM is more common in subvalvular AS.

Presence of supravalvular AS may be suspected in a child with systolic murmur in aortic area invariably accompanied by thrill, with unequal pulses at wrist, who is mentally retarded and has characteristic facies with or without defective teeth or strabismus. ECG shows LVH but may show combined hypertrophy.

Muscular subaortic stenosis is characterized by late appearance of murmur several years after birth. Murmur is best heard at apex and is associated with MDM. There is rapid upstroke of pulse at wrist or carotid artery. Heart may be enlarged but aorta is small on X-ray. ECG may show Q-waves in left precordium and commonly delta wave. Cardiac catheterization outlines site of obstruction.

Pulmonary stenosis murmur may at times simulate AS murmur over upper end of sternum. It may also be accompanied by ejection click but in PS click is louder and apex beat is related to RV rather than LV. Pulmonary component of second heart sound is fainter in PS. ECG shows evidence of RVH. In severe cases there may be cyanosis. Cardiac catheterization differentiates PS from AS. Small VSD has harsher systolic murmur heard best over LICS 3 or 4 which may be ejection type and associated with thrill. In early life similar findings occur in AS. Later the murmur shifts to appropriate aortic area in AS. Presence of ejection click, dilatation of aorta, a murmur that is best heard in aortic area, T-wave changes suggesting LV strain, hilar shadows that are within normal limits all favor diagnosis of AS.

AS may occur with PDA, coarctation of aorta, PS, VSD, interrupted aortic arch and tricuspid stenosis. Signs of associated lesion will be found then. Cardiac catheterization is definitely indicated in them.

PROGNOSIS

Factors affecting prognosis are site of stenosis, severity, presence of associated defects, CHF, Infective endocarditis, angina, syncope and response to surgery.

Those who die of CHF in infancy have evidence of endocardial fibroelastosis involving LV, aortic valve and mitral valve. Incidence of sudden death in AS ranges from 4 to 18%. AS is the commonest cause of sudden death in patients who had sudden unexpected death from cardiac causes. Clinically all of them have criteria of severe AS. They may be asymptomatic and have normal resting ECG. Prophylactic surgery after cardiac catheterization is advisable in them.

Aortic regurgitation eventually occurs in 20% of patients over 1 year of age. There is tendency for this finding to increase with increasing age. EDM can also occur with onset of infective endocarditis which is more commonly a complication of valvular AS.

Syncope incidence increases with age. It occurs in patients with marked gradient across aortic valve, usually more than 50 mm. These patients have ECG evidence of LVH with LV strain and majority have cardiomegaly.

Angina on effort increases seriousness of prognosis and denotes severe AS. It may occur with normal ECG with gradient less than 15 mm Hg and at times in association with syncope. In these cases sudden death may occur. Calcific aortic stenosis on a bicuspid aortic valve may develop in children.

Perforation cr destruction of aortic valve by infective endocarditis may precipitate fatal CHF. Urgent surgery for replacement with prosthetic valve is indicated.

Natural History

A progressive increase in severity occurs with age. Increased gradient with time is due to increased flow across fixed stenotic area. Increased flow being due to normal increase in cardiac output due to growth. Progression is more marked in patients with discrete subvalve or supravalve stenosis. Aortic stenosis is a progressive condition even when originally mild and such patients should be followed closely. Symptoms and an abnormal ECG at rest or on exercise are indications for investigation.

Treatment

Aortic valvotomy in childhood is a palliative procedure. Primary indication for operation is presence of severe obstruction. A peak systolic gradient exceeding 75 mm Hg with normal cardiac output or an effective aortic orifice less than 0.5 cm²/m² of body surface area represents severe or critical AS. Surgery should be considered urgent for patients with critical AS because they may die suddenly. Until surgery activity should be restricted. Preventive measures for infective endocarditis should be done at time of tonsillectomy, dental extraction or oral surgery. A second operation may be required in many patients as they progress into adult life because of restenosis.

Management of as in First Year of Life

The infant is critically ill with CHF. Majority have systolic murmur in aortic area. Apex beat is forceful and arterial pulse is of small amplitude. ECG shows LVH or combined hypertrophy. LV strain pattern of T-wave flattening or inversion in V6 is present. Cardiac catheterization is required to confirm diagnosis. If gradient is less than 30 mm Hg and CHF is present it is likely that aortic stenosis is associated with endocardial fibroelastosis. In such cases digoxin or other decongestive therapy is indicated.

30

Subaortic Stenosis

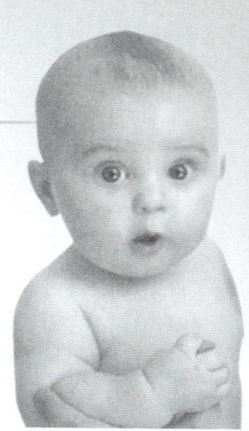

1. Idiopathic hypertrophic subaortic stenosis.
2. Hypertrophic obstructive cardiomyopathy.
3. Asymmetric septal hypertrophy.
4. Obstructive cardiomyopathy.
5. Functional subaortic stenosis.
6. Familial hypertrophic subaortic stenosis.
7. Functional left ventricle outflow tract obstruction.

Definition

By Mac Kinney in 1974. Massive asymmetric hypertrophy of septal portion of LVOT and diffuse hypertrophy of LV walls.

Etiology

Disease is transmitted as autosomal dominant trait with high degree of penetration. Chromosomes are normal. Hypertension may coexist. Role of catecholamines is controversial.

Association with other congenital anomalies:

Fixed LVOT obstruction, ASD, endocardial cushion defect, pulmonary stenosis, dextrocardia.

Association with infiltrative disease particularly Pompe's disease and in infants of diabetic mothers is documented.

Association is noted with Friedreich's ataxia.

Polany and Moynahan in 1972 described a syndrome of multiple symmetric lentigenes, obstructive cardiomyopathy, growth retardation and intellectual impairment. A genetically triggered abnormality of neural crest element was postulated. Subclinical skeletal muscle dysfunction usually generalized is present in 65% of cases. Progressive muscular dystrophy is present in relatives of these patients.

Incidence

Commoner than previously thought. Affects all age groups from newborns onwards. Males predominate. Both sexes are probably equally affected. Black Africans are rarely affected.

PATHOLOGY

Gross anatomical features are:
1. Disproportionate hypertrophy of ventricular septum.
2. Small or normal size of RV or LV cavities.
3. Endocardial mural plaque in LVOT.
4. Thickened mitral valve leaflets.
5. Dilated LA and RA.
6. Hypertrophied free walls of all four cardiac chambers.
7. Normal aortic valve cusps.
8. Normal size ascending aorta.

Histology

Disorganization of muscle cell bundles and abnormal orientation of myofibrils and myofilaments of muscle cells. Perinuclear halo due to accumulation of glycogen. Increased amount of fibrous tissue is present.

Pathophysiology

Asymmetric abnormal septal hypertrophy displaces anterior mitral valve leaflet. Papillary muscles and chordal alignment of mitral valve are also affected. Myofibril disorganization results in an abnormal pattern of contraction.

Narrowing of LVOT by abnormal systolic anterior motion of anterior mitral valve leaflet results in an afterload being imposed on LV late in ejection phase. Disease is dynamic one and obstruction may both develop and regress with progressive advance and deterioration of disease.

Mitral regurgitation frequently occurs and its severity is related to severity of outflow obstruction.

Clinical Features

Symptoms

Patients with this disease may be completely asymptomatic or they may be completely crippled. Usual age of presentation is 3rd or 4th decade.

Exertional dyspnea, fatigue, angina pectoris, dizziness on standing are common. Syncope and palpitation secondary to arrhythmia may be noted. Symptoms of CHF with edema and orthropnea occur as disease progresses.

Physical examination: Peripheral pulses have rapid upstroke with bimodal flow pattern. Apex beat is forceful and double in that the atrial contraction produces a palpable presystolic expansion wave.

First heart sound is normal. Systolic click occurs rarely. A delayed systolic murmur is present in all patients maximally audible over lower LSE inside apex. This murmur decreases in intensity on squatting and increases when patient stands. Amyle nitrite increases intensity and phenylephrine or methoxamine decreases it.

Second heart sound may vary from wide splitting to complete reversal. An MDM right or left sided in origin is present. An EDM due to minimal AR is rare.

ECG

A progression of changes is seen over several years of observation. Electrical axis is usually between 0 and + 90. Features of WPW syndrome notably a short AV conduction time and delta wave are seen. Deep Q-wavess due to septal hypertrophy are seen with normal or small R-waves over left precordium. Over years typical LVH pattern appears. T-wave is upright initially but tends to flatten or become depressed and inverted over a period of several years. Pattern suggestive of myocardial infarction possibly due to myocardial fibrosis may be present. Ectopic beats and atrial fibrillation occur in one-third of patients. P-wave abnormality showing atrial hypertrophy is seen in 50% of cases.

Radiology

Heart is normal or only slightly enlarged. Occasionally massive cardiomegaly occurs in symptomatic infants. Left atrium is large. Ascending aorta normal. RA and RV may be enlarged. Hilar shadows and pulmonary vascularity are normal. Serial X-ray show progressive enlargement over several years.

ECHOCARDIOGRAPHY

1. Asymmetric septal hypertrophy with a ratio of septum to LV wall of 1.3 or more.
2. Diminished left septal surface excursion.
3. Abnormal systolic anterior motion of anterior mitral valve leaflet.
4. Premature systolic aortic valve leaflet closure when obstruction to LVOT is present.

Echocardiography is also useful in:

1. Detecting asymptomatic relatives of affected patients.
2. Repeated follow-up of individual patient.
3. Diagnosis of coexistent dynamic and fixed LVOT obstruction.

Myocardial Imaging

Myocardial perfusion scanning following IV infusion of thallium 201 is noninvasive method of evaluation. Addition of gated cardiac pool scan using technitium 99 m electrolytically labelled human serum albumin allows confirmation of shape of interventricular septum as a negative image. An analysis of regional myocardial wall motion and systolic cavity obliteration can be made.

Cardiac Catheterization

Gradient may be demonstrated across RVOT and LVOT. Gradient across LVOT may be evoked or reduced by use of drugs and maneuvers. An increase in afterload on LV, a decrease in contractility or increase in end diastolic volume will tend to reduce gradient. Gradient is worsened by a reduction in afterload or increase in contractility.

Isoproterenol, digoxin, amylnitrite, Valsalva maneuver, postextrasystolic beat increase gradient.

Alpha adrenergic stimulation, beta adrenergic blockade and infusion of volume expanders reduce gradient.

Cineangiography

Visualization of septum can be made by biventricular cineangiography. Other features of abnormal mitral valve motion, irregular muscular hypertrophy, small cavity, mitral regurgitation and dilated coronary arteries may be appreciated by left ventriculography.

Differential Diagnosis

1. Fixed LVOT obstruction.
2. Primary mitral valve disease usually incompetence but stenosis occasionally.
3. VSD
4. Ischemic heart disease with papillary muscle dysfunction.

Occasionally fixed LVOT obstruction may coexist with idiopathic hypertrophic subaortic stenosis.

Treatment

1. Ventriculomyotomy or myomectomy relieves obstruction and reduces incidence of sudden death in this disease.
2. Prosthetic replacement of mitral valve.
3. Propranolol results in initial improvement that may last some months but symptoms and gradient return. Propranolol is useful for nonobstructed patients or those with labile obstruction. Neither long-term prognosis nor risk of sudden death appear to be influenced by propranolol.

Complications

1. *Atrial fibrillation*: Paroxysmal or sustained.
2. Systemic or pulmonary embolization.
3. Bacterial endocarditis.
4. Progressive cardiac dilatation with onset of CHF.

Prognosis

Sudden death is more common in children. This results from ventricular fibrillation or asystole. Mortality is 15% at 5 years, 35% at 10 years. It does not appear to be altered by either surgery or drugs. Average age of onset of symptoms is 28 years.

31

Supravalvular Aortic Stenosis

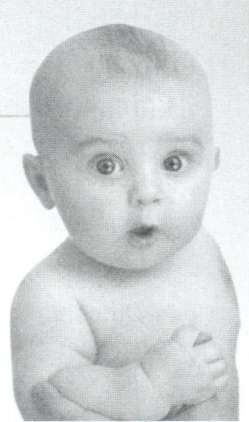

PATHOLOGY

A narrowing in ascending aorta of variable degree and by definition is localized just above sinuses of Valsalva.

There are two main appearances:

1. An hourglass narrowing of aorta (66%)
2. Diffuse narrowing of aortic lumen beginning just above aortic sinuses and extending throughout ascending aorta (20%) Histologically there is an angulation and unfolding of aortic wall with focal disorganization of media capped by a zone of intimal thickening or hypertrophy showing some degenerative changes with calcification.

Two gross forms described are only a reflection of differing degrees of generalized involvement of whole of aortic wall. Diffuse hypoplasia has smaller aortic lumen because intimal changes are extensive. There is a trend towards more frequent stenosis of origin of aortic arch branches in hypoplastic form.

Most patients with supravalvular AS fit into a spectrum of generalized disease of conducting arteries rather than into narrower problem of localized aortic abnormality, such as coarctation of aorta. Pulmonary arterial stenosis is frequently associated with supravalvular AS.

Aortic valve cusps are thickened in a third of patients. Upper margin of aortic cusp may be adherent to aortic wall at stenotic site and may rarely involve coronary ostium. Coronary arteries are often large, dilated and tortuous. Vessels are thick walled and intima shows atherosclerotic changes. Patchy myocardial fibrosis with calcification is reported. Angina occurs in older patients. LVH is often present. RVH when present reflects severity of associated pulmonary stenosis.

True cardiac malformations associated with supravalvular aortic stenosis are VSD, ASD and subaortic stenosis.

Other associated vascular defects could be secondary to major supravalvular obstruction in aorta or pulmonary artery or to basic vessel wall abnormality. Vascular defects are pulmonary and aortic valve stenosis, aortic regurgitation, coarctation of aorta, PDA, aortic aneurysm, hypoplastic descending aorta and carotid, renal and mesenteric arterial stenosis.

MVP may also occur.

Pathogenesis

There is strong circumstantial evidence of fetal disturbance in calcium storage and postnatal expression of idiopathic hypercalcemia.

Abnormal facies in older children with aortic disorder are related to facies of children seen in idiopathic hypercalcemia. Idiopathic hypercalcemia may occur when milk formula are highly fortified with vitamin D or stoss dose of vitamin D given to mothers.

Increased sensitivity to vitamin D on part of mother or child could be considered a cause.

Evidence from skeletal and dental X-ray suggest that children with eventual supravalvular stenosis can have major abnormalities of calcium homeostasis during fetal life. Whether this is due to excessive intake or absorption of vitamin D before and during pregnancy or to a failure of regulatory mechanism for blood calcium in pregnancy is uncertain.

Only one-third of patients with elfin facies are found to have supravalvular AS. Hypercalcemia is seldom demonstrated in infancy for patients who later develop supravalvular AS. For these reasons the syndrome is called William elfin facies syndrome of unknown etiology.

A second group of supravalvular AS occurs in individuals who have normal facies and normal mentality. This group is sporadic in nature and unrelated to disturbance in calcium metabolism. A third group is smaller one with familial aggregation of patients. It is transmitted through an autosomal dominant gene with variable expression.

CLINICAL FEATURES

Birth weight is within lower normal range. Postnatal feeding problems and slow weight gain during infancy are common. Many children show growth retardation. Cardiac symptoms are rare in infancy and childhood. Older children may have dyspnea on exertion, syncope or angina. Facial appearance described in infancy as elfin becomes coarser and easily recognized in older child. There is periorbital fullness, epicanthal folds, anteverted nares, long philtrum, thick lips with an open mouth. There is usually a marked difference between facial appearance of affected subjects and their sibs. Mental retardation with discordant extroverted personality is typical. Minor skeletal abnormalities, strabismus and inguinal hernias are also seen.

Cardiac Signs

There is an ESM maximal in aortic area and conducted to carotid vessels. Murmur is grade 3 to 4 out of 6 in intensity. Usually detected during infancy. Thrill is always present in suprasternal notch even when the murmur is of lower order of intensity. Aortic closure sound is accentuated. EDM is not heard. An additional soft ESM may be heard peripherally over lungs suggesting presence of associated pulmonary arterial stenosis. This and murmur due to MR and coarctation of aorta may be difficult to recognize separately due to louder aortic murmur. Arterial pulse is more prominent in right arm and systolic blood pressure is higher there than in left arm due to high velocity jet of blood from aortic obstruction being preferentially directed into innominate artery called 'Coanda effect'.

Excessive tortuosity of retinal and cerebral vessels is seen. Early appearance of secondary sex characteristics in girls may occur due to vitamin D estrogenic effect.

ECG

Precordial leads show LVH. Occasionally RVH when there is associated pulmonary stenosis or pulmonary arterial stenosis. LVH, wide QRST angle in frontal plane or strain pattern are seen in severe AS as compared to mild AS. An abnormally broad, tall and notched T-wave is found in standard and left chest leads of over 90% cases of infantile hypercalcimia.

Radiology

Most patients have normal size heart. Only one-third patients show cardiomegaly of slight degree. LV is most commonly hypertrophied. In severe PS or PAS associated there is RVH. Some patients with hourglass obstruction show mild to moderate dilatation in ascending aorta. In hypoplastic form aortic knob is small. Lung vascular markings are normal despite PAS. Osteosclerosis is seen in patients with idiopathic hypercalcimia.

Echocardiography

This confirms site of obstruction. Decrease in aortic dimension at level of ascending aorta can be demonstrated.

Cardiac Catheterization

Peak systolic pressure gradient across stenosis range from 10 to 190 mm Hg. Normal amplification of arterial pressure pulse as it proceeds from aorta to periphery may be abolished in patients with hypercalcemic syndrome. Aortography and angiocardiography are methods of choice for definition of this disorder.

Treatment

Preventive measures for limiting infantile hypercalcemia include that no pregnant woman should receive vitamin D in excess of recommended requirement.

Early treatment of infantile hypercalcemia is desirable. Operative intervention is advisable for severe supravalvular AS. Aortotomy with insertion of a large prosthetic gusset is done. For diffuse form LV–aortic bypass shunt is done.

32

Coarctation of Aorta

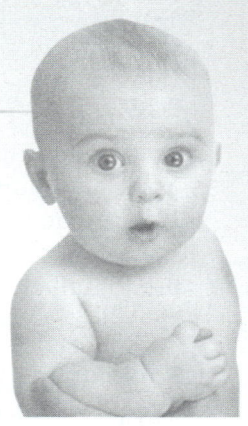

Morgagni 1760: Constriction of aorta a short distance from heart.
Bonnet 1903: Infantile form—coarctation lies above ductus arteriosus. May be localized or diffuse narrowing. Adult form—coarctation is just below entrance of ductus and is localized.
Postductal: When ductus arteriosus is attached above coarctation.
Preductal: When ductus enters below constriction.

Prevalence

- 8th in order of frequency among CHD.
- Approximately 5% cases of CHD.
- More prevalent in males than females. Ratio 2: 1.
- Familial occurrence is extremely rare.
- Other anomalies occurring with coarctation:

In first week of life: Prematurity, RDS, septicemia, atelectasis, tracheoesophageal fistula, pneumonia and CHF. Noncardiac conditions are prime cause of death in this age group.

Under 1 year of age: PDA occurs in 64% of cases, VSD 32%, TGV 10%, ASD 6.5%.

Isolated coarctation of aorta is found only in 18% of infants presenting with signs and symptoms.

Other associated defects are bicuspid aortic valve, hypoplasia of aortic valve, PAPVD into RA, anomalous right subclavian artery, arteriovenous fistula of internal mammary artery, left superior *vena cava* into coronary sinus, complete heart block, endocardial fibroelastosis, Turner syndrome, hypospadius, club foot, mental and ocular defect.

Incidence of associated malformations is 8%.

Etiology

Narrowing whether localized or diffuse is considered a developmental defect.

There can be a localized reactive constriction of aorta following birth. Such constriction may be subsequently followed by hyperplasia and lead to permanent narrowing.

Hutchins in 1971 postulated that position of coarcted segment opposite aortic end of ductus arteriosus suggests it arises as branch point of that channel. In this view the patient with coarctation have a ductal blood flow which exceeds aortic flow during early development.

Talner and Berman in 1975 pointed out that ductal constriction begins at pulmonary artery end and initially this minimizes the effect of Policier aortic shelf or coarctation and permits sufficient flow to transmit pressure to femoral pulsations. During first or second week after birth the aortic end of ductus completes its constriction, aortic flow and pressure are reduced and femoral pulses become diminished or absent.

PATHOLOGY

Postductal type (adult type): There is a localized constriction with aorta reduced in size rather abruptly at site of narrowing. Below coarctation aorta broadens again to a diameter that is greater than aorta above constriction.

Histologically the site of constriction is characterized by a localized medial thickening on which is superimposed new intimal tissue.

LV is usually hypertrophied.

Bicuspid aortic valve is present in 50% of uncomplicated cases. In infancy death is due to CHF or associated cardiac malformation.

Preductal Type (infantile type): Ductus is patent in early life. Blood flow is from aorta towards lung fields. Pulmonary blood flow may be enough to raise pulmonary artery pressure and then direction of flow will depend upon pressure gradient between pulmonary and systemic flow.

There are three types of preductal coarctation:
1. Localized constriction just above entrance of ductus.
2. Diffuse narrowing extending the length of isthmus from entrance of ductus into left subclavian artery.
3. A narrowing that includes not only isthmus but extends further into aortic arch. Associated malformations are commonest with this group.

Collateral Circulation

Dilated and tortuous collateral vessels are chiefly from subclavian artery and its branches. Intercostal, internal mammary, muscular phrenic, superior epigastric, transverse cervical, scapular and lateral thoracic all participate in channeling a more adequate blood flow to lower part of body. Anterior spinal artery also participates in this.

X-ray shows notching of ribs due to continuous pressure of intercostals against posterior or inferior aspect of rib. Scapular vessels may be seen winding in a sinuous fashion beneath skin of back and pulsating visibly.

Collaterals can be demonstrated angiographically in most infants with preductal coarctation.

Higher mortality in preductal type as compared to postductal type is related to more frequent presence of associated heart anomalies.

Cause of Hypertension

1. *Renal hypothesis*: Goldblatt demonstrated in 1939 a renal factor to produce delayed hypertension when blood supply to kidney is impaired.
2. *Mechanical hypothesis*: Besides an increased resistance above constriction there is reduced capacity and distensibility of aortic chambers into which LV empties with each systole.

Current evidence strongly favors a mechanical component playing significant role in infancy.

Surgical Groups

Infants with coarctation can be divided into three groups considering the selection of cases for surgery:

Group 1: Coarctation is found incidentally during an examination. Heart may be slightly enlarged. There is no CHF. Such babies are operated at optimum time.

Group 2: CHF develops after two months of life. There is no evidence of associated defects. These babies are treated medically with digitalis.

Group 3: CHF develops in first two months of life. They usually have an associated defect, e.g. PDA. They are first treated with digitalis rapidly, oxygen and lasix. When improvement occurs the baby should be operated in improvement stage. Ductus is closed at the same time coarctation is resected. VSD may be repaired or palliated with pulmonary artery banding.

If endocardial fibroelastosis accompanies coarctation as indicated by inverted T-waves in lead V6 and positive mumps antigen skin test prompt surgery is required.

Recurrent coarctation of aorta or restenosis of coarctation of aorta:

Various causes are:

1. Inadequate repair in previous operation.
2. Failure of growth of anastomosis when performed in a small child.
3. Restenosis in region of original suture line due to fibrosis, thrombosis or granuloma.
4. There is residual ductal tissue in aorta well above and below actual site of coarctation, unless this is removed actually reactive hyperplasia may occur after correction and may result in restenosis.

Optimum time of surgery is around 5 years of age.

COARCTATION OF ABDOMINAL AORTA

Causes

1. Fusion error in development of paired dorsal aortae.
2. Primary aortitis.
3. Infantile hypercalcemia.
4. Rubella.
5. von Recklinghausen disease.
6. Takayasu pulse less disease.
7. Infections.
8. Periaortic fibrosis.
9. Nonspecific aortitis.

PREDUCTAL COARCTATION (UNDER ONE YEAR OF AGE)

Two-third of cases seen in first year of life are of preductal type, usually presenting in first six weeks of life. Early appearance of heart failure and higher mortality appear to be related to frequent presence of associated anomalies chiefly noncyanotic heart disease including PDA. Coarctation of aorta is second leading cause of heart failure in childhood.

Clinical Features

Dyspnea occurs in 48 hours of life in 80% of cases.

Cyanosis is present from birth intermittently in 20% cases. All have severe associated heart disease, such as TGV or common ventricle. Cyanosis may be present with marked respiratory distress or heart failure.

In 50% cases no heart murmur is heard. When murmur is present it is maximum between LICS 2 and 3 but may also be heard in pulmonary area or LICS 3 and 4 and occasionally at apex in 10% cases. VSD may be associated when murmur accompanied by thrill appears in LICS 3 and 4.

Heart failure is present in 70% of babies. Dyspnea is constant symptom. Liver enlargement occurs. Rales in chest occasionally. Pulmonary edema in few cases. Cardiomegaly always occurs. Femoral arteries are not palpable in two-third of cases. Blood pressure is higher in arms than legs but when marked failure is present blood pressure in upper limbs fall to normal. With administration of digitalis hypertension in arms become evident.

ECG

In first two months of life RVH is present if ductus is patent. LVH appears between 6 months to 1 year of life. If ductus remains patent RVH pattern persists. When a marked left heart strain pattern appears with inverted T-waves over left precordium association of coarctation with endocardial fibroelastosis should be suspected.

Radiology

Cardiomegaly is invariable. In most cases left border is full associated with raised apex. Both hilar shadows and lung fields are congested if CHF is present. In PDA hilar shadows are pulsating. Barium swallow reveals indentation of left aortic arch and beneath it a second indentation due to poststenotic dilatation of aorta immediately below the coarctation. A general displacement of aorta to right is common.

Aortogram reveals whole area of aorta or great vessels arising from it. Coarctation and descending aorta and collateral circulation is visible. This procedure differentiates between postductal and preductal type. Diffuse hypoplasia of aortic arch is in favor of preductal type. Filling of ductus can be seen. Direction of flow in ductus may be seen.

Diagnosis

Should be suspected in any baby with dyspnea, heart failure or cyanosis. Femoral pulses are faint or absent. Blood pressure is higher in arms than legs. ECG has RVH. X-ray shows cardiomegaly with congestion of lung fields. Aortogram confirms diagnosis. In patients under 6 months PDA is always associated. Ductus always enters below coarctation. High mortality is due to heart failure which appears earlier due to hypertension and left to right shunt. VSD, ASD, TGV are also associated.

In differentiating between preductal and postductal coarctation during infancy following features are useful:

1. Failure occurs in first month of life in preductal type.
2. LVH in ECG appears in postductal type.
3. Diffuse hypoplasia in aortogram suggests preductal type.

Treatment

Preductal type has poorer prognosis and requires prompt treatment. When coarcted segment is localized it is resected and two ends of aorta are anastomosed.

POSTDUCTAL COARCTATION

Clinical Features

Children over one year age. Usually have no symptoms. Defect is identified accidentally during routine medical examination. Presenting feature in most cases is finding of heart murmur or systolic hypertension. Only 5% children present with dyspnea or CHF. Majority presenting at 4- to 5-year age.

Normal Anthropometry

There is a visible pulsation in sternal notch.

Pulsating collaterals around scapula are rarely seen. Blood pressure in arms is raised. There is hypotension in legs. Femoral artery pulsations are feeble.

Heart murmur systolic of moderate intensity down the LSE, transmitted to back and apex. Less harsh and less widely transmitted than murmurs due to VSD or PS. There is no thrill. Murmur is best heard in LICS 2 and 3.

ECG

Majority show LVH. When VSD is associated combination may lead to Eisenmenger complex. Also with PDA. In these RVH with RV loading pattern is seen.

Radiology

Heart size is enlarged in 50% cases. Gross cardiomegaly in 5% cases. 45% cases have normal size heart.

Left border is full or bulging. Apex protruding down and out. Cardiomegaly is more with associated defects.

Notching of ribs in coarctation of aorta is due to dilated internal mammary collaterals.

Other causes of notching of ribs are:

- Thrombosis of abdominal aorta.
- Blalock-Taussig operation.
- Tetralogy of Fallot.
- Ebstein anomaly.
- Unilateral absence of pulmonary artery.
- Superior *vena cava* obstruction.
- Intercostal arteriovenous fistula.
- Pulmonary arteriovenous fistula.
- Hyperparathyroidism.
- Intercostal neurinoma.
- Idiopathic.

X-ray chest in coarctation of aorta shows visible indentation at site of coarctation producing E sign in left anterior oblique view. Ascending aorta may be dilated. There may be hypoplastic aortic arch.

Barium filled esophagus shows alteration in contour that corresponds with level of aortic arch and another wider indentation at site of poststenotic dilatation of aorta. A bulge due to left subclavian artery with prominent pulsations is seen just above aortic knob.

Angiocardiography

Aortogram reveals aortic arch and coarctation in lucid fashion. Ductus can be visualized. Collateral circulation can be seen. Associated defects can be visualized by combination of cardiac catheterization with selective angiocardiography.

Diagnosis

Absent or weak femoral pulses, lower blood pressure in legs, pulsations in sternal notch should arouse suspicion. Most common associated defect is PDA. A continuous murmur in pulmonary area identifies its presence. Rarely pulmonary hypertension of severe degree reverses flow through ductus. Cyanosis is then noted in toes but not in fingers.

Left subclavian artery may arise from aorta below coarctation. Blood pressure in left arm then may be low.

Atresia of left subclavian artery may occur. In this case no pulse or blood pressure is recorded in left arm.

When coarctation and atresia of left subclavian artery is combined with an aberrant right subclavian artery arising from aorta below coarctation pulses will be absent in all four extremities.

Complications

Premature coronary artery disease may occur and cause sudden death.

- Cerebral hemorrhage, cerebral thrombosis.
- Rupture of aorta.
- Necrotizing arteritis.
- Infective endocarditis near site of coarcted segment may cause rupture of aorta.
- Endocarditis of aortic valve may occur because aortic valve is often abnormal in coarctation of aorta.
- Aortic regurgitation usually develops because of underlying bicuspid aortic valve.

Treatment

Resection is more safely done after first year of life and before the age when aneurysms and atherosclerotic changes become apparent.

Direct union between resected segments is done but a homograft may be inserted between two segments. Anastomosis grows with child.

Associated large VSD causes irreversible pulmonary vascular changes. These children should be operated upon early. When PDA is associated it is preferable to operate upon ductus and coarctation together.

Postoperative paraplegia may occur due to thrombosis of spinal artery. It may be associated with prolonged occlusion of aorta. Hypothermia reduces its incidence.

Optimum age for surgery is 4 to 5 years. This avoids vascular catastrophes and aorta is elastic and pliable for surgery. Postoperative complications:

Paradoxic or reactive hypertension.

Abdominal pain due to necrotizing arteritis.

Both above are often associated. Hyperactive adrenal glands and vasospasm are possible causes for both. There is initial flooding of lower part of body that causes a blood vessel reaction that can be traumatic. Temporary hypertension developing in postoperative period may be due to reflexes from pressure set at a high level before operation which may continue after relief of obstruction.

33

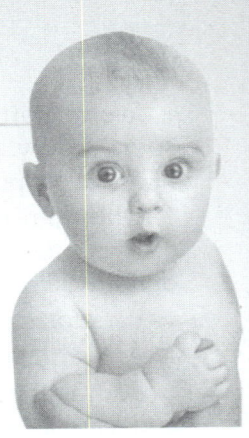

Pulmonary Stenosis

Pulmonary stenosis with normal aortic root (Wood 1951). The term includes simple PS, PS with AV shunt and PS with venoarterial shunt.

More generally accepted term is PS with intact ventricular septum.

PREVALENCE

10% of CHD.

Different seasonal peaks of birth rate have been found for patients with PS. Males peaking in fall and females in spring.

2.2% of siblings of patients of PS have a cardiac malformation usually PS. Familial pulmonary stenosis is known.

Anatomy

Obstruction to Pulmonary Blood Flow

1. *Valvular PS*: In severe form there is fusion of cusps to form a dome projecting within pulmonary artery. Dome has small central perforation 1–3 mm in diameter at its apex. Eccentric position of orifice may occur. Bicuspid pulmonary valve is found in 20% of cases. Calcification of pulmonary valve is rare. About 10 to 15% of patients show abnormally thick leaflets—so called dysplastic valves seen in Noonan's syndrome most commonly.
2. *Infundibular PS*: Incidence 2 to 7%. Many cases are a development secondary to associated VSD that later closes.

3. *Combined valvular and infundibular stenosis*: A reduction in size of infundibulum accompanies severe valvular stenosis due to marked muscle hypertrophy particularly in anterior wall and crista region of right ventricle.

Right Ventricle

Muscular hypertrophy is present in varying degree. Cavity size is reduced. Myocardial infarcts are found in subendocardial region of free wall and papillary muscle of right ventricle.

Pulmonary Artery

Poststenotic dilatation. Circumference of trunk exceeding that of aorta. In severe infundibular stenosis hypoplasia of pulmonary artery is usual. In very young infant with severe valvular stenosis poststenotic dilatation is not evident. There is an inverse relationship between severity of stenosis and degree of pulmonary artery dilatation.

Right Atrium

In severe stenosis right atrial hypertrophy is usual. An anomaly dividing right atrium into two chambers is described. Coronary sinus opens into medial chamber which opens into tricuspid orifice. Small lateral chamber receives both *vena cavae* and appendage and opens into medial chamber through a wide orifice.

Septa

Atrial septum may be completely closed. A wide defect is common with moderate PS. Ventricular septum is closed in most cases. Upper one-third of muscular septum bulges convexly into cavity of left ventricle. This reduces width of LVOT seen in severe PS.

Cirrhosis of Liver

Alteration in liver architecture, such as central lobular atrophy or marked congestion may be seen in infants. Cardiac cirrhosis is rare.

Aorta and Left Ventricle

Aorta is normal in size and arises from LVOT. Occasionally ductus is patent. Left ventricle is dilated. Hypertrophy of wall is seen only when severe PS is associated with hypoplastic right ventricle and right to left shunt. Parachute mitral valve is reported in association.

Widespread Cardiovascular Disease

- Myocardial dysplasia and necrosis.
- Coronary arterial occlusion.
- Higgledy-piggledy aortic wall histology.
- Hypertrophic cardiomyopathy.
- There is an association with Noonan's syndrome.

HEMODYNAMICS

Severe stenosis: There is elevation of right ventricular pressure. This may exceed systemic levels in systole. Right ventricle hypertrophies concentrically and enormously as does right atrium. End result is right heart failure. In presence of patent foramen ovale there may be right to left shunt causing cyanosis.

Mild to moderate stenosis: There is moderate elevation of right ventricle pressure. Systemic values are never reached. Right ventricle hypertrophy is moderate. When ASD or VSD are present direction of shunt is left to right. Cyanosis is not usual. Right heart strain is not severe to cause right ventricle failure.

Clinical Features

1. **Mild to moderate stenosis:** There is lack of cyanosis at any age. Physical development is normal except with arteriovenous shunt who may be dystrophic. Dyspnea on effort is rare. Squatting never occurs. Familial occurrence has been reported. There are no features of CHF.

   There may be precordial bulge in cases with AV shunt. Moon face is rare (20%). A few show a tapping right ventricular type of apex beat. Those with VSD may have left ventricle type of apical thrust.

Ejection systolic murmur is always present. Murmur is moderately loud and ends before aortic valve closure. In mild stenosis murmur is relatively short and soft whereas in severe stenosis murmur is louder and longer. Murmur increases in intensity after inhalation of amyl nitrate. Murmur is usually maximal in LICS2. In infundibular stenosis murmur is best heard in LICS4. Intensity is grade 3. Thrill is unusual. Mid-diastolic murmur may be heard at apex in cases with large left to right shunt. An ejection click loudest in expiration in LICS2 and 3 is heard in trivial and moderate stenosis. Click is related to sudden doming of pulmonary valve and results from opening motion of pulmonary valve being checked. When diastolic pressure in pulmonary arteries consistently exceeded right ventricle end diastolic pressure a click is present in all phases of respiratory cycle. If on inspiration right ventricle end diastolic pressure exceeded diastolic pressure in pulmonary artery no click is found. Second heart sound in pulmonary area is distinctly split and normal in intensity. Occasionally second heart sound is widely split and fixed in presence of intact atrial septum in patients with mild stenosis. In these cases there is marked poststenotic dilatation and deficiency in vessel recoil plays a role.

2. **Severe Stenosis:** 25% are asymptomatic. Generalized cyanosis is seen in patients with venoarterial shunt. Some severe cases with patent foramen ovale have no shunt. Some show minute shunt insufficient to cause cyanosis at rest or with exertion. Some show cyanosis only with exertion and some are cyanosed at rest.

15% cases are markedly cyanosed.

20% have clubbing. Some limitation of exercise tolerance is reported. All cyanosed cases have exertional dyspnea. There is no squatting. In older children episodes of fainting and precordial pain may occur. Sudden death is reported.

Physique is normal. Moon face is common. Increased amplitude of 'a' wave in JVP is visible. Enlarged liver occurs in CHF in severe stenosis. Apex beat is tapping in character. Right ventricle heave is noted in sternal border. Thrill in pulmonary area extends to carotid or suprasternal notch always. Systolic murmur is loud, harsh and long, heard maximally in LICS2. Murmur may be atypical in Noonan's syndrome due to dysplastic valve. In neonate with severe stenosis who present with tricuspid regurgitation loud presystolic murmur is heard at lower left sternal edge and no murmur in pulmonary area.

Diastolic murmur may occur in progressive poststenotic dilatation of pulmonary artery or due to infective endocarditis. Continuous murmur is found in associated PDA. In patients with hypoplastic pulmonary valve paradoxic reverse splitting of second heart sound occurs.

ECG

1. *Mild to moderate stenosis*: In pulmonary valve stenosis of mild severity and right ventricle pressure less than 80 mm Hg normal ECG is reported or equivocal signs of right heart overload.

   QRS conduction delay is characteristic of mild stenosis. Right axis deviation and inversion of R/S ratio in V1 and discrete P- and T-wave changes of right ventricular hypertrophy are seen in moderate severity stenosis.
2. *Severe Stenosis*: RVH is striking. Characteristic features are RAD, abnormally tall peaked P-waves, inverted R/S ratio in V1 and V6, deep inversion of T-waves in lead 2 and 3 and precordial leads as far to the left as V4. qR pattern is present in 50% cases. This is a strong evidence of severe RVH and may be related to myocardial ischemia and infarction of papillary muscles in RV.

Unusual features: Occasional cases in infancy show LVH and RA overload, and LAD due to conduction abnormality in left bundle which may be related to Noonan's syndrome.

ECG Correlations

1. *Changes with age*: Moderate type of RVH seen with moderate stenosis does not change with age. Severe cases show progression in ECG changes with age. Height of P- and R-waves increase over the years. T-wave inversion may extend

from V3 V4 to V6 or it may become deeper with age. In cases with venoarterial shunt Q-waves appears in left chest suggesting a degree of LVH or dilatation.

2. *Hemodynamic relationship*: *P-wave*: P-waves are abnormal and indicative of right atrial hypertrophy in 25% cases with right ventricle pressure less than 100 mm Hg. *qR in V1*: This pattern is associated with a mean right atrial pressure of more than 8 mm Hg.

R in V1: When R is more than 30 mm severe stenosis is certainly present and an RV systolic pressure of at least 150 mm Hg is found. R in V1 correlates better with valve area than with pressure gradient across the valve. While mean QRS axis correlates better with pressure gradient. When R in V1 is more than 35 mm Hg, frontal plane QRS angle is 180°, no S-wave in V1 valvotomy is required.

T-wave: When RV pressure exceeds 100 mm Hg in systole deep T inversion as far as V4 occurs.

Diagnostic importance: In severe form of PS with normal aortic root ECG is characteristic in its inhibition of RVH and RAH which is not seen in TOF. Moderate PS has ECG changes similar to TOF.

There is no cyanotic case of PS with moderate RVH.

Prognostic Importance

Progression of T inversion in short interval is an indication for surgery. Stationary and deep T-wave inversion indicates severe RVH and strain. PR interval of 0.21 to 0.31 sec is associated with poor prognosis due to underlying myocardial ischemia.

RADIOLOGY

1. *Cardiac contour and size*: Cases of mild to moderate severity show no cardiomegaly unless there is an associated AV shunt. Cases with severe stenosis have cardiomegaly. Tricuspid regurgitation contributes to right atrial enlargement and overall cardiomegaly. A distinctive feature of cardiac contour is pulmonary artery bulge present in 90%

of cases. An increase in size of left main pulmonary artery branch in contrast with normal size of right pulmonary artery is characteristic of this anomaly.

RV enlargement and forward projection are obvious in lateral chest films. Marked anterior bulging of RV and spinal overlapping of LV are indicative of RVH.

Barium swallow confirms aorta of normal size with left aortic arch.

2. *Lung vascular markings*: Usually normal regardless of severity of stenosis unless there is venoarterial shunting, then lung vascularity is reduced. When markings are increased the shunt is arteriovenous from ASD or VSD associated with moderate PS.

ECHOCARDIOGRAPHY

Posterio leaflet of pulmonary valve moves to its open position earlier than expected during atrial systole. In moderate to severe PS posterior leaflet motion in late ventricular diastole is exaggerated above normal. Increased right ventricle wall thickness is additional diagnostic aid in severe cases. LVH is present in 25% cases of Noonan's syndrome.

Cardiac Catheterization

1. *Pressures*: In valvular stenosis of severe degree there is obliteration of usual pressure pulse in pulmonary artery branches. On entering MPA distortion of pressure record with large negative deflections is constant. On entering RV an abrupt rise in pressure occurs.

   In mild to moderate PS pulmonary artery pressure pulse is preserved and pulmonary artery pressure is higher. RV pressure is less than 70 mm Hg. RA pressure curve shows giant 'a'waves in all severe cases and none of moderate PS. A slow rate of 'Y' descent in atrial pulse with severe muscular infundibular obstruction and a normal 'Y' descent in those with moderate PS are helpful diagnostic points.

2. *Pressure flow relationship*: Small pressure gradient exist across valve until orifice area is reduced to less than 1 sq cm.

Patients with valve area in range of 0.8 sq cm should undergo surgical treatment. Result of exercise on pressure flow characteristics show that severe PS is associated with fixed or lower stroke volume, elevated right ventricle end diastolic pressure and suboptimal responses of cardiac output on exercise. These changes are reflection of altered right ventricle compliance. They improve within an year of valvotomy.

3. *Shunts*: *Venoarterial shunts*: Right to left shunts are obvious by presence of clinical cyanosis by some arterial oxygen desaturation in those with smaller shunts or by indicator dilution curves showing varying degrees of early appearance of indicator in systemic curves following injection in vena cavae. Right to left shunt occurs in presence of severe pulmonary stenosis with an atrial communication of either widely stretched foramen or true secundum atrial septal defect. Very rarely there is a minute VSD present. There is a right to left atrial pressure differential in ventricular diastole with an left to right atrial pressure differential throughout ventricular systole.

Arteriovenous shunt: Oxygen analysis will localize an AV shunt to atrial or ventricular level in moderate PS or to pulmonary artery in all degrees of stenosis. Detection of smaller volume AV shunt is assisted by use of hydrogen electrode or by indicator dilution techniques.

ANGIOCARDIOGRAPHY

Selective cineangiocardiography gives good indication of right ventricle cavity size, tricuspid valve orifice and dynamic changes in right ventricle outflow, thickness and mobility of pulmonary valve and its size of orifice. Poststenotic dilatation is visible. In newborn babies with papillary muscle dysfunction tricuspid regurgitation may be quite severe. Levophase is particularly useful in determining presence and site of any left to right shunting, particularly at atrial level and may show abnormalities of LV musculature in patients with Noonan's syndrome. In this condition pulmonary valve is dysplastic. On basis of ventricular volume studies it is seen that right and left ventricular function is normal in patients with isolated pulmonary valvular stenosis. But when major right to left shunt is present ventricular function is depressed to variable degree.

Diagnosis

Simple pulmonary stenosis can be recognized in noncyanotic patient of normal physique who may or may not have fatigue and dyspnea with exertion and who has a pulmonary ejection click and an ESM between grade 3 and 6 in intensity with or without thrill maximum in LICS2. Pulmonary component of second heart sound may be normal, reduced, delayed or absent. An RV lift and prominent 'a' wave in JVP will be seen if stenosis is moderate or severe. Except in very severe cases heart size is normal though a prominent pulmonary artery bulge is present. ECG may be normal or show varying degree of RVH. Diagnostic difficulty arises in Noonan's syndrome, newborn with critical PS and in mild form of PS.

Differential Diagnosis

1. *Idiopathic dilatation of pulmonary artery*: There is a debate whether this condition represents a mild form of pulmonary stenosis or is truly a congenital anomaly of pulmonary artery alone. RV pressure is normal. Clinically such patients have a pulmonary artery lift, loud pulmonary ejection click and wide splitting of second heart sound. The distinguishing feature from significant PS is that pulmonary valve closure is loud and EDM can be detected in up to 80% of patients. Radiologically pulmonary artery segment is very prominent. ECG is frequently normal but may show RVH and variety of conduction disturbances.

2. *Straight back syndrome*: This condition may mimic mild pulmonary stenosis by virtue of a normal second heart sound and an ESM of grade between 2 and 3 out of 6 intensity in pulmonary area. It is usually unassociated with a click. Presence of pectus excavatum deformity with narrow AP diameter of chest is helpful in diagnosis.

3. *ASD secundum*: Cases with small defect where pulmonary to systemic flow ratio is less than 2 may show wide but variable splitting of second heart sound, no MDM, normal heart size and a modest increase or normal lung vascular markings. Echocardiogram is very useful in differentiating since right ventricle is always enlarged with small ASD of this sort.

4. *Mitral valve prolapse*: Click and murmur may be audible maximally in pulmonary area because transmission of transients and mitral regurgitation is directed towards left atrial appendage.

5. *Pulmonary arterial stenosis*: This is associated with mild PS and physical signs are similar. In bilateral form of disease most significant clue to associated arterial anomaly lies in wide transmission of systolic murmur to axillae and to back. There is rubella background and a history of siblings with pulmonary stenosis or presence of intrahepatic biliary dysgenesis.

6. *Congenital absence of pulmonary valve*: This condition can produce features of severe PS. Presence of EDM distinguishes this malformation from simple valvular obstruction. Such a to and fro murmur in presence of signs of severe PS is always pathognomonic. CHF is common in first few months of life and secondary compression effects of aneurysmal dilatation of pulmonary artery branches can produce severe respiratory dysfunction.

7. *Aortic valve stenosis*: In young infants murmur of AS can be confined to LSE and ECG shows signs of RV dominance. Ejection click is apical in position and uninfluenced by respiration. These features may be less conclusive in older infants.

8. *VSD*: Some cases of PS have murmur in lower LSE. Administration of amyl nitrite will reduce length and intensity of murmur of VSD but will intensify murmur of PS.

9. *Combined PS and AS*: This rare association may occur as either valvular stenosis alone, infundibular and subaortic stenosis in combination or both valvular and subvalvular obstruction.

ECG shows LVH and LAD through combined hypertrophy to RVH alone.

DIFFERENTIAL DIAGNOSIS
PULMONARY STENOSIS SECONDARY TO OTHER DISEASE

1. *Left ventricle myocardial disease*:
   - Myocarditis.
   - Glycogen storage disease.
   - Obstructive muscle disease.
   - These produce infundibular stenosis.

2. *Tumors*: Right ventricle or pulmonary valve myxomata.

   Neurofibromatosis.

   Little Leopard syndrome is a disorder of pigmentation in association with infundibular stenosis due to right sided hypertrophic muscular disease.

   A syndrome of pulmonary stenosis, cafe au lait spots and dull intelligence has been described by Watson.

3. *Noonan's syndrome*: About half the cases have CHD and most of them have PS. Characteristic facial features and other phenotypic stigmata should be the clue to association. Those with PS have dysplastic valves. Ejection clicks are absent. ECG may show LAD. There is a paradoxical low intensity of systolic murmur when obstruction is severe. Hypertrophic LV disease occurs in a proportion of patients.

4. *Carcinoid cardiovascular disease*: This disease may be associated with PS. Patients develop abdominal pain, diarrhea, weight loss and paroxysms of flushing. There are facial telangiectasia, wheezing, hepatomegaly and an organic murmur over pulmonary or xiphisternal area. X-ray and ECG evidence of RVH of variable severity is found. Cardiac catheterization confirms presence of PS. Death occurs from CHF. Autopsy shows carcinoid of small bowel with liver metastasis and pulmonary or tricuspid valvular stenosis. CVS phenomenon are related to excretion by tumor cells of excessive amount of serotonin.

Pulmonary Stenosis with Arteriovenous Shunt

These stenoses are always moderate in severity. Symptoms are more frequent. Cyanosis is absent. Murmur and thrill are either in pulmonary area or LSE in lower chest due to associated VSD or infundibular stenosis. Second heart sound may be closely or widely split and apex beat may be tapping or thrusting. Cardiomegaly is the rule. A pulmonary artery bulge is visible and lung vascularity appears slightly increased. ECG shows moderate RVH or incomplete RBBB.

Pulmonary Stenosis with Venoarterial Shunt

This defect has effort dyspnea but no squatting. Cyanosis is slight to marked with clubbing. Moon face is often present. A long harsh systolic murmur. Thrill in pulmonary area. Absent or single reduced second pulmonic component is found. Giant 'a' waves are seen in neck. Liver may be enlarged and firm. Occasional infant develops CHF or develops severe anoxic spells. Moderate to gross cardiomegaly, distinct pulmonary artery bulge, down pointing apex and reduced lung vascularity on X-ray chest. ECG has evidence of extreme RVH and occasionally RAH. Cardiac catheterization indicates a pointed RV pressure pulse exceeding systemic levels in systole and low PAP.

1. *Tetralogy of Fallot*: Differentiated by history of squatting, loud single second heart sound and absence of 'a' waves in JVP. Heart size is normal in X-ray chest. Apex is uptilted and not down pointing. Pulmonary artery bulge may occur. Most helpful in presence of cyanosis is only moderate RVH in ECG of TOF, a feature never seen in cyanotic cases of PS with normal aortic root. RV pressure pulse in TOF has a plateau whereas in PS with normal aortic root it is rounded, symmetric and greater than systemic levels in systole. Severe PS with a small VSD may cause diagnostic confusion with TOF.

2. *Transposition of great vessels*: L transposition with PS and complex intracardiac anatomy and patients with D transposition and VSD with pulmonary valvular

obstruction create diagnostic difficulties radiologically but here the low grade intensity of systolic murmur would be incompatible with severity of cyanosis in PS with intact VS and R to L. atrial shunt.

3. *Right heart hypoplasia*: LAD and LVH differentiate tricuspid atresia from PS. Occasionally a newborn with cyanosis, no murmur, large heart and reduced lung vascularity with LVH will be found to have critically severe PS with normal size RV. Often those findings are indicative of pulmonary atresia or critically severe PS with hypoplastic RV. Rarely isolated RV hypoplasia will present in similar manner. In older infants and children with small RV and PS paradoxic splitting of second heart sound may be a helpful point in diagnosis.

4. *Ebstein disease*: It produces a cyanotic infant with systolic murmur of moderate intensity situated over sternum or apex, a grossly enlarged heart with absence of pulmonary artery bulge and reduced lung vascularity. ECG shows reduced voltage and complete RBBB a finding never encountered in PS.

5. *Pulmonary vascular disorders*: Heart may be enlarged, ECG shows moderate LVH, there is a systolic murmur of tricuspid regurgitation, RV lift along LSE and prominent 'a'-waves in jugular venous pulse. The main differentiating points from PS lie in character of second heart sound. Pulmonary valve closure is notable and splitting of second heart sound is narrow. These signs suggest pulmonary hypertension.

6. *Pulmonary vascular obstruction*: Primary pulmonary hypertension may be associated with cyanosis from a venoarterial atrial shunt. Extreme RVH in ECG and reduced lung vascular markings. Absence of murmur and presence of loud click and closely split or single second heart sound help indicate the real cause for pulmonary bulge and right heart hypertrophy.

7. VSD of Eisenmenger type having major R to L shunt has absent murmur and loud click, closely split or single second heart sound.

ASSESSMENT OF SEVERITY

The judgment is based on resting pressure difference across pulmonary valve and/or the peak systolic RV pressure levels.

Cutoff points for mild stenosis are differential pressure of less than 50 mm Hg and peak RV systolic pressure of less than 70 mm Hg.

For severe stenosis differential pressure of 80 mm Hg and peak RV systolic pressure of more than 100 mm Hg.

Severe stenosis can be assumed to be present in those patients where at least one of following features is present:

- Cyanosis.
- CHF.

S-wave in lead 1 of ECG equal to or greater than 15 mm, Q-wave in V1, inverted T-wave in avF and sum of RV1 + SV6 equal to or greater than 35 mm. In such patients the pressure difference across pulmonary valve averages 110 mm Hg. Higher gradient occurs when more than one criterion is present.

In US joint study of CHD prediction equations using universally available items were derived:

Pressure gradient RV – PA mm Hg = 10.5 (ISM) + 2.6 (S1) + S2 score + T score.

ISM = Intensity of systolic murmur graded 1 to 6.

S1 = S in lead 1 in mm, where 1 mm = 0.1 mv.

S2 Score = – 10 if P2 is normal.

+ 2 if P2 is audible but diminished.

+ 15 if P2 inaudible.

T Score = + 15 if T is biphasic in V1 when RV1 is greater than 10 mm, otherwise T score is 0.

If established gradient is under 35 mm the cardiac catheterization would measure a gradient less than 65 mm Hg. If estimated gradient lies between 35 and 50 mm Hg a small proportion show a higher gradient.

If the estimation is more than 50 mm Hg a cardiac catheterization should probably be performed.

COMPLICATIONS

1. *CHF*: All of these patients have right ventricular pressure in excess of 80 mm Hg.

2. *Hypoxic spells*: Cyanosis occurs with pressure gradient between 50 and 70 mm Hg.
3. *Infective endocarditis*: Incidence is 3%.
4. *Tuberculosis*: Common complication of severe PS.
5. Sudden death due to myocardial ischemia.

Clinical Course

In patients with right ventricle to pulmonary artery gradient under 40 mm Hg there is over a period of 4 to 8 years either no change or a decrease in gradient. Whereas in those with severe obstruction with a gradient in excess of 80 mm Hg there is never any improvement. It is apparent that truly mild PS never increases in severity but moderately severe stenosis commonly does so. Majority of these potentially severe cases can be identified by analysis of auscultatory data and ECG in patients with initial RV pressure levels at borderline between mild and moderate PS.

Treatment

A. *Medical management*: During early childhood mild cases do not require surgical management. Aim of pediatrician should be to ensure first that the cases are, in fact really mild in degree and second that the child is protected against infective endocarditis by penicillin prophylaxis at times of special risk.

B. Surgical management:
   1. *Indications for operation*: A right ventricle strain pattern in ECG is an urgent indication for operation. RV pressure over 100 mm Hg in systole is the level by which operation is recommended.
   Patients under 1 year age constitute surgical emergency.
   2. *Results of successful valvotomy*: Cyanosis due to a right to left shunt is abolished, exercise tolerance improves, heart size reduces, ECG evidence of severe RAH and RVH become replaced by moderate hypertrophy or RBBB, RV pressure falls considerably on catheterization and pulmonary valve incompetence occurs in 50% cases which may cause chronic overloading of RV in diastole.

34

Pulmonary Arterial Stenosis

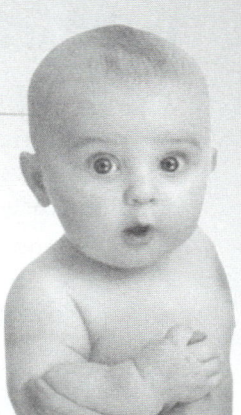

TYPES

A. Simple pulmonary artery stenosis:
    1. Isolated PAS.
    2. PAS associated with simple intracardiac or extracardiac anomalies, e.g. PS, PDA, VSD.

B. Complex PAS: Part of a basically complex intracardiac anomaly, e.g. TOF, TGV, mitral atresia.

Each of these two groups can be further subdivided to indicate position within pulmonary arterial system of major obstruction:

1. *Central*: Localized constriction within MPA usually at origins of either right or left pulmonary artery or both branches.

2. *Peripheral*: Localized constriction at secondary branching of major pulmonary artery divisions.

3. *Intermediate*: Hypoplastic segment of pulmonary artery usually commencing at either distal end of MPA or at its origin of major divisions extending for a significant distance into either or both branches.

Finally the condition may be unilateral or bilateral.

PATHOLOGY

Primary disorder is an anomaly of medial elastic tissue with intimal proliferation at bifurcation of lobar arteries. Thrombotic changes may be a late cause of subsequent increase in degree of obstruction to blood flow at these points. Systemic conducting vessels may also be involved. Secondary changes in severe cases are RVH and enlargement of bronchial arteries.

PAS is commonly associated with other CVS anomalies, e.g. PDA, PS, AS, VSD, ASD, TOF, TGV, TAPVD, coarctation of aorta, aorticopulmonary septal defect and mitral atresia.

ETIOLOGY

Clinical associations in simple PAS:
  A. Functional PAS:
      1. Infants of low birth weight:
          – Prematurity.
          – Racial.
      2. Patients with high pulmonary blood flow:
          – ASD.
          – VSD in infancy.
  B. True PAS:
      1. Familial.
      2. Inherited.
          – Noonan's syndrome.
          – Dolicho ectasia.
          – Cutis laxa.
          – Ehlers-Danlos syndrome.
          – Keutel syndrome.
      3. Prenatal infection:
          – Rubella.
          – Hepatitis.
          – Intrahepatic biliary dysgenesis.
      4. Metabolic:
          – Idiopathic hypercalcemia.
          – Maternal diabetes.
          – Mucopolysaccharidosis.
          – Hypothyroidism.

5. Hemodynamic:
   – Pulmonary AV fistula.
6. Uncertain:
   – Mitral regurgitation.
   – Hypertension.

HEMODYNAMICS

In normal individuals even in term infants where variation in pulmonary flow might be expected the average pressure difference across the pulmonary bifurcation is not more than 5 to 15 mm Hg.

Diastolic pressure difference between main trunk and a branch of pulmonary artery is directly proportional to severity of obstruction.

In unilateral disease there is no major change in cardiac dynamics unless there is atresia of opposite pulmonary artery. Where bilateral stenosis exists RV work increases depending upon severity of obstruction.

In isolated anomaly this is reflected in varying degrees of RV and MPA hypertension.

In patients with associated anomalies the extent of obstruction may not be easy to assess. Particularly in patients with TOF arterial stenosis may appear relatively innocent before correction of more proximal obstruction.

In TGV and VSD arterial stenosis is beneficial in that it protects distal pulmonary vascular bed.

Cyanosis when present is often due to associated cardiac anomalies and rarely due to venoarterial interatrial shunting in isolated types.

Clinical Features

Overall incidence of PAS is 2 to 3% of total CHD.

Murmur caused by PAS is most important diagnostic feature. It is systolic in time, ejection in nature. 10% cases have continuous murmur. Murmur tends to peak in late systole, maximal in pulmonary area, transmitted widely especially to axilla, lower anterior and posterior aspect of chest. Second heart sound is usually normal in intensity and its width of splitting. Pulmonary closure sound may be delayed in presence of associated PS and ASD. With isolated form of disease ejection clicks are absent. A transient murmur resembling that of PAS is heard frequently in healthy premature infants during first 6 weeks of life. Similar observation is made in term small for date infants. Association of these signs with an infant born between October and February in northern hemisphere should raise the possibility of rubella background. Family history should be assessed more closely for presence of heart murmur in relatives and the possibility of transmitted anomaly, such as Noonan's syndrome.

Associated lesions tend to distract the examiner from usually important but less obvious arterial anomaly. Nevertheless it is possible to maintain high index of suspicion if due attention is paid to distribution and character of murmur.

Symptoms may vary from being absent to gross CHF. It is usual for moderate fatigue and dyspnea to develop on exertion in isolated cases. In severe cases signs of RV overwork are evident from prominent 'a' of JVP and parasternal thrust, while accentuation of pulmonary valve closure is indicative of main pulmonary hypertension. Hemoptysis may occur as terminal event.

Radiology

Heart size is affected only minimally in isolated forms unless obstruction is severe when cardiomegaly and prominence of pulmonary artery segment on left border is seen. Associated anomalies usually dictate X-ray appearance.

ECG

In severe bilateral isolated PAS, RAD and RAH with RV loading pattern is seen. Change from RV overload to strain pattern is reported. In mild PAS the ECG may be normal in young children. In cases with associated anomalies the clinical picture varies greatly.

In patients with Noonan's syndrome there may be left anterior hemiblock in ECG.

Cardiac Catheterization

Aim is to detect a pressure gradient within MPA or its branches. Pressure gradient in severe isolated PAS shows normal pulmonary artery wedge pressure and high pressure beyond the proximal obstruction. Sometimes venturi effect is seen.

The peculiar appearance of MPA pressure pulse is that the appearance of systolic portion of MPA pulse is identical with that of RV, while the diastolic level is normal dicrotic notch is deep and diastolic descent following pulmonary valve closure is flattened increasingly with increasing degree of obstruction. At birth major branches of MPA are small relative to MPA. It takes several months to achieve the older child size relationship. In patients with rubella syndrome a more obvious degree of smallness or hypoplasia of pulmonary artery branches is evident at birth. In severe arterial stenosis at early age the factors that lead to death are hemoptysis due to rupture of thin walled distal vessels in lung or thrombosis in these dilated channels.

Angiography

This is essential to provide a complete picture of anomaly. It classifies various types of obstruction. In complex types it may be the only method of detecting unsuspected stenosis or confirming the clinical impression of presence of associated anomaly. Association of PAS with systemic arterial disease necessitates angiography of aorta and its branches.

DIAGNOSIS

Most helpful sign is wide transmission of systolic murmur into anterolateral chest including axillae. In bilateral disease which is the only clinically important type the diagnosis will seldom be missed if a careful auscultation is made over whole of right thorax. History of maternal rubella in pregnancy, familial CHD or finding of features and facies suggestive of Noonan's syndrome or idiopathic hypercalcemia syndrome should alert one to possibility of diagnosis.

The functional type of PAS seen in preterm infants or in patients with septal defects are easily distinguishable from true stenotic disorders.

In those patients with a continuous murmur from PAS the diagnosis will resolve round other causes of continuous murmur distributed widely over chest. Seldom will this include simple PDA, coronary arterial anomalies or sinus of Valsalva rupture and more often will concern lesions with diffuse collateral blood flow to lungs or in various forms of pulmonary atresia or in truncus arteriosus.

In isolated anomaly apart from murmur distribution the degree of prominence of jugular 'a' wave, parasternal RV heave and accentuation of second heart sound will provide clinical indices of severity.

Murmur situation in idiopathic pulmonary hypertension or pulmonary hypertension secondary to intracardiac lesions is different from murmur situation in PAS.

Prognosis

Unilateral PAS of mild central type or mild stenosis immediately above the valve has good prognosis.

Peripheral stenosis carry a poor prognosis due to secondary thrombotic lesions.

Majority are asymptomatic or have mild symptoms in first decade. Only rare cases with calcific changes deteriorate in infancy. CmHF is uncommon in infancy.

Treatment

In supravalvular obstruction, central obstruction at pulmonary branch origin treatment is surgery.

The problem is important for patients with TOF undergoing corrective surgery. Residual pulmonary and RV hypertension will jeopardize the end result. In these patients if the associated PAS is not remedied simultaneously.

Anticoagulants might prove useful as a prophylactic measure against pulmonary arterial tree thrombosis.

35

Mitral Stenosis

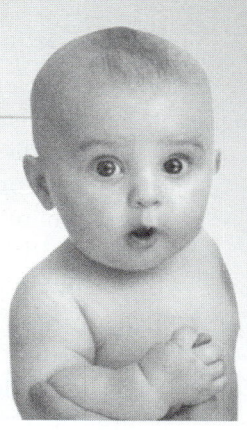

ANATOMY

There are four major components:

1. *Leaflets*: There is a continuous circumferential rim of leaflet tissue in orifice of mitral valve. Separation of these into anterior and posterior leaflet occurs at posterolateral and anteromedial commissures. These commissures may be identified by tips of papillary muscles and chordae tendineae that inserted into these commissures. Anterior leaflet extends much further into orifice of valve than does posterior leaflet, but is attached to only one third of annulus. It is continuous with left and part of noncoronary cusps of aortic valve. Together with adjacent portion of ventricular septum it forms borders of LVOT. There is rough zone into which chordae tendineae insert and a clear zone. Posterior leaflet has several clefts along its free margin and usually divided into 3 scallops. Rough and clear zone are identified. There is also a basal zone into which chordae tendineae that originate directly from trabeculae corneae of LV myocardium insert.

2. *Chordae tendineae*: These arise from two papillary muscles and insert into ventricular surfaces of rough areas of both leaflets, basal area of posterior leaflet and commissural areas. They branch several times from their origin, increasing in number from 25 to 120. Blood passes through interchordal spaces. Fusion will narrow effective mitral orifice.

3. *Papillary muscles*: These are two in number and are related to commissures on their ventricular surface. Anterolateral usually consist of a single muscle belly. Its arterial supply is from many branches of LCA. Posteromedial papillary muscle is usually bifid. Its arterial supply is from terminal branches of right and left coronary arteries.
4. *Annulus*: This is part of fibrous skeleton of heart. Anteromedial leaflet attaches to its anterior third and posterior leaflet to its posterior two-third. Cross sectional area of annulus is about 80% of cross sectional area of leaflets allowing for considerable overlap during closure.

PATHOLOGY

1. *Leaflet abnormalities*: Thickened and fibrotic leaflets are combined with rudimentary and fused commissure. Valve is funnel shaped. An accessory mitral valve tissue has been described which is attached to atrial aspect of posterior leaflet. This tissue can obstruct orifice of mitral valve on basis of its size.
2. *Chordae tendineae*: Thickened and shortened chordae tendineae often matted together may obstruct LVOT. Laymen and Edwards in 1967 described a bridge of fibrous tissue continuous with free aspect of anterior mitral leaflet resulting in direct continuity of mitral valve leaflet with papillary muscle. Three papillary muscles:
   Shone in 1963 described developmental complex of parachute mitral valve, supravalvular ring of left atrium, subaortic stenosis and coarctation of aorta. Mitral valve in this situation consists of two mitral valve leaflets and commissures but chordae converge to insert into one major papillary muscle.
4. *Compound involvement of mitral valve mechanism*: Leaflets are thickened as well as chordae tendineae are shortened, thickened and atrophic to a variable degree.
5. *Mitral stenosis associated with other congenital anomalies*:
   – Coarctation of aorta. Parachute mitral valve. Components of mitral valve may be small compared to normal.

Abnormalities of papillary muscles and chordae tendineae primarily may be present.

– TGA. Minor chordal anomalies. Slight reduction of mitral annulus size. Fusion of papillary muscles and abnormal mitral valve leaflet attachment.

– DORV. Incidence of severe mitral valve anomalies in 28% in group with subaortic VSD without PS.

– Single or primitive ventricle, VSD, DOLV. Straddling AV valve orifices are often associated with hypoplastic valves and abnormal valve tissues. DILV is also associated with functional MS.

– ASD (Lutembacher's syndrome). Association of MS with ASD may result from rheumatic endocarditis. Congenital deformity of mitral valve has also been described.

Pathophysiology

Isolated MS: Transmission of high left atrial pressure through bronchial veins results in edema of bronchial mucosa and increased airways resistance. Elevated left atrial pressure is also transmitted through pulmonary veins and pulmonary capillary bed. Pulmonary edema occurs when hydrostatic pressure in capillaries rises above oncotic pressure of blood and lymphatics are unable to drain increased amount of tissue fluid formed. Vascular congestion results in decreased static and dynamic compliance of lungs. Severe pulmonary vascular disease and marked interstitial fibrosis occurs in young patients. Compensatory mechanisms develop in lung vascularity which enable one to tolerate greater elevation of left atrial pressure than one could acutely.

These mechanisms are:

– An increased capacity of lymphatic system.
– Development of pulmonary bronchial collaterals.
– Reflex pulmonary arteriolar constriction.
– Possibly altered pulmonary capillary permeability.

MS with other defects: Finding of large left to right shunt at atrial level or greater pulmonary hypertension than would otherwise be expected may lead one to suspect coexistence of abnormal mitral valve. Hemodynamic diagnosis may be difficult with complicated associated defects.

CLINICAL FEATURES

Dyspnea occurs in almost all cases. Effort intolerance is usually marked. This may be due to disproportionate rise in PVR on effort. PND and orthropnea are seen. RVF with peripheral edema may occur. Cyanosis may occur in otherwise uncomplicated MS due to decreased oxygen saturation of blood due to pulmonary edema. There may also be a disturbance of ventilation perfusion ratio of lungs secondary to abnormal capillary blood flow.

Examination of heart reveals visual or palpable features of RVH.

Auscultation Findings

1. *MDM*: An apical rumble is often best heard when patient lies in left lateral position.
2. *Presystolic accentuation*: This is due to increased velocity of blood flow across stenotic valve following atrial contraction. It is also noted in atrial fibrillation particularly after short diastolic pause.
3. *Loud and delayed mitral component of first heart sound*: This indicates pliable mitral valve leaflets and mobile chordae. Soft first heart sound common in congenital MS suggests immobile leaflets with thickened and short chordae.
4. *Opening snap*: Presence of this sound indicates that mitral leaflets are mobile. This is frequently absent in congenital MS.
5. *Systolic murmur*: Due to associated MR or if PHT is present tricuspid regurgitation.
6. Other cardiac defects will modify clinical picture.

ECG

Mean frontal plane QRS axis is between + 90 and + 150°. RVH and bilateral hypertrophy are common.

Radiology

Cardiomegaly with LA and RV enlargement. Severe stenosis may be indicated by presence of Kerley A and B lines.

Echocardiography

Best diagnostic aid when MS complicates other defects. There is a decreased EF slope of valve, decreased amplitude of excursion. In congenital MS when chordae tendineae are fused there is a reduced amplitude of opening, reduced EF slope, abnormal posterior leaflet motion in that the posterior leaflet moves anterior and parallel with anterior leaflet echo instead of away from it. EF slope may be normal if the only valvular pathology is small annulus. Enlarged LA is seen in uncomplicated MS.

Radionuclide Angiography

Using ^{99m}technetium pertechnetate shows enlargement of LA with prolonged visualization and persistent visualization of LA and LV in tight MS.

Cardiac Catheterization

LAP is elevated with diastolic gradient across MV. There may be PHT. Cineangiography may show a large LA with delayed emptying, reduced mobility of MV mechanism and a jet of blood entering LV may be seen. RAO view is best in children.

Differential Diagnosis

Other anomalies resulting in LVIT obstruction are:
1. Pulmonary venous stenosis.
2. Cor triatriatum.
3. Anomalous pulmonary venous return.
4. Atrial tumors.

LVIT obstruction may coexist at two different sites, e.g. parachute mitral valve with supravalvar stenosing ring, and also at pulmonary venous level.

Management

Conservative decongestive therapy. Digitalis is indicated. Diuretics must be used cautiously as low output states may be produced. Systemic emboli occur with AF and increasing age. Rarely in pediatric age group. Anticoagulants may be used on individual basis. Surgery is the only effective method of treating severe obstruction. Valvotomy or fenestration of fused leaflets gives good palliation. Possibility of valve replacement should be considered.

Prognosis

Depends upon severity of obstruction and nature of associated lesion. Most children with severe disease die in first year of life. Complications of endocarditis and emboli are rare in children. All surgery is palliation. There are long-term problems of prosthetic valve replacement in children.

Complications

1. Chronic obstructive lung disease.
2. Hemoptysis due to rupture of bronchial veins, pulmonary edema and pulmonary emboli.
3. Chronic RVF leading to cardiac cirrhosis, significant proteinuria and protein losing enteropathy.
4. *Atrial fibrillation*: This may give rise to pulmonary edema.
5. *Systemic embolization*: TIA, CVA, convulsions, myocardial infarction, renal or splenic infarction, superior mesenteric embolization, acute hypertension due to large renal artery embolism, paraplegia due to aortic embolism.
6. Massive atrial thrombus.

36

Mitral Valve Prolapse

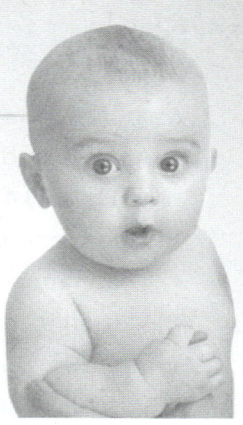

SYNONYMS

- Floppy mitral valve.
- Ballooning mitral valve.
- Billowing mitral valve.
- Doughnut mitral valve.
- Systolic click—late systolic murmur syndrome.
- Myxomatous mitral valve.

HISTORY

Barlow in 1963 first demonstrated angiographically association of mitral regurgitation with clinical syndrome of systolic click and late systolic murmur.

Osler in 1880 had described clinical constellation characteristic of mitral valve prolapse.

INCIDENCE

MVP is ubiquitous in general population. A significant proportion of pediatric population referred for cardiac evaluation is composed of patients with MVP.

Symptoms tend to manifest in mid childhood and early adolescence.

There is female preponderance.

Association with Congenital Heart Disease

- ASD secundum 15%.
- VSD, ASD + VSD, Ebstein anomaly.
- Membranous septum aneurysm.
- Coarctation of aorta.
- Marfan's aortic regurgitation.
- PS, PAS, TGA, TOF, AS.
- Vascular ring.
- Cardiomyopathy.

Etiopathogenesis

Two hypotheses:

1. *Valvular theory*: Myxomatous degeneration of valve tissue is primary event. As degeneration advances valve area increases due to its redundancy. During systole increased surface area of valve results in transmission of increased tension to chordae and papillary muscles. Such tension could produce local ischemia, account for chest pain and ECG changes and serve as arrythmogenic focus.

2. *Myocardial theory*: Segmental or regional myocardiopathy is responsible for prolapse by allowing chordae to become slack during systole. Morphologic changes in valve structure are secondary to abnormal stresses generated.

   Prolapse of mitral valve has been documented in patients with:

   - Turner syndrome.
   - Homocysteinuria.
   - Ehlers-Danlos syndrome.
   - Muscular dystrophy.
   - Tuberous sclerosis.
   - Cardiomyopathy.
   - Acute rheumatic fever.
   - Arteriosclerotic coronary artery disease.

Relationship of myxomatous degeneration of mitral and aortic valves with Marfan's syndrome:

- Mitral regurgitation is present in 47% cases of Marfan's syndrome. More frequent among girls.
- Isolated forms of MVP may be a forme fruste of Marfan's syndrome.
- Marfan's syndrome is known to occur sporadically or in families as Mendelian dominant trait.
- Familial occurrence with dominant inheritance is documented in isolated MVP.

There are frequent occurrence of skeletal abnormalities particularly thoracic, increased joint laxity and increased aortic root diameter demonstrated by echocardiography.

These findings suggest that idiopathic MVP represents connective tissue disorder of subtle degree the extremes of which constitute classic Marfan's syndrome.

Pathology

Mitral valve is thickened and redundant bulging into annulus. Hemorrhoidal appearance of posterior leaflet is result of its normally triscalloped configuration.

The pathologic process may be limited to posterior leaflet or isolated scallops.

Advancing severity is characterized by involvement of rough zone extending toward base of valve.

Rupture of chordae is noted.

Microscopically there is myxomatous degeneration of leaflet characterized by replacement of collagen fibers of fibrous and spongiosa by loosely organized relatively acellular material. Ground substance is a protein acid mono polysaccharide complex. These findings are indistinguishable from Marfan's syndrome. Since focal myxomatous changes can be seen associated with a variety of conditions, diffuse involvement of central plate must be demonstrated to support diagnosis of MVP.

SYMPTOMS

Majority of patients are asymptomatic. Symptoms are nervousness, emotional instability and tachycardia, chronic fatigue, shortness of breath and palpitations.

Clinical entities known in past as neurocirculatory asthenia, soldiers heart, Da Costa syndrome represent cases of MVP. SOB accompanied by cardiomegaly is a manifestation of CHF and related to significant MR.

Acute onset CHF suggests rupture of chordae tendineae. Spontaneous rupture is age related occurring in adult life. Such an occurrence in childhood would suggest an infectious process and demand careful investigation for bacterial endocarditis. Transient neurological manifestation of cerebral embolization may occur without bacterial endocarditis.

Palpitation may be manifestation of arrhythmias but may occur without any ECG changes. Syncope and near syncope may occur with ventricular fibrillation.

Chest pain of anginal type have been reported accompanied by biphasic flat T-wave changes in ECG and apical honk. Sharp stabbing precordial pain, pleuritic in character is a common complaint in adolescent.

AUSCULTATION

When associated with other CHD auscultatory findings of MVP are masked. An apical systolic click or murmur of MR may appear only after surgical correction, e.g. ASD secundum.

In uncomplicated MVP findings are variable within the same patient. Murmur and clicks may differ from one examination to the next in regard to their presence, timing or combination. Patients with classic findings (apical mid diastolic click followed by late systolic murmur or honk) may go through short or prolonged silent periods. This intermittency is highly characteristic. Often the diagnostic findings will be absent when the patient is examined resting in supine position but will be uncovered with manipulations, such as auscultation in held expiration, in left lateral supine, sitting and standing position.

Variability also occurs in terms of natural history. A patient who starts with an isolated mid systolic click may be found to have a click and late systolic murmur at a later date and pan systolic murmur still later.

Further variations exist in relation to degree of valvular deformity. With minor form of prolapse there is a high incidence of atypical findings namely mid systolic murmur of variable quality resembling functional murmur. Their suspicious nature is underscored by an apical location and by frequent association with apical clicks. Angiographically there is no MR hence, these murmurs are attributed to anomalies of chordae tendineae. An attempt is made to correlate physical findings with degree of prolapse. Apical murmurs produced by MR are more frequent (78%) in the group with severe prolapse than in the group with slight prolapse (34%), however, the minor type of deformity does not preclude occurrence of all classic findings.

In general the auscultatory findings are located over cardiac apex. Infrequently the classic late systolic murmur, mid diastolic click or late multiple systolic clicks are heard over pulmonary area and not over the apex. Basal location of auscultatory findings occur when mitral deformity of anterolateral commissural region is dominant and clicks and murmurs are transmitted into an enlarged left atrial appendage.

Systolic click is usually single. It is best heard over apex, occurs during middle third of systole and precedes a late systolic murmur. It marks onset of prolapse and is attributed to sudden tensing of chordae tendineae (chordal snap) or sudden billowing of prolapsed valve (sail sound).

Clicks may be multiple, occurring in grating showers, mimicking a friction rub.

An isolated click may become multiple with held expiration, in left lateral supine posture or when sitting. It may disappear with inspiration.

Clicks may occur in early systole or migrate towards first heart sound with sitting, standing, head up tilt position, the strain phase of Valsalva maneuver, tachycardia or administration of vasodilators. With these maneuvers valve prolapse occurs earlier in systole. This phenomenon is related to reduced left ventricle end diastolic volume. The click occurs in any individual patient at a constant ventricular volume and migration of click in systole is dependent on combination of EDV and contractile state of ventricle.

Squatting, vasoconstrictors and bradycardia have opposite effect. Click is delayed, diminished or abolished. Murmur becomes shorter and fainter and honks disappear. Pregnancy by increasing blood volume tends to diminish or abolish auscultatory features. They return in postpartum period.

Differentiation of these clicks from ejection clicks occurring in semilunar valve stenosis or with aneurysm of membranous septum is established by producing migration with appropriate posturing or drugs. Multiple clicks result from asynchronous tautening of individual chords or asynchronous prolapse of individual scallops.

The late systolic murmur is typically initiated by a click best heard over apex and of a crescendo or decrescendo quality. It may become audible only when provoked by held expiration or posturing in left lateral supine, sitting or standing. The same maneuvers may increase its intensity or produce a honk or whoop, on occasion they may be so loud that they are heard by child's parents across a quiet room or by patients themselves. These beeping hearts are source of parental alarm and may be sole reason for referral to cardiologist. Same maneuvers will make already audible murmur longer and may change its acoustic quality into a grating, scratchy noise by superimposition of multiple clicks. Infrequently a late systolic murmur becomes pansystolic. Pansystolic murmur occurs less frequently. Systolic click is commonly absent or obscured. It signifies a high degree of regurgitation and may in time substitute a late systolic murmur. Under these circumstances clicks may be obscured or occur very early in systole, rendering it inaudible. Diagnosis of MVP can be established by echocardiography or left ventricular angiography. Systolic ejection murmurs are atypical for disease but occur in

18% of cases. Commonly they have vibratory quality of Still's murmur. They may be recognized as suspicious of MV deformity when they are heard over cardiac apex and diagnostic when preceded or interrupted by clicks. It is postulated that unlike the late systolic murmurs they are not produced by MR, rather they are of chordal origin and produced by tautening of chordae tendineae which are abnormal.

Early diastolic murmurs are infrequent. They may be long and decrescendo when produced by AR in Marfan syndrome. Early diastolic scratches are not related to aortic valve disease. They are similar to diastolic scratch occurring in Ebstein anomaly of tricuspid valve and may be attributed to sudden relaxation of abnormal chordae tendineae.

Radiology

Cardiac size and contour are normal except in patients with significant MR. In these LA is also enlarged. LA appendage appears dilated.

Calcification of mitral valve is reported.

When MVP is complicated by associated CHD, e.g. ASD, Ebstein anomaly X-ray features of these disorders will be dominant. Association with thoracic skeletal anomalies is noted. 75% cases have thoracic boney deformities, e.g. pectus excavatum, straight back syndrome (abnormally narrow AP diameter of chest) and scoliosis. Presence of these thoracic deformities on chest X-ray justifies a deliberate search for MVP.

Pseudoheart disease traditionally associated with pectus excavatum and other deformities is likely to represent bonafide MVP.

ECG

Abnormal ECG pattern occurs in 53% cases.

They are of three groups:

1. Disorders of repolarization.
2. Disorders of conduction.
3. Arrhythmias.

Commonest ECG abnormality is partial or complete reversal of T-wave polarity in inferior limb leads 2, 3, AVF. These changes are less frequently seen in lateral precordial leads as well. Such repolarization disturbances are variable in degree and may resolve entirely. Accentuation of T-wave changes may occur spontaneously and are precipitated on effort, inhalation of amyl nitrite and assumption of erect posture. T-wave changes suggesting anterior myocardial infarction have been reported and are confined to anterior precordial leads and seen in combination with inferior lead changes. Alteration in ST segment are usually absent or show mild depression in inferior limb leads. Such changes may be induced by exercise.

Electrophysiologic basis for these observations:

1. Abnormal tension on papillary muscles creating local ischemia.
2. Tension may alter myocardial membrane characteristics that become manifest as abnormalities of repolarization. Arrhythmias may be supraventricular tachycardia, ventricular tachycardia, premature ventricular contractions, occasional or persistent and multifocal ectopic beats, may be uncovered on exercise.

Conduction disturbances:
- Detected in 10% cases.
- First degree heart block.
- Complete heart block.
- Complete RBBB.
- Left axis deviation.

Selective chamber hypertrophy:
- RVH, LAH, LVH.
- LV strain pattern may be seen.

Echocardiography
This is capable of detecting abnormal mitral valve motion when auscultatory findings are absent, so called silent prolapse.

There are two characteristic patterns of MVP in echo:

1. Mid-diastolic posterior motion of valve leaflets with a discrete late systolic dip towards left atrial wall.
2. Pansystolic posterior bowing or hammocking consists of gradual posterior motion during systole.

There is a high incidence of aortic root dilatation.

Angiography

LV angiography is the single definite diagnostic method for MVP, either isolated or associated with CHD. The RAO projection is best analysis of posterior leaflet.

DIAGNOSIS

Clinically MVP may be suspected in girls who are tall, slender, have skeletal thoracic deformities and who complain of palpitation, unjustified fatigue or chest pain. With a family history the index of suspicion is heightened.

Examination should be carried out in all body postures. Recumbent, left lateral supine, sitting, standing and withheld expiration.

Systolic clicks should be differentiated from ejection click of semilunar valve stenosis, bicuspid aortic valve and membranous septum aneurysm with small VSD.

Mild systolic sounds may also occur with pericarditis, atrial myxoma, subvalvular ventricular aneurysms and restrictive cardiomyopathy.

Late systolic honks have been heard with ventricular aneurysms.

Blowing late systolic murmur occurs with coarctation of aorta. Best heard over cardiac apex. Their extension over left and right lateral chest and over back indicates nature of anomaly. Differentiation from Ebstein anomaly becomes difficult in cases showing ECG evidence of RBBB or RV overloading, loud systolic clicks and early diastolic squeaks.

When presenting feature is an arrhythmia the search for a possible organic substrate should include MVP, myocardiopathies, idiopathic hypertrophic subaortic stenosis, Ebstein anomaly, myocardial tumors, catecholamine producing tumors or metabolic disturbances, such as hypokalemia.

With palpitation and tachycardia hyperthyroidism needs exclusion.

In presence of physical findings of MR without history of rheumatic fever cardiac catheterization is required to differentiate from congenital MR.

Anginal or typical anginal chest pain may require selective angiocardiographic studies although the probabilities of detecting coronary anomalies in young patients is minimal.

Prognosis

Majority of patients remain symptom free and have a good prognosis.

Those without MR tend to produce good valvular function. Those with slight MR develop progression.

Spontaneous rupture of chordae tendineae may occur with infective endocarditis.

Complications

1. *Infective endocarditis*: Incidence is 1: 500 cases. Common in association with ASD secundum. Presence of endocarditis without apparent evidence of pre-existing heart disease requires a systematic search for MVP or bicuspid aortic valve.

2. *Sudden death*: Presence of ST – T abnormalities in association with ventricular premature beats has predictive value. Hence an effort to detect arrhythmias at rest and with exertion in patients with repolarization defect is justified.

3. *Cardiac failure*: Chronic intractable CHF due to MR occurs. Acute severe CHF is a feature of rupture of chordae tendineae.

4. *Cerebral embolism*: With TIA is attributed to thrombosis. It could also occur with infective endocarditis as a result of septic embolization.

Management

1. Asymptomatic patients need no active treatment. Cardiac re-evaluations at rare intervals are justified in order to detect new and significant findings and to ascertain that ECG remains free of repolarization defects and arrhythmias. Customary measures for prevention of infective endocarditis at appropriate times are indicated.

2. Severe degree of MR will require treatment of CHF and surgical therapy. Abundance of mitral leaflet substance and absence of ruptured chordae tendineae in young patients offers good opportunity for annuloplasty or suturing of pseudoclefts. Surgical approach is contraindicated in Marfan syndrome. Three presence of chest pain, syncope and palpitation requires ECG studies including long-term monitoring. Occasional benign ventricular ectopics require no treatment. Ectopic activity of significant nature, such as early premature ventricular beats (R on T phenomenon), bifocal or multifocal beats, repetitive firing, exercise induced ectopy or ventricular tachycardia requires chemotherapy in effort to suppress these potentially fatal disturbances, particularly in patients who have repolarization abnormalities. Propranolol, quinidine and procainamide are useful.

   Chest pain does not respond to coronary dilators. Propranolol is helpful in such cases.

   Excision of papillary muscles and replacement of mitral valve for control of disabling chest pain has been considered.

3. Emotional support of symptomatic individual is most important and may occasionally be required in patients who have no objective findings.

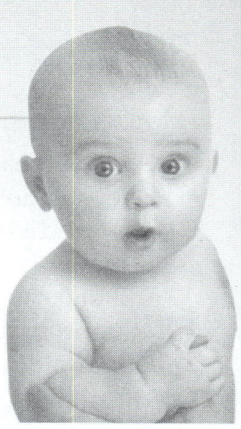

37

Congenital Mitral Regurgitation

Most frequently it is associated with some other cardiac lesion and may be part of a well known syndrome or a combination of defects, e.g. atrioventricularis communis, ostium primum, corrected TGV, endocardial fibroelastosis, aneurysmal dilatation of left atrium or left ventricle and coarctation of aorta.

MR can result from papillary muscle dysfunction from ischemia or infarction due to coronary artery abnormalities and also from mitral valve dysfunction.

Transient changes in myocardial perfusion in neonate may lead to mitral valve incompetence.

Prolapse of mitral valve may also result in MR.

A group of cases in which MR is the only defect is characterized by such anomalies as cleft leaflet of mitral valve, anomalous chordae, perforated valve, shortened or defective valve tissue, double orifice thickening and deformities, Ebstein type of valve anomaly and dilatation of annulus.

Pathology

Character of mitral valve offers opportunity for developmental defects in fetal life. Posterior or lateral leaflet is attached to the annulus of mitral valve at junction of left ventricle and left atrium while anterior or medial leaflet extends its attachment up into aortic root and is continuous with portions of aortic valve above. Leaflets in closed position are suspended by chordae tendineae and papillary muscles which insert into ventricular wall just below commissure.

Congenital anomalies are identified according to component of mitral valve involved, e.g. leaflets, commissure, chordae tendineae and papillary muscles.

Abnormalities of papillary muscles is most common. MR may also result from anomalous mitral arcade. In this condition there is connection of left ventricle papillary muscle to anterior mitral leaflet either directly or through interposition of abnormally short chordae tendineae.

In endocardial fibroelastosis thickening of mitral valve occurs at times making it less mobile and if process involves chordae tendineae these structures become stiff, preventing full excursion of leaflets. Shortened chordae tendineae and deformed valve leaflets frequently coexist and accentuate insufficiency that either one may produce.

Calcification of mitral valve is rare.

Dilatation of left atrium from any cause can proceed to a degree that enlarges mitral ring and prevents anterior and posterior cusps from approximating in systole leading to serious degree of MR. A cleft in anterior leaflet is associated with AV canal defect. In atrioventricular communis where both mitral valve and tricuspid valve are cleft chordae tendineae may be inserted into unusual sites, such as margin of VSD. MR will persist postsurgery unless chordae are cut.

In coarctation of aorta mitral valve has leaflet abnormalities (cleft, perforation, myxomatous change) and chordae abnormalities (short, long, ruptured, deficient chordae). In corrected TGV mitral and tricuspid valve are transposed and valve on left side of heart may be defective. There may be anomalous insertion of chordae or Ebstein type anomaly of left AV valve.

Accessory commissures may lead to a localized leak in mitral valve.

Double orifice of mitral valve may cause progressive MR. Congenital MR may be found in patients with congenital polyvalvular disease. Valves are involved in dysplastic process characterized by increase in valvular spongiosa with vacuolar and lacunar degeneration. These cases are often associated with trisomy 18 or 13–15. Usually dysplastic valves are stenotic but in some valves are severely incompetent.

With enlargement and dilatation of left ventricle that characterizes MR, chordae tendineae spread out in lateral fashion until in some cases a situation may be reached where valve leaflets cannot approximate each other and a further degree of MR occurs. Thus mitral insufficiency begets insufficiency.

CLINICAL FEATURES

History and clinical findings vary according to underlying associated pathology and degree of severity of MR.

In isolated congenital MR there is a history of fatigue and retarded growth and frequent respiratory infection. There is no previous history of rheumatic fever. ESR and ASO titre within normal limits. PR interval may be normal or lengthened.

CHF is common in congenital MR.

On examination there is usually an apical thrust due to enlarged LV, a mitral systolic murmur, third heart sound and as a rule an apical diastolic murmur. Systolic murmur is frequently accompanied by thrill at apex. Diastolic murmur is inflow type. Pulmonary second sound is likely to be accentuated due to elevated pulmonary artery pressure.

In ostium primum apical systolic murmur indicative of MR is present in 80% of cases. Apical systolic murmur is not a feature of corrected TGV since signs of associated anomaly, e.g. VSD dominate, a PSM is recorded at apex, apparently due to MR.

ECG

In isolated MR axis is in quadrant from 0–90°. Broad bifid P-wave is present with evidence of LV overloading characterized by a tall R in V6. An increased conduction time is associated with Q-waves in right precordium in corrected TGV.

Echocardiography

MVP is readily diagnosed. MR secondary to ruptured chordae tendineae gives specific echo findings. Most characteristic echo finding in nonrheumatic MR is marked increase in diastolic slope and opening and closing heights of mitral valve.

Radiology

LAH and LVH, recognized in AP view as diffuse cardiomegaly. A double atrial contour may be recognized with LA protruding through right margin. A barium swallow will confirm LA enlargement. Large LA may elevate and spread mainstem bronchi. Pulmonary vascular markings are increased especially shadows at right apex due to back pressure in pulmonary veins. LAO view outlines LV enlargement. Kerley lines may be present. When corrected TGV is present aorta can be seen coming up the left cardiac border.

In common AV canal since an ASD is present excessive LA flow due to MR is not forced into a confined LA but is allowed to escape through ASD, thus enlarging right side of heart rather than left. When ASD is less than 1 cm diameter, LA will enlarge like in isolated MR.

Angiography

Catheter in LV will show regurgitant flow of contrast material sweeping back with each systole into LA. It will also show immense dilatation of LA with each systole. LV enlargement is seen. Selective aortic root angiography will exclude an anomalous origin of LCA from pulmonary artery as etiology of MR.

Cardiac Catheterization

High EDP in LV and high mean diastolic pressure in LA. LA pressure pulse is characterized by tall peaked V-wave followed by rapid descent. LV pressure pulse shows a rapid fall after ejection peak. Pulmonary artery wedge pressure is always elevated with significant MR. RV and PAP are elevated to some degree.

Diagnosis

Obvious hemodynamic defect in MR is flux of blood back into LA at a time LV is attempting to empty its contents out into aorta. This augments volume of LA during next diastole and results in abnormally large quantity of blood entering LV producing diastolic overload. At same time blood is forced back into pulmonary veins. LV then gradually increases in size and dilates to greater capacity in both systole and diastole. Dye dilution curve will show prolonged disappearance time that is suggestive of MR (Two catheter double dye).

DIFFERENTIAL DIAGNOSIS

1. Atrioventricularis communis and septum primum are always associated with some degree of MR.
2. Corrected TGV may be associated with minor MR.
3. Rheumatic heart disease in absence of history of acute rheumatic fever.
4. Congenital MR without associated anomalies. Patient does not have AV communis, corrected TGV or RHD but he may have associated PDA, ASD or small VSD. Hemodynamics are dominated by MR.
5. Congenital MR with coarctation of aorta. Coarctation aggravates severity of MR.
6. Anomalous LCA originating from pulmonary artery may have MR due to ischemic damage to LV and papillary muscles.

    Typically the patient is an infant with cardiomegaly, MR and characteristic ECG changes, i.e. abnormal Q-wavess in lead 1, avL and evidence of LV ischemia. Aortic root angiography will provide conclusive evidence of this anomaly.
7. Varying degrees of MR may accompany MVP. Atrioventricularis communis and ostium primum group can be identified by ECG and cardiac catheterization findings. 95% cases have axis between – 50° and – 150°. Systolic murmur is apical.

In corrected TGV X-ray shows an aorta that traverses left cardiac border and can be confirmed by an angiogram by retrograde injection into LVOT.

In RHD patient may have history of rheumatic fever but if this is lacking the ECG shows LV overloading of considerable degree. LA is usually not enlarged dramatically. ASO titre and ESR may be elevated.

In congenital MR without ASD group anomalies history of CHF is common and is often associated with failure to grow, bifid P-wave in ECG, large LA and apical systolic murmur transmitted to axilla. There is absence of cyanosis and at cardiac catheterization tall V-wave is apparent in LA pressure tracing. Angiocardiogram shows regurgitant flow when injection is made into LV.

In AS or AR one may have some enlargement of LA or LV but LA enlargement is not marked. Pressure curve in LA will be different.

Chronic myocarditis of nonrheumatic origin may give apical systolic murmur with MR due to dilated mitral ring. Such cases usually have history of onset with acute illness, ECG characteristic of myocarditis and disease is likely to be associated with progressive improvement if medically treated in early stages. In late stages patient may run a progressive downhill course with further cardiac enlargement and CHF. Chronic myocarditis with fibrosis and hypertrophy of myocardium may be associated with cardiac enlargement and MR.

Acquired disturbances of coronary arteries may result in coronary insufficiency and MR. Infantile periarteritis nodosa may result in coronary arteritis, myocardial infarction and papillary muscle dysfunction. Mucocutaneous lymph node syndrome may have significant coronary artery disturbance, e.g. aneurysms.

Unusual congenital defects of mitral valve with defects of membranous portion of ventricular septum causes injection of blood from left ventricle into right atrium rather than right ventricle and presents with mitral regurgitation.

Treatment

Most useful procedure in presence of dilated ring or mitral annulus has been placing of many through and through silk sutures in region of one or both commissures in order to narrow the opening.

Mitral valvuloplasty has been carried out in rheumatic MR but there is little experience with congenital MR.

When mitral valve is deformed in the spectrum of endocardial cushion defect Rastelli modification of repair has been used. Plication and narrowing of mitral valve can be done in children. Indication for surgery:

CHF and cardiomegaly which is progressive.

Prognosis

Patients with severe chronic MR can remain asymptomatic for many years despite a significant regurgitant volume. Myocardial mechanism that allows MR to be tolerated needs appreciation. In patient with chronic MR cardiac index is usually nearly normal and total left ventricle output to left atrium and aorta exceeds the normal. MR reduces the radius of ventricle more than normal during systole resulting in significant reduction in myocardial wall tension. Reduced tension of loading on ventricle allows a larger proportion of contractile energy of myocardium to be expanded in shortening than in tension development. The striking reduction in LV tension that occurs in MR allows LV to increase its total output and accounts for the observation that patients with severe MR can sustain enormous regurgitant volumes for prolonged periods without clinical deterioration.

38

Congenital Aortic Regurgitation

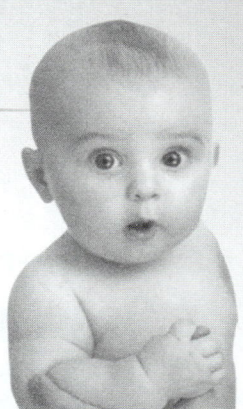

CAUSES

1. Bicuspid aortic valve with stenosis.
2. Congenital aortic stenosis.
3. Prolapse of aortic valve with VSD.
4. Coronary AV fistula.
5. Dilatation of aortic annulus in Marfan's syndrome and relapsing polychondritis.
6. Rheumatic, syphilitic, bacterial endocarditis.
7. Rupture of aortic cusp.

Aorto LV tunnel is most unusual form of congenital aortic runoff and must be considered in differential diagnosis of congenital AR. This tunnel represents an abnormal communication that begins in ascending aorta above origin of coronary arteries, bypass aortic valve and terminates in LV. The condition should be suspected in any infant with features suggestive of severe AR particularly if the murmur is loud in first month of life.

Chest X-ray shows dilatation of ascending aorta, LVH and disproportionate dilatation of right aortic sinus.
Ascending aortography will confirm diagnosis.

Treatment is closure of aortic ostium of tunnel. Early surgery is indicated to prevent aortic valve deformity secondary to ring dilatation.

Differential diagnosis should include VSD with AR, PDA, AR accompanying bicuspid aortic valve, ruptured sinus of Valsalva and coronary AV fistula.

39

Congenital Pulmonary Regurgitation

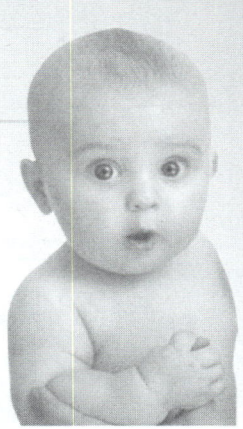

Causes

A. Low pressure pulmonary artery:

1. Isolated congenital PR (idiopathic dilatation of pulmonary artery).

2. Isolated pulmonary stenosis.

3. Absence of pulmonary valve:

   – Infantile form associated with TOF, symptoms develop secondary to bronchial compression caused by aneurysmal dilatation of pulmonary arteries.

   – Associated with VSD or other intracardiac lesion.

4. Postoperative PR:

   – After pulmonary valvulotomy for PS.

   – After outflow reconstruction in TOF or other conotruncal anomalies.

B. High pressure pulmonary artery:

1. Eisenmenger syndrome (pulmonary vascular obstructive disease).

2. Primary pulmonary arterial hypertension.

3. Obstruction distal to pulmonary capillary bed:

   – Mitral stenosis.

   – Cor triatriatum.

- Pulmonary vein stenosis.
- Pulmonary vein occlusive disease.
- Obstructed TAPVD.
- LVOT obstruction.
- Miscellaneous left heart lesions.

4. Cor pulmonale.

40

Congenital Pulmonary Arteriovenous Aneurysm

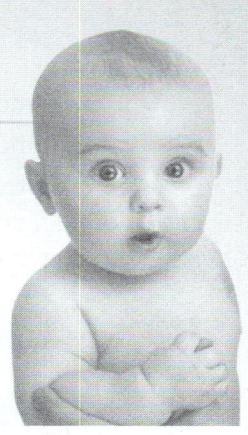

PREVALENCE

80% cases present with signs and symptoms in infancy and childhood. This is not a common disease.

Pathology

Aneurysm is seen incorporated into lung tissue with an enlarged pulmonary artery entering it and equal size vein emerging. Vascular channels of aneurysms are tortuous and lined with endothelium. Wall is thin. Rupture may occur into lung parenchyma or bronchus. Size of aneurysm may be from a pinpoint to small orange. 50% patients have 2 or more. Telangiectatic form occurs in 10% cases. In most instances the shunt is from pulmonary artery to pulmonary vein. Occasionally communicating artery may arise from aorta directly or as branch of bronchial artery.

Hemodynamics

A dilated branch of pulmonary artery carries venous blood into aneurysm and quickly recirculates it through tortuous channels permitting it to return to pulmonary vein without being oxygenated. There is a shunt of venous blood into systemic circulation producing cyanosis and polycythemia. From 18% to 89% of RV output may pass through aneurysm. Usually cardiac output is not significantly increased. Cardiomegaly is uncommon (10% cases). Blood pressure, heart rate and circulation time are within normal limits.

Clinical Features

Small aneurysms remain asymptomatic. Majority of patients have characteristic dyspnea, nose bleeds, cerebral manifestations, hemoptysis and chest pain. On examination there may be cyanosis, clubbing or a murmur over involved lung. Hemangiomas of skin and mucous membrane occur in one-third to half of patients and association with Rendu-Osler-Weber disease is now well established. Heart is usually within normal limits of size. Dyspnea appears on exercise. Cyanosis is associated in 80% cases. Epistaxis occurs in 32% cases due to associated telangiectasia in nasal mucosa. Numbness, dizziness, convulsion occur in 25% cases due to cerebral anoxia or localized thrombosis. Hemoptysis occurs occasionally due to rupture of aneurysm into bronchus, may be massive and fatal. Cyanosis and clubbing occur in 80% cases without obvious signs of CHD. Murmurs of varying type are heard over chest at site of aneurysm, sometimes continuous, increases in intensity with deep inspiration. Children look well nourished and are not underdeveloped. ECG shows slight RVH.

Radiology

Rounded or nodular lung opacity in either lung fields in lower lobes most frequently. Borders of aneurysm are well defined. Two cord like strands may be seen proceeding from shadow to hilum of lung. They are dilated artery and vein. Fluroscopy reveals pulsation in aneurysmal shadow. Mass increases in size with Valsalva maneuver (which increases pulmonary pressure). In telangiectatic type X-ray may be normal.

Echocardiography

Appearance of echoes in LV are delayed for several cardiac cycles.

Angiography

Reveals anatomic details of lesion. Mass is well delineated and dilated vessels are clearly seen. Tortuous channels show up as nodular prominences in and at margin.

Treatment

Excision is method of choice. This is carried out by lobectomy or segmental resection. Symptomatic patients are most suitable for surgery.

COMPLICATIONS

- Brain abscess.
- Massive hemoptysis.

41

Ebstein Disease

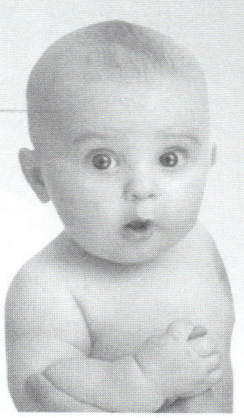

First reported by Wilhelm Ebstein in 1866 in autopsy finding in a man aged 19 years who had a malformation of tricuspid valve and right ventricle.

Pathology

RA is greatly enlarged. Tricuspid valve is prolapsed into body of RV in such a manner that its cavity is greatly reduced in size. Septal and posterior cusps of tricuspid valve are grossly deformed and shortened with their chordae tendineae appearing like small trabeculae in reduced RV. Attachment of these deformed valves and trabeculae produces two chambers in RV, one towards apex and other towards infundibulum, with relatively small opening in between. Wall of RV is thin while pulmonary conus is slightly hypertrophied. Wall of RA shows hypertrophy in young patients and fibrosis in old patients.

In 3/4 cases either foramen ovale is patent or fossa of valve is fenestrated. Defective RV cannot handle returning blood adequately so large proportion is shunted across foramen into left ventricle and systemic circulation. Thus, this anomaly is classified into cyanotic group although onset of cyanosis is frequently delayed.

Conduction system is normally situated but AV node may be compressed and RBB may be fibrotic.

Associated lesions with Ebstein anomaly:
- PDA.
- Pulmonary atresia.
- VSD.

Current opinion emphasizes spectrum of involvement of entire tricuspid apparatus and of RV.

Clinical Features

Males and females are equally affected. Majority are sporadic but familial cases have been reported. Mothers exposed to lithium gave birth to babies with Ebstein anomaly. Children are thinner than average. Dyspnea is commonly present especially in those with cyanosis but it may precede onset of cyanosis or CHF.

Cyanosis

3/4 patients have right to left shunt through foramen ovale or ASD. In 2/3 cyanosis is present since birth or early infancy. In most other patients cyanosis will appear insidiously between 3 to 12 years of age. It is characteristic of this condition that cyanosis may be absent or minimal at birth but appear later in childhood. At birth there may be simple dyspnea and then dyspnea and cyanosis.

Pulse

Radial pulse is usually small not brisk. BP is within normal limits. There is relatively small pulse pressure.

Thrill

There may be slight precordial bulge. Occasionally a thrill can be palpable at precordium.

Cardiac Impulse

Over lower precordium cardiac impulse is quiet and subdued. Over conus area where RV muscle is sometimes thick a more powerful heart beat may be felt. Thus a localized impulse over conus helps to differentiates this anomaly from pulmonary stenosis with patent foramen ovale where cardiac impulse is felt over whole precordium. Impulse is associated with coarse systolic thrill.

Heart murmurs

A systolic and short diastolic murmur are present in 50% cases. Most of rest have only systolic murmur. Murmur is best heard over lower precordium and may be loud or faint. It is described as scratching or crunching. Majority have diastolic murmur. This may be presystolic or mid diastolic. It is usually accentuated in inspiratory phase of respiration suggesting a tricuspid valve origin. To and fro murmurs are also heard. The effect may simulate precordial friction rub.

Heart Sounds

Third heart sound is heard giving a triple rhythm. It occurs commonly in those patients who have a diastolic murmur. Heart sounds are of normal intensity but at times they may be faint. Consistent finding on phonocardiography is abnormally wide splitting of first heart sound which has been shown to be caused by delayed closure of large anterior tricuspid valve leaflet.

RADIOLOGY

There is an impression of generalized enlargement with prominence of both left and right heart borders. Convex left border is due primarily to dilatation of RVOT but it is further displaced by abnormal development of RV. Prominent right border is due to enlargement of right atrium which is affected by rise in internal pressure. Cardiac outline is highly suggestive of underlying pathology.

In newborn heart may be within normal limits. Pulmonary vascular markings are either normal or decreased. Under fluroscope there is lack of movement of cardiac borders more likely in older cases. There is close correlation between degree of cyanosis and decrease in hilar markings.

Left atrial enlargement is not seen in children with Ebstein disease. Calcification of mitral valve and ring has been demonstrated.

ECG

Most striking feature is association of complete RBBB with abnormally low R- and S-waves over right precordium. This is an unusual combination in CHD and should immediately arouse suspicion. QRS is long and multiphasic. P-waves are abnormal showing increased amplitude or duration. PR interval is increased to 0.16 second or more. QRS axis ranges between – 30 and – 170°. WPW syndrome is identified with Ebstein disease. With this association cases can be divided into two groups. Those with right axis deviation and those with left axis deviation. Second group suggest LBBB. Right precordial leads show deep S and left tall R-waves. Tall peaked P-waves are also present. Although conduction tissue is normally sited electrophysiology studies reveal conduction delays at several levels of system. Dysrrhythmia of paroxysmal nature may occur in patients.

Echocardiography

An abnormally anterior position of anterior leaflet during entire period of diastole together with delayed closure of tricuspid valve are consistent echo features in Ebstein disease. Septal motion may also be abnormal. Ability to record anterior tricuspid leaflet farther to left of LSE than in controls is a useful sign.

Cardiac Catheterization

Catheter may be coiled up in RA to reveal an abnormally large chamber. RAP is slightly raised. There may be difficulty in entering RV. RVP is within normal range. PAP is similar to that of RV or slightly lower. Oxygen content of RA is identical with that of RV and pulmonary artery. Systemic arterial blood shows undersaturation. Catheter may pass through atrial septum opening into LA and LV.

Value of intracavity electrode catheter in diagnosis of Ebstein anomaly:

On withdrawal of catheter from RV to RA, QRS and P-wave change. Fluroscopy control will show this change when catheter tip is in area one would expect to be in body of RV, thus suggesting one of the diagnostic features of Ebstein anomaly.

ANGIOCARDIOGRAPHY

The technique defines displaced tricuspid valve and its relation to tricuspid annulus as two notches at inferior cardiac border. Fenestration of anterior leaflet can be identified. In all cases there is evidence of large right atrium occupying half of cardiac shadow. There is late emptying time of RA and RV. Right to left shunt through atrial opening can be demonstrated.

Prognosis

Largest proportion die in second and fourth decade of life. Degree of interference of blood flow to lungs is most important prognostic factor. When it is marked there is progressive cardiac enlargement and early death. Pediatric mortality is highest during first year of life.

Treatment

1. Patients should live within their exercise tolerance and avoid dyspnea, excessive fatigue and excessive cyanosis.
2. Suitable antibiotic should be given for respiratory illness.
3. Antiarrhythmic therapy is frequently successful.

Surgical Treatment

1. In presence of marked cyanosis Glenn anastomosis between superior *vena cava* and right pulmonary artery allows systemic venous system to provide the slight pressure required to pass blood through right lung. This may relieve the load on abnormal right atrium and right ventricle.
2. Blalock-Taussig shunt is useful in presence of pulmonary stenosis but not recommended in average type of Ebstein disease.
3. Prosthetic replacement of tricuspid valve in grossly defective valve.
4. Tricuspid valve annuloplasty is preferred and currently a Carpentier ring would be preferred method.
   Indications of surgery:
   1. Presence of intractable CHF.
   2. Repeated arrhythmias difficult to control.

42

Right Aortic Arch

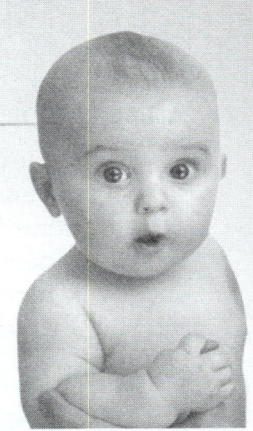

Classification

A. With mirror image brachiocephalic branching and:
   1. Left ductus arteriosus connecting left pulmonary artery to
      - subclavian portion of left innominate artery.
      - upper descending aorta.
   2. Right ductus arteriosus.
B. With aberrant left subclavian artery and:
   1. Left ductus arteriosus connecting left pulmonary artery to
      - Aberrant subclavian artery.
      - Upper descending aorta.
   2. Right ductus arteriosus.
C. Aberrant left innominate artery.
D. With isolation of left subclavian artery from aorta.
   Incidence in CHD:
   1. In TOF: 14–34%
   2. DORV: 20%
   3. Truncus arteriosus: 31%
   4. Isolated VSD: 2.3%
   5. Tricuspid atresia: 5%
   6. Complete TGV: 2.3%
   7. Congenitally corrected TGA: 1%

Radiology

Right aortic arch is visible where it indents the trachea slightly just above right tracheobronchial angle and there is mild displacement of trachea to left. Arch is larger than normal. Upper descending aorta can be seen to right of spine. Cardiac shape is determined by associated intracardiac anomaly.

43

Tetralogy of Fallot

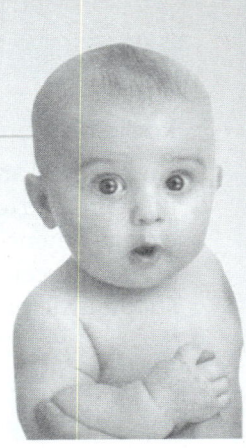

ANATOMY

TOF consists of stenosis of RVOT at one or more of various levels, VSD, RVH and aorta that straddles the septal defect at its origin.

VSD is large. There is always anatomic abnormality of pulmonary infundibulum. There is fibrous continuity of aortic and mitral valves.

Primary anatomic considerations:

1. *VSD*: Defect is large and only rarely there is more than one. It is situated in anterior part of ventricular septum and frequently involves membranous septum. Defect is confluent with aortic ring and lies beneath posterior part of right and anterior part of posterior aortic cusp. In almost two-third the ventricular defect is bounded posteriorly by muscle or fibrous band possibly representing an inferior division of embryonic infundibular septum that separates it from membranous ventricular septum.

2. *Aortic relationship*: There is maintenance of normal fibrous continuity between mitral and aortic valves. Aortic root is rotated to a variable degree so that the noncoronary cusp of aortic valve lies more or less to patient's right and more anteriorly than normally. Thus, whereas anterior leaflet of mitral valve is normally directly related to noncoronary cusp, in TOF it has more continuity with aortic cusp.

3. *Pulmonary stenosis*: There is disturbance in RV muscle bundle architecture, therefore all patients of TOF narrowing of infundibulum of some degree. Van Praagh in 1970 called it monology of Fallot. Small size of conus muscle made-up by parietal band and adjacent free wall of infundibulum are primary cause of all other major parts of malformation. Crista supraventricularis is rotated into more vertical position. Septal band is hypertrophied and parietal band is deviated anteriorly away from base of tricuspid valve. Chordae are abnormally placed and are inserted at lower edge of VSD. Thus ventricular communication is located between posteriorly displaced papillary muscle of conus and displaced crista. Degree of abnormality of crista determines the size of ostium infundibuli at birth and whether or not the newborn will exhibit pronounced cyanosis. Although obstruction to pulmonary blood flow is intracardiac and subvalvular additional obstruction may occur at pulmonary valve and beyond.

More than 70% cases with pulmonary valve stenosis in TOF have bicuspid pulmonary valve.

Valvular atresia is extreme form of obstruction at valve. It may be present as thin diaphragm occluding the ring but commonly exists as thick portion of ventricular wall with no obvious connection with pulmonary artery. Some patients acquire atresia over the course of years at previously stenotic site. Such atresia may develop at infundibulum itself as well as at valve where calcification is an important component. Absence of pulmonary valve occurs in 3% cases of TOF. Pulmonary artery beyond is aneurysmal. There is associated infundibular stenosis. Left pulmonary artery may be absent.

4. *Distal pulmonary tract*: Main pulmonary artery and its major divisions are hypoplastic in 82% cases. Pulmonary artery stenosis occurs in 3% cases of TOF. Obstruction occurs in distal portion of MPA and involves a segment extending into origin of both main divisions. Diffuse forms of pulmonary artery stenosis occurs in patients with rubella syndrome and TOF. Pulmonary artery stenosis is also seen in Noonan's syndrome and TOF. Single pulmonary artery

with absent left pulmonary artery and a vessel connecting MPA with left subclavian artery is described. Absence of right pulmonary artery occurs rarely. Hemitruncus (right pulmonary artery from ascending aorta) may occur.

SECONDARY ANATOMIC CONSIDERATIONS

Associated cardiovascular anomalies reported in TOF:

1. Right aortic arch.
2. Absent innominate artery (subclavian and carotid arteries arising separately)
3. Right aortic arch, left subclavian retroesophageal.
4. Double aortic arch (vascular ring)
5. Left aortic arch, right subclavian retroesophageal.
6. PDA arising from subclavian artery (not connected to aorta).
7. Unilateral absence of pulmonary artery.
8. Patent ductus arteriosus.
9. Pulmonary artery stenosis.
10. Partial anomalous pulmonary venous return with mitral atresia.
11. Persistent left superior *vena cava*.
12. Bronchial arteries entering pulmonary arteries.
13. Abdominal aorta to pulmonary artery connection.
14. Multiple VSD.
15. Patent foramen ovale, ASD primum or secundum.
16. Absent pulmonary valve.
17. Coronary artery anomalies.
18. Aortic valve with unequal sized cusps or a small fourth cusp. Right atrium is hypertrophied. Tricuspid valve shows varying degrees of mitralization. Left superior vena cava entering coronary sinus is found in 5–8% cases.

Interatrial communication exists which causes residual right to left shunt after correction of TOF.

Main bundle of His is related to posteroinferior margin of defect. Right bundle a direct continuation of the main travels beneath free margin of inferior portion of defect.

Right ventricle is enlarged and hypertrophied. Left ventricle is usually normal. Biventricular hypertrophy occurs in Noonan's syndrome associated with TOF. These children respond poorly to shunt procedures and die of myocardial ischemia after shunt operation.

Supravalvular mitral stenosis, cor triatriatum and abnormal chordae tendineae have been reported.

Aortic valve may be bicuspid. Right coronary—noncoronary commissural deficiency with right coronary cusp prolapse into VSD are reported.

Coronary Arteries

Changes in position of coronary ostia due to counterclockwise rotation of aortic root, increase in vascular branching of right coronary artery over right ventricular outflow tract and anterior descending coronary artery from right coronary artery are reported.

Single coronary artery and origin of RCA or LCA from pulmonary artery are less common.

Aortic arch is right sided and right descending in 20% cases. Retroesophageal subclavian artery aberrant or absent innominate artery and double aortic arch may occur.

Ductus Arteriosus

Incidence of patency is high during infancy and is seen with pulmonary atresia. Persistence beyond 15 months is unusual. Partial persistence of ductus (aortic end closed) occasionally occurs.

Other Collateral Pathways

Brochial arteries are increased in size and provide collateral circulation to pulmonary artery.

Pulmonary vascular bed is normal in patients with mild pulmonary stenosis at birth. With age changes appear. Small pulmonary vessels show obstruction by thrombosis. Medial atrophy and intimal fibrosis secondary to thrombotic lesions occur. Variation in arrangement of elastic tissue in MPA of children with TOF is consistent with the view that there is a group of patients in whom pulmonary stenosis develops after birth.

Etiology

Actual cause of arrested cardiac development is unknown. In few cases there is definit history of Rubella in first trimester of pregnancy. Tetralogy also occurs in Down syndrome and Noonan's syndrome. Prematurity and low birth weight is associated with TOF.

Frequency

Most frequent cyanotic congenital heart disease. 9.7% of all CHD. Risk of recurrence in siblings if there are no other affected first degree relatives is 3%.

CLINICAL FEATURES

1. *Cyanosis*: At some period in first 6 months cyanosis is noted in vast majority of cases. Cold and exertion increase degree of cyanosis. Clubbing of moderate degree is present with minimal cyanosis and is related to effort oxygen arterial desaturation.

2. *Dyspnea*: Prominent at first with feeding and crying, later with walking. Paroxysmal dyspnea associated with marked cyanosis is common during infancy. Such blue spells may occur without warning during infection or in summer months but are most likely to occur around time of breakfast or early evening hours. These incidents become frequent and prolonged between 9 and 18 months. During a severe blue spell an infant may become unconscious and develop paralysis. There is a tendency to reduction in frequency of blue spells between 18 months to 2 years due to development of collateral circulation. Appearance of blue spells are indication of major therapeutic moves. Etiology of blue spells is unclear. They result from a periodic marked reduction of already decreased blood flow to lungs. During these spells life is supported by collateral blood flow to lungs. There is disappearance of systolic murmur, reduction in arterial oxygen saturation, reduction in pulmonary vascularity and

increased voltage of P-wave with ST segment depression in standard limb lead of ECG during such spells. Development and morphological appearance of muscle in RVOT make it unusually susceptible to spasm. Most likely exciting stimulus is reflex. This is supported by fact that during spell an ESM ordinarily present and due to infundibular stenosis disappears to return on recovery. Circumstances precipitating such spells are many:

- Release of norepinephrin by increasing myocardial contractile force might create a temporary complete obstruction in a previously markedly narrowed and hypertrophied RVOT.
- Any situation that stimulates hyperpnea may precipitate an episode. Hyperpnea increases oxygen demand and cardiac output. Because pulmonary blood flow is relatively fixed in TOF a lowered oxygen saturation will result from increased venoarterial shunt. Low arterial oxygen tension and pH as well as high CO_2 tension combine to stimulate respiratory center to further hyperpnea especially when respiratory control has been rendered normally sensitive by benefit of sleep. A vicious cycle then result to be broken only when respiratory responses are depressed by exhaustion, sedation or general anesthesia.
- Some of these episodes may be related to severe metabolic acidosis.
- About 25% of patients with absent pulmonary valve will present with symptoms off severe airways obstruction due to bronchial compression.

3. *Squatting*: Closely allied to periodic dyspnea is postural change these subjects undertake. Infants prefer lying on one side hunched up like a fetus or in knee chest position. Older children avoid standing upright for long without movement of some sort or squat after effort. Oxygen saturation falls in these subjects even on quiet standing. Squatting enables return to previous levels and avoids any falls. Unfavorable postures by reducing venous return cause returning venous blood to contain lower level of oxygen. Thus less saturated

systemic venous blood mixing with saturated pulmonary venous blood results in an arterial mixture of lower saturation. Squatting acutely angulates lower limb blood vessels and so reduces blood flow to legs. An increase in cardiac output confined to upper portion of body results and arteriovenous oxygen difference consequentely lessened. Hypoxia to vital centers thereby reduced. Increase in cardiac output, blood pressure and PaO_2 occurs with reduction in right to left shunt during squatting. These effects may be due to gravity effect on circulation since this effect was not observed with squat lying. The explanation is that the posture adopted shifts blood from legs to lungs and heart and so increases left ventricle output. Beneficial effect of increased LV output is related to anatomic and functional relationship of VSD to aorta in TOF. Such change is not observed in pulmonary atresia, single ventricle with PS, PS with VSD placed lower in septum than in TOF or PS with interatrial communication.

Recent theory: Blood flow in IVC is decreased in squatting equivalent position. Beneficial effect of squatting is that this posture:

– Avoids syncope.
– Prevents blood of low PaO_2 reaching heart from legs so elevating arterial PaO_2 even if right to left shunt volume is unchanged.
– Increased pulmonary blood flow through an increase in systemic vascular resistance.

4. *Development*: Infants with TOF gain weight slowly. Physique is never optimal. 75% cases fall below average. Moon face suggestive of PS with normal aortic root also occurs. Mild thoracic deformities are common. Slight precordial bulge occurs in older infants. Scoliosis is much common.

Cardiovascular Findings

In average case apex beat is tapping and not displaced. Precordium is quiet. Second heart sound in pulmonary area varies in intensity. It is often loud. Exceptionally it is split. Single second heart sound is due to aortic valve closure. Delayed pulmonary valve closure is rarely heard. Aortic ejection sound is noted in cases with very severe PS or pulmonary atresia. Murmur may also be absent when obstruction is considerable but incomplete and at infundibular or valvular level or at both sites. Commonest murmur is a short, moderate intensity ESM at LSE due to infundibular stenosis. 75% cases have murmur in LICS 3–4. 25% in pulmonary area due to valvular stenosis.

Systolic murmur is accentuated within 15 minutes of administration of 0.25 to 0.5 mg phenylephrine. In rare case of absent one pulmonary artery murmur is best heard on the side opposite the absent main branch. Because most frequently left pulmonary artery is absent murmur is heard on right of sternum. In related absent pulmonary valve syndrome a to and fro murmur is commonly heard, there being a systolic ejection murmur and an early diastolic murmur widely distributed over chest. Continuous murmur in pulmonary area occurs in 10% cases. Soft continuous murmur means pulmonary atresia with marked collateral circulation through bronchial vessels. In infants PDA is responsible for continuous murmur but even in them aortopulmonary collateral flow is responsible for soft, diffuse continuous murmur. Diffuse continuous murmur is more likely to be due to numerous large collateral vessels and not a PDA. Continuous murmur over right upper chest is associated with right aortic arch and large collateral vessels to right upper lobe. Diastolic murmur may arise from bicuspid aortic valve. Thrills are not common during infancy. CHF never occurs in classic form of this malformation.

CHF may occur under following circumstances with TOF:

– Anemia.
– Systemic hypertension.
– Infective endocarditis.
– Single pulmonary artery.
– Absent pulmonary valve.
– Mild pulmonary stenosis.
– Subendocardial fibrosis.

Fundus

There is distension of veins in markedly cyanotic cases. Dilated tortuous retinal vessels and occasional papilledema correlates with low PaO_2 and high hematocrit values and is independent of age.

Atypical TOF

Infants presenting with clinical signs of large VSD, frequent respiratory infections, rasping systolic murmur with thrill at LICS4, split second heart sound and lack of cyanosis. ECG shows combined ventricular hypertrophy with QRS of + 90°. X-ray shows moderate cardiomegaly with increased lung vascularity. Right aortic arch is present. Cardiac catheterization reveals large left to right shunt at ventricular level, systemic systolic pressure in right ventricle, valvular pulmonary stenosis, normal pulmonary artery pressure, direct entry into aorta from right ventricle and absence of any right to left shunt by arterial sampling, dye dilutional studies, selective ether test and angiocardiography. Transformation from simple VSD without PS to TOF has occurred during infancy in most cases by age 4 years. A high incidence of this development in patients with VSD, right aortic arch and narrow RVOT has been noted. Relative hypoplasia of pulmonary valve ring is also present. Reason for development of increasing infundibular stenosis is an abnormal muscle bundle (Gasul phenomenon). Watson in 1971 described a syndrome of very severe right ventricle hypertrophy due to increasing infundibular stenosis with reduction in size of VSD.

Radiology

Most important constant findings are normal or near normal cardiac size and reduction of lung vascular markings.

Contour: Young infants in AP view contour is extremely variable especially when thymus contributes to mediastinal opacity. Tipped up apex may be a pointer but even this is found in some normal infants. Left heart border is normal at this age.

Older infants and children—clinical cases have been divided into four groups:

1. *Those with right aortic arch (30%)*: normal heart size, aortic knob or sweep up on right high border and no evidence of concavity on left middle arc.
2. *Those with infundibular chambers of moderate size (30%)*: These show a slight or distinct bulge along lower left middle arc. Aortic knob is not necessarily prominent.
3. *Those with slight bay shape in left middle arc (30%)*: Fluroscopy shows concavity better than AP X-ray. Aortic knob is clearly visible.
4. *Those with marked concavity of middle arc, large ascending aorta and aortic knob (10%)*: These usually represent pulmonary atresia, most severe type of malformation.

Rarely gross cardiac enlargement is found. Diagnosis is then impossible without further investigation.

Lung Vascularity

Study of lung vascular markings particularly at hilum permits an approximation of amount of blood flow to lungs.

Most cases have normal or slightly decreased vascular markings. Rib notching due to extensive collateral development in intercostal arterial system is rare in children preoperatively except in patient with absent usually left major branch of pulmonary artery. Unilateral pulmonary artery atresia when associated with absent pulmonary valve gives rise to tremendous increase in vascular markings in opposite lung.

Absence of pulmonary valve shows gross dilatation of major pulmonary arteries with reduced peripheral lung vascular markings. Signs of lung collapse and obstructive emphysema can be seen in this variant.

Sometimes left pulmonary artery is visibly enlarged and these cases almost invariably have systolic murmur in pulmonary area with associated valvular stenosis.

Hypovascularity of left upper lobe due to rotational effect on heart in severe degree of malformation whereby outflow jet of blood is directed more towards right pulmonary artery is seen in 20% cases of cyanotic TOF.

Barium swallow confirms side of aortic arch.

Barium will also reveal abnormality of aortic area branches such as retroesophageal subclavian vessel. In older cases enlarged bronchial arteries may indent barium filled esophagus. Approximately 50% of patients with severe uncorrected cyanotic heart malformation between 12 and 29 years will be found osteoporotic. A change accompanied by delayed skeletal maturation.

ECG

Common findings are right axis deviation and right ventricle hypertrophy.

1. *QRS axis*: moderate to marked RAD is present in all except in atypical group with increased pulmonary blood flow. In rare case of Pentalogy and Noonan's syndrome LAD has been recorded.
2. *P-wave*: RAH with tall P-waves occurs with increasing age.
3. Pattern of RVH with inverted R/S ratio is found (predominant R over right precordium, predominant S over left precordium). Transitional complex is situated in V1 or V2. This is characteristic ECG finding (40% cases).

   Incomplete RBBB occurs in 20% cases.

   Predominant LVH is extremely rare but electrical evidence of associated LVH is not infrequent. This may occur without any associated anomalies.

   When a deep Q is found in leads over left precordium LVH may be assumed to be present if RVH is present. This is seen in patient with left superior vena cava entering left atrium. Associated PDA also gives rise to LVH.

   Combined ventricular hypertrophy with predominant LVH occurs in atypical TOF with increased PBF.
4. *T-wave*: T-wave in V1 is only normally upright in first 24 hours of life and thereafter constitutes evidence of abnormal RVH. Inversion of T-wave in V1 is never normal in infants with TOF and when present it indicates that degree of RVH is more marked than usual.

   Frontal plane vector is inscribed in clockwise direction. Horizontal vector is more often clockwise

DIAGNOSIS: BLOOD GASES AND METABOLIC CHANGES

Arterial oxygen desaturation present at rest in most cases increases slightly with standing alone and markedly with exercise. Considerable rise occurs on inhalation of 100% oxygen. Arterial pH is below normal range in 1/3rd of cyanotic patients. Blood lactate and puruvate levels are inversely related to arterial oxygen tension.

Under ordinary resting conditions cyanotic patient with TOF has normal arterial pH and PaO_2.

During hypoxic spell there is profound drop in PaO_2 and marked metabolic acidosis may develop rapidly.

Blood Changes

Polycythemia is a common finding. Hematocrit is abnormally high. In polycythemic patients there is delicate balance between intravascular thrombosis and bleeding diathesis. Abnormalities of platelet function most frequent hemostatic disturbance. This is important for patients in whom open cardiac surgery is contemplated. Routine evaluation of common hemostatic factors is done prior to surgical intervention and appropriate therapy with epsilon amino caproic acid 48 hours before surgery is advised. In postoperative bleeding diathesis administration of fresh plasma with steroids is advised.

Echocardiography

Main variables are amount of PBF and degree of aortic overriding. LA size is normal except when there is increased PBF due to mild PS or there are collateral sources of PBF.

Mitral aortic valve continuity is necessary finding for diagnosis. Overriding of ventricular septum by aorta can be visualized. The more severe the PS larger will be aortic diameter.

In very severe TOF it is difficult to visualize pulmonary valve because of marked hypoplasia and rotation of RVOT.

Cardiac Catheterization

PBF is reduced and there is collateral bronchial arterial blood flow in older children with TOF.

In usual cyanotic form of this disorder LV pressure rise during isovolemic contraction precedes RV pressure rise so in this phase of cardiac cycle left to right shunt occurs.

During ventricular ejection both ventricles eject into aorta. In isovolemic relaxation when pressure in LV falls right to left shunt occurs across VSD.

RAP is normal. Prominent atrial 'a'-wave is unusual in young children but may develop in older patients and reflect increasing RVH and ventricular compliance change. RV pressure is equal to that in aorta. PAP is low.

Passage of catheter from RV to aorta is invariable. Isoproterenol increases right to left shunt and reduces arterial oxygen saturation in TOF. Propranolol in infants particularly can abolish this response as well as effect of exercise.

Angiocardiography

Determines site and degree of PS, size of pulmonary ring and MPA and presence of pulmonary arterial stenosis or hypoplasia. Additional information: whether there is a large VSD or single ventricle, mitral aortic valve continuity, mitral valve abnormalities, coronary artery anomaly and source of collateral PBF. In absence of pulmonary valve the most striking feature is an aneurysmal dilatation of right and left pulmonary artery with sharp narrowing distal to secondary arterial branches.

DIFFERENTIAL DIAGNOSIS: NEWBORN

For TOF to produce serious symptoms in newborn period is unusual. In serious TOF cyanosis presents in second week of life. Murmurs are absent or if present are continuous in these children. TGA may be confused but cyanosis is more marked and early in them and X-ray chest shows increased vascular markings. In tricuspid atresia and Ebstein anomaly ECG has characteristic LAD and LVH or RBBB with large P-waves respectively. Pulmonary atresia with normal aortic root has a larger heart and frequently develops CHF, normal axis with LVH in ECG. Asplenia syndrome presents with fatal hypoxia within 48 hours of birth. Diagnosis is with Howell Jolley bodies. CHF develops in some TOF with absent pulmonary valves. Characteristic loud to and fro murmur widely transmitted through the chest is diagnostic of this variant.

Older Children

Acyanotic forms of TOF are mistaken for isolated VSD or isolated PS depending upon degree of outflow tract obstruction that is present. Presence of right aortic arch should arouse suspicion of TOF. Murmur is long ejection systolic, second heart sound is normal and precordium quiet. ECG shows RVH invariably. In isolated PS murmur is usually upper along LSE and ejection click is heard.

Cyanotic forms of TOF are to be differentiated from:

A. Simple cyanotic malformations:

1. *Pulmonary stenosis with normal aortic root*: In severe form (Grandes Trilogy) onset of cyanosis is early. Squatting is exceptional. Prominent RV heave is present along LSE. Harsh ESM in LICS 2 and 3 is accompanied by thrill. Moon face is common. The 'a' wave is prominent in JVP. Heart is enlarged and although lung fields are clear a pulmonary artery bulge is visible. No right aortic arch. Extreme RVH in ECG. Cardiac catheterization localizes shunt at atrial level. RV pressure pulse above systemic level. Angiocardiography reveals wide RVOT and valvular stenosis with contrast entering a dilated main and left pulmonary artery.

   In pentalogy of Fallot (TOF with ASD) heart may function in some cases as tetrad hemodynamically and in other cases like severe PS with normal aortic root and venoarterial shunt. Right to left interatrial shunt occurs in Pentalogy only when there is severe PS, tricuspid valve deformity or Partial anomalous pulmonary venous drainage.

2. *Severe PS with small VSD*: This gives rise to profound cyanosis, prominent 'a'-wave in JVP, RV parasternal heave, single second heart sound and severe RVH in ECG. X-ray picture may remind of TOF more than PS.

3. *PS with VSD with hypoplastic RV*: Cyanosis is common from birth or early infancy. Large jugular 'a'waves are visible in neck. There is long loud ESM maximum in pulmonary area. Heart is slightly enlarged. X-ray picture resembles TOF. However, there is no RV parasternal heave and no RVH in ECG. Second heart sound may be paradoxically or reversed split.

4. *Anomalous muscle bundles in RV with VSD*: Clinical picture may resemble TOF. Obstruction is in mid RV and is a consequence of muscle bands other than parietal band. Selective RV angiogram with patient in RAO position shows a wide slanting filling defect within body of ventricle.

5. *TOF with unusual ECG signs*: LAD is occasionally seen. This is related to changes in conduction pathways of a primary or secondary nature, e.g. TOF with type B WPW syndrome, Noonan's syndrome, congenital rubella. Differentiation from Tricuspid atresia is based on RVH seen in ECG despite LAD.

B. Complex cyanotic malformations:

1. *DORV with PS*: Squatting is uncommon, ESM is longer and harsher. Chest X-ray shows a larger heart. ECG shows LV potentials but clinical picture may be very similar to TOF. RV selective angiogram shows aorta to be anteriorly placed in lateral view, parietal band of crista is missing in this projection and prominent in AP frames. Aortic mitral discontinuity is present. Clear distinction from TOF is not always possible and diagnosis is often evident at operating table.

2. *Complete TGV with PS*: Clinical picture may be identical with tetrad particularly in regard to cyanosis and clubbing, response at oximetry, ECG, small heart size and reduced lung vascular markings. Cyanotic spells and squatting are less frequently seen. Aortic bulge high on left heart border with downpointing apex may allow recognition of condition. Selective angiocardiography is the critical investigation.

3. *Single ventricle with PS*: X-ray contour of heart and ECG are different. Echo and angiocardiography separate the condition from TOF.
4. *Asplenia syndrome*: More likely in smaller infant but should be considered in all cyanotic children with reduced pulmonary blood flow. Plain X-ray may show ambiguous situs, symmetric liver shadow, central stomach or bilateral SVC. Howell-Jolly bodies in peripheral smear are seen. Liver and spleen scan are useful pointers to diagnosis.
5. *Rare conditions like double inlet left ventricle or mitral atresia with PS*: In older cases ECG may show certain differences, such as RBBB or LVH and dense hilar vascularity due to development of collateral circulation, all of which can argue for angiocardiography as the best means for confirming diagnosis.

PROGNOSIS

Average case becomes progressively more cyanosed and dyspneic after first 6 months. Many will have a period of blue spells during infancy. Developmental mile stones are delayed. After 2 years of life squatting or lying are common. At puberty dyspnea and cyanosis occur. Average age of survival is 12 years. Severe cases have early cyanosis, feeding difficulty and severe and prolonged blue spells often proceeding to CVA. They frequently die of anoxia in first year of life. Such cases have pulmonary atresia. Occasionally severe stenosis is associated with large PDA. These cases are not obviously cyanotic and therefore tend to present as isolated form of PDA. Such presentation is common in severe TOF in rubella syndrome. Major clue to underlying defect is RVH in ECG.

Cases with increased lung vascular markings: These may have markedly increased PBF or merely more than in mild cases of TOF.

1. *Atypical TOF*: Cases may die in infancy from infection or CHF. Extreme dystrophy is the rule. Those surviving develop classic TOF picture.

2. *Single pulmonary artery*: They have unilateral pulmonary plethora. Cyanosis is delayed in mild PS.

3. *Large PDA*: Cardiac enlargement is present in addition to increased lung vascular markings. ECG shows combined ventricular hypertrophy with LV dominance.

4. *Absent pulmonary valve*: Pulmonary artery has aneurysmal size. Compressing bronchus and may prove fatal in this account rather than cardiac disability.

Complications

Causes of death in TOF: Hypoxia, infection, thrombotic episode, cerebral abscess, CHF, infective endocarditis and heart block.

1. *CVA*: Venous sinus thrombosis, arterial thrombosis or embolism, widespread embolic episodes, gangrene of limbs. There is a relationship between development of hemiplegea and presence of relative anemia than with high hematocrit levels. In fact specific occlusions are rarely found and most infarcts are probably anoxic in nature.

2. *Cerebral abscess*: Uncommon in first two years of life. Headache, fever, lethargy are common symptoms with abrupt onset. Persistent vomiting and convulsions are late features. Insidious onset or sudden hemiparesis is less common. Embolus from infective endocarditis is practically never the cause of abscess. More likely explanation is that a small cerebral infarct is infected by one of transient, frequent systemic bacterimias in TOF. Treatment is with antibiotics and aspiration of abscess.

3. *Infective endocarditis*: Incidence is 14% of cyanotic cases. Streptococcus viridans and staphyllococcus are causative organisms.

4. *Tuberculosis*: There is an increased liability for cyanotic cases with PS to develop tuberculosis. Arterialization of blood in pulmonary artery aggravates pre-existing tuberculous lesion. Lung apical fibrosis in patients with long standing cyanosis should be considered before infective label is applied.

5. *CHF*: Rare in children with TOF but can occur in circumstances already mentioned under clinical features. It never occurs in classic case with usual anatomy and high hematocrit level.

6. *Pheochromocytoma*: Among 5 cases of this tumor in association with cyanotic CHD 2 cases were TOF (Folger 1964). Death may occur during shunt surgery in a patient without symptoms of adrenal tumor.

TREATMENT

Aim is to avoid recurrent hypoxic spells.

Anemia and dehydration should be corrected to avoid CVA and cerebral abscess.

Drugs in use for acute blue spell:

1. *Morphine*: 1 mg/5 kg body weight in combination with oxygen administration.

2. *Propranolol Intravenous*: reduces infundibular spasm.

3. *Phenylephrine infusion*: by acutely raising systemic resistance it improves systemic arterial oxygen level and has been advocated for protracted spells as medical treatment of choice. Treatment of developed cerebral thrombosis is by IV fluids and heparin.

Surgical treatment is necessary for symptomatic infant. Operation can be palliative or corrective at that age.

Palliation

1. *Blalock Taussig shunt*: This consists of anastomosis between a branch of aorta and one of pulmonary arteries. End to side anastomosis is conducted on side of chest opposite to that where aortic arch is situated. This crossed operation is more effective in young patients.

2. *Pott's operation*: This procedure consists of direct anastomosis between descending aorta and left pulmonary artery.

3. *Waterston shunt*: Ascending aorta is anastomosed to right pulmonary artery.

4. *Pulmonary valvulotomy and infundibulectomy* by incision into right ventricle.

5. *Glenn procedure*: *Vena caval* pulmonary artery shunt. Anastomosis of superior *vena cava* with distal end of divided right pulmonary artery. Useful in treatment of uncorrectable cyanotic malformations with pulmonary stenosis or pulmonary atresia.

Most palliative surgery is done under hypothermic conditions or normothermic conditions with hyperbaric oxygen.

Corrective

Closure of VSD by prosthetic patch, resection of infundibular stenosis and valvulotomy or relief of pulmonary arterial stenosis have become standard optimal treatment for TOF. Circulatory support during surgery is maintained by cardiopulmonary bypass combined with profound hypo-thermia.

Selection of Patients

Correction of TOF should be objective in every instance. Immediate correction at about 8 to 9 years is done regardless of nature of obstruction. Best results occur in children who are mildly cyanotic or acyanotic and in those with low infundibular stenosis or where anomalous muscle bundle is creating obstructive lesion.

Infants with severe symptoms of blue spells which are frequent and unrelated to anemia or who have faint murmurs when out of spell and for whom use of propranolol is contraindicated or not effective, surgical treatment is indicated. Shunts are performed in infancy. Correction is done in infancy only if shunt fails.

Complications of shunt procedure:

1. CHF and pulmonary vascular disease.
2. Infective endocarditis.
3. Subclavian steal syndrome.
4. Development of pulmonary hypertension.
5. Unilateral rib notching because collateral channels develop to supply affected areas following surgical interruption of subclavian artery.

6. Gangrene of arm.
7. Horner syndrome.
8. Diaphragmatic paralysis.
9. Vocal cord paralysis.
Hemothorax and atelectasis.

Complications of corrective surgery:

A. Immediate:
1. Bleeding requires surgical exploration.
2. Complete heart block requires myocardial pacing electrodes.
3. Respiratory distress due to pulmonary edema requires diuretics, ventillatory support and steroids.
4. Reduction in cardiac output due to ventriculotomy or ischemia due to cross clamping of aorta. Isoproteronol infusion is given. Digoxin may be added.

B. Late
1. Postpericardiotomy syndrome.
2. CHF due to residual ventricular shunt or tricuspid valve dysfunction.
3. Complete right bundle branch block.
4. Pulmonary regurgitation with right to left shunt at atrial level.
5. Outflow tract aneurysmal formation from patching.
6. Intrapulmonary shunts.

44

Persistent Left Superior Vena Cava

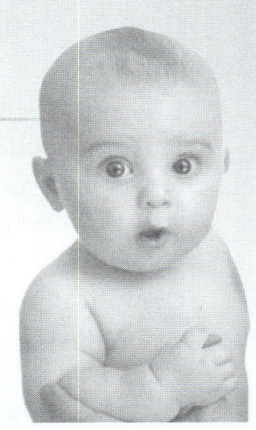

INCIDENCE

Once in 200 of general population. In CHD patients 3 to 5%.

Anatomy

Failure to atrophy of left anterior cardinal vein below origin of brachiocephalic vein. Thus after union of left jugular and left subclavian veins left superior *vena cava* descends vertically in thorax to left of spine.

Group A: Proximal connection of left superior *vena cava* to coronary sinus. Most frequent. Isolated anomaly. No functional disturbance. ASD and PAPVD may be associated. Anomalies of inferior *vena cava* may be associated.

Group B: Proximal connection of left superior *vena cava* to left atrium. Isolated anomaly. There may be mild cyanosis.

Group C: No proximal connection of left superior *vena cava*. Two types:

1. Union of left superior *vena cava* and pulmonary veins. In PAPVD and TAPVD pulmonary veins unite and enter left superior *vena cava* that has a connection with systemic venous circulation at left innominate vein only.

2. Left superior *vena cava* associated with atresia of ostium of coronary sinus. Venous blood from heart reaches right atrium indirectly through left superior *vena cava*, left innominate vein and right superior *vena cava*. Other cardiac malformations may be present.

Diagnosis

One-third of patients with left superior *vena cava* draining into coronary sinus and congenital intracardiac defect show LAD of P-wave.

Abnormal left jugular pulsations may be first physical clue to persistence of left superior *vena cava*.

An X linked recessive form of Pierre Robin syndrome with left superior *vena cava* and ASD has been described.

In X-ray chest a vertical venous shadow is seen along left border of supracardiac portion of mediastinum. This sign is present after 6 months of life in association with total anomalous pulmonary venous drainage into left superior *vena cava*. Nuclear angiography confirms these arrangements.

During cardiac catheterization from left antecubital vein catheter enters left superior *vena cava* and right heart via coronary sinus in group A cases. Left atrium and left ventricle in group B cases. Pulmonary veins in group C.

In complicated cases angiocardiography is useful.

Treatment

Group A: No treatment.

Group B: Simple ligation of left superior *vena cava* provided a superior *vena cava* exists on right side. Alternatively anastomosis of anomalous vessel to right atrium may be performed.

Group C: Treatment of anomalous pulmonary venous drainage.

45

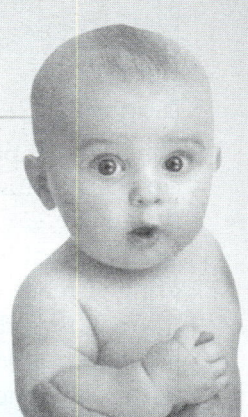

Total Anomalous Pulmonary Venous Drainage

PATHOLOGY

A. *Complicated form*: A variety of associated intracardiac defects have been described:

- Cor biloculare
- Single ventricle
- Transposition of great vessels
- Truncus arteriosus
- Ventricular septal defect
- Tetralogy of Fallot
- Tricuspid atresia
- Asplenia
- Gross systemic venous anomalies.
- In 25% of these cases pulmonary veins communicate with right heart through connection below diaphragm.
- In 10% direct connection into right atrium.

The remainder insert in superior *vena cava* or left superior *vena cava* or have multiple insertions of which one is superior *vena cava* and other either innominate vein, portal vein or inferior *vena cava*.

Less common sites of insertion are right innominate, left gastric, hepatic or azygous veins and sinus venosus. Two-third of cases have heterotaxy. Associated pulmonary atresia and complex intracardiac malformations are common.

B. *Isolated form*: Commonest variety is where all four pulmonary veins drain into left innominate vein through left superior *vena cava*.

Next commonest is drainage of all four pulmonary veins into coronary sinus, followed by infradiaphragmatic connections and drainage into right atrium and superior *vena cava*.

Darling in 1957 classified TAPVD into four groups:

Group 1: Supracardiac

Group 2: Cardiac

Group 3: Infracardiac

Group 4: Mixed

Most commonly all four pulmonary veins unite to form single large sinus like channel which then joins systemic circulation at particular level.

Pulmonary venous obstruction may occur either because the connecting vein is obstructed at some point in its course prior to the site of connection to systemic circuit or because the orifice of anomalous connecting vein is small at site of insertion into right side.

Right ventricle and right atrium are strikingly enlarged and dilated. Left ventricle cavity is compromised by severe septal displacement with a reduced left heart inflow which contributes to low systemic output in these cases.

There is an interatrial communication due to patent foramen ovale or large secundum ASD.

- PDA is present in 25% cases.
- Pulmonary artery is dilated.
- Tricuspid valve ring is larger than mitral.
- Pulmonary vascular disease is present in presence of pulmonary venous obstruction.
- Subendocardial infarction is found in many cases during infancy affecting right ventricle papillary muscles.

Frequency

1 to 3% of all cardiac malformations. Male preponderance is seen.

Hemodynamics

In isolated form oxygenated blood returning from lungs enters right atrium directly or indirectly usually by means of a single common pulmonary vein. Thus pulmonary venous blood with high oxygen saturation mixes with systemic venous blood of low oxygen saturation in right atrium. Blood then passes from right atrium through a defect in interatrial septum to left heart and aorta and through tricuspid valve to right ventricle and pulmonary artery.

CLINICAL FEATURES

A. *Complicated form*: In those cases complicated by major intracardiac malformation life expectancy is prolonged by TAPVD which acts as a natural partial correction.

B. *Isolated form*: Clinical picture is determined by four variables:

   1. Factors that govern pulmonary blood flow, e.g. level of pulmonary arteriolar resistance and tone of ductus arteriosus.

   2. Degree of pulmonary venous obstruction—anatomic obstruction at connecting site, within pulmonary vein, external compression of anomalous vein or relative pulmonary venous obstruction associated with torrential pulmonary blood flow.

   3. Nature of atrial communication—patent foramen ovale, ASD secundum.

   4. State of right ventricle myocardium—whether or not there is infarction.

Clinical presentation occurs in three main forms:

1. Infant with low PVR, huge PBF, small foramen ovale, no organic pulmonary venous obstruction but with subendocardial infarction of RV muscle.

2. Infant with pulmonary venous obstruction.
3. Asymptomatic or mildly symptomatic older child with normal PVR, ASD secundum and no pulmonary venous obstruction.

Infant with High PBF

Earliest sign encountered is tachypnea and cyanosis. Cyanosis is obvious in perinatal period. It tends to diminish or even clear in half of cases. In majority a muddy discoloration of equivocal cyanosis is more usual at rest. More obvious cyanosis or intense cyanosis though can be seen at late stage is most often an indication that pulmonary venous obstruction coexists. Clubbing is rare. Tachypnea is always present. At this stage cyanosis is absent, infant does not look ill. Over next few weeks infant fails to gain weight and becomes dusky intermittently. Failure to thrive is invariable. Striking dystrophy is present after a day or two. Inevitably liver becomes enlarged, precordium bulges, heart obviously overactive and gallop rhythm and cardiac murmur develop. These signs of right ventricle failure are present in 50% cases in first month of life.

CHF in first week of life occurs in 60% of all cases. First heart sound is very loud. Second heart sound is closely split. Splitting is fixed. Third heart sound is common.

Commonest murmur is soft ESM over LSE. A blowing ESM along lower LSE due to tricuspid regurgitation is characteristic in perinatal period. Loud regurgitant murmur of this sort present very serious prognosis because it indicates major subendocardial damage of RV muscle and appreciable interference with tricuspid valve apparatus.

An MDM of tricuspid origin is common and is more frequent in patients with less severe pulmonary hypertension. Continuous murmur due to turbulence along anomalous venous channel is common in cases with pulmonary vascular obstruction.

Infant with Pulmonary Venous Obstruction

These have a brief and stormy life characterized by early appearing and intense cyanosis worsened during feeding.

Marked dyspnea is a feature and liver is usually enlarged. Murmurs are inconspicuous. Death occurs due to pulmonary edema or anoxia. Mildly symptomatic older child:

Mild exertional dyspnea is chief complaint. Long-term survivors behave like patients with simple secundum defect.

ECG

There is moderate RAD. P-waves are abnormally tall and peaked after one to two months of age. RVH is of marked degree. Most striking feature is presence of Q-waves in right precordial leads. This is due to large right atrium and possibly indirectly of papillary muscle infarction. Complete RBBB and type B WPW syndrome are reported. T-waves are upright in first two weeks of life and become inverted with increasing age. With increasing RV strain T-waves inversion extends across left chest leads. This reflects ischemic change.

In patients with left to right shunt in PDA biventricular hypertrophy is noted.

RADIOLOGY

In patients with pulmonary venous obstruction heart is usually normal in size. Lung fields show fluffy opacification due to pulmonary venous congestion. Presence of Kerley B lines is useful sign of pulmonary venous obstruction especially in newborn. Other types have increased lung vascularity.

Progressive cardiomegaly occurs in first few months of life. RVOT enlargement obscures pulmonary artery dilatation. This appearance of left cardiac border gives rise to box like contour. Box like contour is also seen in:

- Atrioventricularis communis
- Partial anomalous pulmonary venous drainage (TAPVD) with ASD with VSD.
- Aorta is left sided and small.
- A localized indentation of anterior aspect of barium filled esophagus just above diaphragm in lateral films has been described as additional characteristic of infradiaphragmatic type of connection.

Snowman appearance or figure of 8 appearance:

A specific cardiac contour first described by Snellen and Albers in 1952. The contour takes sometime to develop. Occasionally being evident before age of 4 months. This contour is present when all four pulmonary veins drain into innominate vein via a persistent left superior *vena cava*. Dilatation of left superior *vena cava*, left innominate vein and right superior *vena cava* then produce a rounded supracardiac shadow which with rest of the heart results in figure of 8 appearance.

Differential diagnosis of snowman appearance:

- Expiration chest film of normal children.
- Partial anomalous pulmonary venous drainage into left superior *vena cava*.
- Mediastinal neoplasm.
- Large thymus.
- Severe pulmonary stenosis with left superior *vena cava* draining into coronary sinus with development of CHF.
- Unilateral emphysema from compression of left main bronchus between left vertical vein and left pulmonary artery occurs rarely.

Echocardiography

Large RV chamber with abnormal septal motion is described. Normal septal motion with pulmonary hypertension is also seen. LA dimensions may be minute. LV mitral valve and aortic measurements are at lower limit of normal for patient's age. Common pulmonary venous channel may be identified behind LA posterior wall.

Cardiac Catheterization

1. *Blood oxygen saturation*: Level of insertion of pulmonary veins can be established by noting the site at which high blood oxygen saturation is obtained.

    Oxygen saturation of blood from RA and systemic arteries remains high as long as high PBF is maintained. In high PVR oxygen saturation of blood from RA and systemic arteries is reduced.

2. *Pressures*: In infants PHT is found in all cases. In older children PAP is normal or slightly elevated.

   In presence of pulmonary venous obstruction pressure differences across obstructed point within pulmonary vein range as high as 30 to 60 mm Hg.

3. *Exploration with catheter*: It is usually possible by manipulation with catheter tip to pass into anomalous pulmonary veins attached to left innominate vein through persistent left superior *vena cava*.

   If left pulmonary vein can as well be entered from superior vena the evidence is strong for total anomaly.

4. *Indicator dilution*: A short appearance time with a double tip characteristic of right to left shunt and prolonged disappearance time or flattened curve when shunt patterns are obscured.

Angiography

Selective contrast injections into MPA result in visualization of all four pulmonary veins and resultant connection to systemic circuit.

DIAGNOSIS

Failure to gain weight may be presenting symptom in infants. Tachypnea, precordial bulge and mild cyanosis on crying occurs. After several months obvious signs appear, such as heart murmur, cyanosis and CHF.

Diagnosis at this stage of TAPVD unassociated with major intracardiac defects is based on general dystrophic appearance, mild cyanosis, absent or nonspecific murmur, cardiac enlargement with increased lung vascularity on chest X-ray and QR pattern in right precordial leads indicating RAH and RVH in ECG. Exception to this general picture occurs in pulmonary venous obstruction where there is intense cyanosis at birth, normal heart size and death by 3 months age from anoxia or CHF.

Differential Diagnosis in Newborn

1. Mitral or aortic atresia: Very early CHF.
2. Congenital mitral stenosis.
3. Cor triatriatum: This rare malformation consists of an accessory chamber that lies within LA and receives pulmonary veins. The abnormality results from entrapment of LA ostium of common pulmonary vein by that tissue of right horn of sinus venosus from which septum primum develops. This entrapment leads to failure of common pulmonary vein to be incorporated into LA during 5th week of fetal life.
4. Individual stenosis of pulmonary veins.
5. Lymphangiectasis.
6. Transient tachypnea of newborn.
7. Transient myocardial ischemia
8. Ostium primum ASD: Produces large heart and CHF. ECG shows LAD and LVH. LA is enlarged.
9. ASD secundum associated with anomalous insertion of right pulmonary vein.
10. Complete TGV: Early cyanosis. egg shaped heart in chest X-ray.

TAPVD in Older Children

Closely resembles isolated ASD.

Differentiation of Types of TAPVD

In 25% cases of persistent left superior *vena cava* a continuous murmur is audible in pulmonary area. Figure of 8 contour is present in X-ray chest.

Echocardiography is useful in confirming diagnosis.

Prognosis

Over 80% cases die in infancy. Worst prognosis is with insertion of anomalous channel at infradiaphragmatic level.

In absence of pulmonary venous obstruction a large ASD will enhance patient survival by permitting easy, e.g. ress of mixed venous blood to systemic circulation.

Adverse factors are anatomic pulmonary venous obstruction, early development of low PVR and right ventricle myocardial infarctions.

Treatment

Indications for surgery:

1. Organic pulmonary venous obstruction producing severe symptoms in infancy.
2. Infradiaphragmatic connection.
3. Chronic CHF.

Techniques

1. Anastomosis of common pulmonary vein to LA.
2. Obliteration of connection between common pulmonary vein and systemic venous system.
3. Closure of interatrial communication.

A technique involving anastomosis of common pulmonary vein to both atria and construction of a pericardial conduit across floor of fossa ovalis has been successfully applied to patients with extremely small LA.

Long-term results in survivors are excellent.

46

Approach to Diagnosis in Congenital Heart Disease

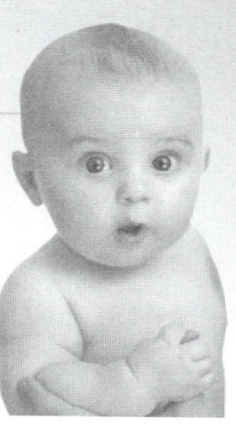

From diagnostic standpoint there are three major cardiac segments also called developmental units or building blocks of heart:

1. Visceroatrial situs (location of viscera and atria).
2. Ventricular loop (location of ventricles).
3. Conotruncus (location of infundibulum and great arteries).

General idea of segmental approach to diagnosis in CHD is:

1. Diagnose anatomic type of each of three major cardiac segments.
2. Mentally put the three major segments together. This is segmental combination or set of atria, ventricles and great arteries.
3. Search for associated malformations within each of three major segments and between them.
4. Assess function or physiologic resultants of system (segmental combination and associated malformations).
5. Assess therapeutic options both medical and surgical. Segmental approach to diagnosis is independent of cardiac position because it rests on basic developmental and anatomical positions and principles. This approach applies to normally located hearts as well as to abnormally located hearts.

There are at cardiac segments or independent units composing the heart:

1. *Sinus venosus*: This forms venous portion of morphological RA, SVC, IVC, coronary sinus, right and left venous valves, inferior limbic band and septum primum.
2. *Primitive atrium*: Forms muscular part of both atria, right and left atrial appendages and septum secundum.
3. *Common pulmonary vein*: Forms right and left pulmonary veins and smooth dorsal wall of left atrium between pulmonary veins.
4. *Atrioventricular canal*: Endocardial cushions of AV canal form tricuspid and mitral valve and canal septum.
5. Ventricle of bulboventricular loop forms morphological left ventricle.
6. Proximal bulbus cordis of bulboventricular loop gives rise to morphological right ventricle.
7. Distal bulbus cordis forms infundibulum.
8. Truncus arteriosus gives rise to ascending aorta and MPA.

ATRIAL LOCALIZATION

Types of visceroatrial situs:
1. Situs solitus (normal)
2. Situs inversus (mirror image of normal)
3. Situs ambiguous (syndromes of asplenia or polysplenia but can occur with normal spleen).

Type of visceral situs and type of atrial situs almost always are the same, e.g. both in situs solitus, inversus or ambiguous. These are visceroatrial concordances.

In X-ray chest location of stomach bubble and liver shadow usually indicate the atrial location:

1. Right liver shadow and left sided stomach bubble indicates situs solitus of atria and viscera.
2. Left sided liver shadow and right sided stomach bubble indicates situs inversus of atria and viscera.
3. An abnormally symmetric liver shadow and a shifting stomach bubble (that can be left sided, midline or right sided

because of a common gastrointestinal mesentery) should suggest asplenia. Bilateral right sidedness is characteristic of asplenia. Right and left sided air bronchograms both have appearance of a right air bronchogram because of presence of an eparterial bronchus bilaterally (bronchus to right upper lobe normally is upon or passes over right pulmonary artery, hence right upper lobe bronchus is eparterial).

In polysplenia bilateral left sidedness is typical.

Normally left main bronchus is hyparterial, it passes beneath left pulmonary artery.

Normally there is no eparterial branch of left bronchus. In high KV films patients with polysplenia often have left airbronchograms bilaterally. They appear long and concave superiorly.

Methods of atrial Localization

1. *X-ray chest*: Provides 3 clues—liver shadow, stomach bubble, air bronchogram.

2. *ECG*: By spatial axis of P-wave. Reliable, except when supraventricular arrhythmia is present. When P-waves suggest situs inversus (negative P-wave in lead 1) one should think of asplenia syndrome.

   In asplenia there is high incidence of bilateral superior *vena cava* with bilateral sinoatrial nodes. Frequent similarity of P-waves in asplenia and situs inversus appears to reflect high incidence of left superior *vena cava* and left sinoatrial node in asplenia. When chest X-ray suggests one type of visceroatrial situs and ECG suggests other this dichotomy suggests possibility of asplenia or polysplenia.

3. *Angiography*: Utilizes *vena cava*e and pulmonary veins and shape of atrial appendages which is usually distinctive and different. Right atrial appendage is large, broad and pyramidal. Left atrial appendage is relatively small, narrow and tubular. Hepatic inferior *vena cava* visualized by reflex of contrast following venous or selective right atrial angiocardiography can be used for atrial localization (in absent inferior *vena cava*, hepatic inferior *vena cava* is present).

4. Surgical inspection: Permits accurate atrial localization by seeing shape of appendages on opening the pericardium. If both appendages are large, broad and pyramidal (bilateral right sidedness) asplenia is present.

   Atrial septal surface morphologies can also be utilized at open heart surgery: Right atrium is that atrium which on its septal surface displays septum secundum.

   Left atrium on its septal surface displays septum primum, the flap valve of foramen ovale.

   Septum primum lies to left of septum secundum in situs solitus, to the right of septum secundum in situs inversus and in asplenia septum primum is poorly lateralized relative to septum secundum or deficient hence situs ambiguous.

5. *Cardiac catheterization*: Inferior *vena cava* to right atrium concordance. When present inferior *vena cava* always returns to right atrium even if it has to switch sides to do so. Thus, the course of catheter through inferior *vena cava* is reliable diagnostic marker of right atrium

VENTRICULAR LOCALIZATION

Types of ventricular loops: Precardiac mesoderm of cardiogenic crescent migrates cephalically and medially to form straight cardiac tube. Normally straight cardiac tube turns to right forming a D loop (dextro or right). Abnormally straight tube bends to left forming L loop. D loop formation places proximal bulbus cordis (future RV) to right of ventricle of bulbo-ventricular loop (future LV) resulting in normally interrelated ventricles.

   L loop formation places proximal bulbus cordis (future RV) to left of ventricle of bulboventricular loop (future LV) resulting in ventricular inversion.

   Ventricular D loop is RV right sided. Ventricular L loop is RV left sided.

   Mechanism underlying D loop formation: Loop formation is due to change in shape of myocardial cells. This change in cell shape depends upon myofibril formation. Myofibrils appear to function as cytoskeleton, controlling shape of cardiac myocytes. This protein dependent change (myofibril dependent) in cell shape is reflected at organ level as D loop formation. Since protein (myofibril) formation is under genetic control, cell shape change depending upon cytoskeletons of various protein types may prove to be one of the mechanisms linking genome to organ morphogenesis.

Method of ventricular localization:

1. *Selective biventricular angiocardiography*: Best method, by direct visualization of distinctive and different internal morphologies of RV and LV. RV is globular in shape, LV is foot shaped in diastole and tail shaped in systole. RV is coarsely trabeculated. LV is finely trabeculated or nontrabeculated. Moderator band of RV can be seen.

2. Arterial method: It involves two main considerations:
   – relationship between great arteries at semilunar valves.
   – origin and distribution of coronary arteries.

   Loop rule summarizes usual relationship between great arteries and ventricles.

   Usual or solitus type of normally related great arteries, D transposition and D malposition of great arteries (transposed or malposed aortic valve to right relative to transposed or malposed pulmonary valve) usually are associated with D loop (RV right sided).

   In inverted or mirror image type of normally related great arteries, L transposition and L malposition of great arteries (transposed or malposed aortic valve to left relative to transposed or malposed pulmonary valve) usually are associated with L loop (RV left sided).

   Usual type of normal relationship between great arteries, usual type of transposition and usual type of malposition of great arteries are associated with normally interrelated ventricles. Inverted type of normally related great arteries, inverted transposition and inverted malposition of great arteries is associated with ventricular inversion.

   Malposition of great arteries indicates an abnormal relationship between great arteries but in which great arteries are not transposed. Example of malposition are DORV, DOLV and anatomically corrected relationship.

With D loop coronary arteries are not inverted.

With L loop coronary arteries are inverted.

Given good coronary visualization by selective coronary angiography distribution of coronary arteries is helpful in localizing ventricles. Periventricular branches particularly marginal branch is characteristic of RV and diagonals to large anterolateral and posteromedial papillary muscle groups is very characteristic of LV.

With D loop anterior descending coronary artery arises from left coronary both with normally related great arteries and with D transposition. But with L loop anterior descending originates from right coronary artery both with inverted normally related great arteries and with L transposition.

3. *Deductive echocardiography*: When aortic valve lies to right of pulmonary valve D loop is present. Aortic valve is to right and posterior with normally related great arteries, to right and side by side with TOF and DORV and to right and anterior with D transposition. Thus both normally and abnormally aorta is right sided with D loop. Aortic valve is left sided with L loop. Posterior and left with inverted type of normally related great arteries, side by side and left with TOF and DORV (left sided) and anterior and left with L transposition.

When aortic valve is to right of pulmonary valve this is called D conotruncus.

When aortic valve is to left of pulmonary valve this is called L conotruncus.

Tricuspid valve septal leaflet normally does not separate far from right ventricle septal surface because septal leaflet of tricuspid valve is attached to RV septal surface. By contrast septal or medial leaflet of mitral valve does separate widely from left ventricle septal surface because normally septal leaflet of mitral valve does not attach to LV septal surface. These differences can be elicited echocardiographically.

Semilunar–atrioventricular contiguity or separation can be appreciated echocardiographically. Since diameter of pulmonary artery is greater than aorta and since component of second heart sound associated with closure of pulmonary valve usually follows component associated with aortic valve closure it may be possible to determine which great artery is which.

In aortic: Mitral contiguity the great arteries are normally related.

In pulmonary: Mitral contiguity there is D or L transposition.

In semilunar: Atrioventricular discontiguity there is bilateral conus with DORV.

Aortic: Mitral and pulmonary—mitral contiguity is seen in DOLV.

4. *Deductive electrocardiography*: Based on morphologies of unipolar QRS complexes which in turn are related to sequence of ventricular activation. Abnormalities of ventricular conduction make ECG unreliable for ventricular localization.

TYPES OF CONOTRUNCUS

1. Subpulmonary truncus is associated with normally related great arteries in situs solitus and situs inversus. Underdevelopment of subpulmonary conus results in TOF. Atresia of subpulmonary conus plus a truncal septal defect results in truncus arteriosus communis. Hypoplasia and leftward displacement of conal septum producing subaortic narrowing is present with interruption of aortic arch. Isolated ventricular inversion is situs solitus of atria and viscera, ventricular L loop and solitus type of normally related great arteries. Isolated ventricular noninversion is situs inversus of viscera and atria, ventricular D loop and inverted type of normally related great arteries. Both isolated ventricular inversion and isolated ventricular noninversion have normally related great arteries and hence have subpulmonary conus with aortic mitral fibrous continuity.

These two entities constitute isolated ventricular discordance: isolated ventricular inversion in situs solitus and isolated ventricular noninversion in situs inversus.

2. *Subaortic conus*: Pulmonary mitral fibrous continuity. Typical TGA has subaortic conus. Anatomically corrected malposition of great arteries also has subaortic conus.

3. *Bilateral conus*: Presence of conal musculature beneath both aortic and pulmonary valves prevents any semilunar atrioventricular fibrous continuity. Bilateral conus occurs in TGA with pulmonary infundibular stenosis and VSD. Occasionally it occurs with TGA and VSD without PS. DORV has bilateral conus, e.g. Taussig Bing malformation. Asplenia syndrome has bilateral conus with pulmonary infundibular stenosis. DORV is the rule in asplenia not TGA. Bilateral conus also occurs in juxtaposition of atrial appendages syndrome, anatomically corrected malposition of great arteries and normally related great arteries very rarely.

4. *Absent conus*: Conal muscle can be absent or rudimentary beneath both semilunar valve but some conal musculature is present above RV.

   Taussig Bing malformation: DORV, bilateral conus and subpulmonary VSD.

ANATOMIC TYPES OF CONGENITAL DEXTROCARDIA

In order of frequency:
1. Normal heart (30%). Solitus normal exceeds inverted normal (classic mirror image dextrocardia)
2. Corrected TGA (28%)
3. Single ventricle (20%)
4. Asplenia (18%)
5. Complete TGA (12%)

There is tendency towards dextrocardia in juxtaposition of atrial appendages syndrome.

20% cases of DORV have dextrocardia. All of these have pulmonary outflow tract stenosis.

Lev's Classification of Dextrocardia

1. *Dextroversion*: Normal type of heart with complete transposition.

2. *Presumptive dextroversion*: Same as dextroversion except that classification of atria as being in situs solitus is not certain due to coexistence asplenia or polysplenia.

3. *Mirror image dextrocardia*: Inverted normal type of heart and complete transposition in situs inversus.

4. *Presumptive mirror image dextrocardia*: Same as above except that situs inversus of atria is anatomically uncertain usually because of coexistence of asplenia or polysplenia syndrome and associated abnormal atrial septal morphologies.

5. *Mixed dextrocardia*: Indicates ventriculoatrial discordance, e.g. corrected transposition, isolated ventricular inversion, isolateral ventricular noninversion and anatomically corrected malposition.

6. *Dextrocardia type undetermined*: Indicates that atria and ventricles cannot be identified morphologically.

Essentially there are three main types:

1. *Dextroversion*: Normal heart in right chest.
2. *Mirror image dextrocardia*: Inverted normal heart.
3. *Mixed dextrocardia*: Heart with ventriculoatrial discordance.

ASPLENIA AND POLYSPLENIA SYNDROMES

When one thinks of dextrocardia one should think of asplenia and polysplenia and of complex CHD. that typifies these syndromes, e.g. common atrioventricular canal, with or without tricuspid or mitral stenosis or atresia, single ventricle, DORV, TGA with pulmonary outflow tract stenosis or atresia, common atrium, bilateral superior *vena cava*, interruption of inferior *vena cava* with azygous extension to superior *vena cava*, TAPVD and ipsilateral PVD.

In view of complex CHD associated usually with asplenia and less frequently with polysplenia such cases have to be assessed very carefully even for palliative shunt surgery, e.g. TAPVD with obstruction will become evident only following a shunt procedure when pulmonary edema develops in association with radiologic picture of pulmonary venous obstruction (butterfly pattern in chest X-ray PA view).

Diagnosis

1. Symmetric liver shadow.
2. Shifting stomach bubble.
3. Bilateral right air bronchogram in asplenia.
   Bilateral left air bronchogram in polysplenia.
4. Howell-Jolly bodies in peripheral smear.
5. Splenic artery angiography (during angiocardiography)
6. Splenic scan.

Dextrocardia, mesocardia and isolated levocardia all are associated with splenic dysgenesis (asplenia, polysplenia, accessory spleen) and visceral heterotaxy.

Asplenia: Congenital absence of spleen.

Polysplenia: Multiple small splenic nodules, i.e. rudimentary or hypoplastic spleen.

Accessory spleen: Normal spleen plus additional splenic tissue.

Heterotaxy: Scrambling. Hetero = other, taxis = arrangement.

Isolated levocardia is 80% splenic dysgenesis plus 20% situs inversus. Consequently isolated levocardia should be regarded as splenic dysgenesis until proven otherwise.

Associated malformations with asplenia syndrome:

- Bilateral trilobed lungs.
- Bilateral superior *vena cava*.
- TAPVD.
- Common AV canal.
- Pulmonary atresia.
- Coarctation of aorta.

Accessory spleens and asplenia frequently coexist. Asplenia has bilateral trilobed lungs (bilateral right sidedness). Polysplenia has bilateral bilobed lungs (bilateral left sidedness). Accessory spleen has normal bronchial pattern in majority. Asplenia has right sided inferior *vena cava*.

In polysplenia suprarenal to subhepatic segment of inferior *vena cava* is absent as also with accessory spleen.

TAPVD is rule with asplenia.

Ipsilateral pulmonary veins are typical of polysplenia. Common AV canal is common to all three groups.

Normal relationship of great arteries is a rule with polysplenia. Transposition is common with asplenia and accessory spleen. Pulmonary outflow tract obstruction occurs with asplenia and accessory spleen.

Antibiotic prophylaxis for asplenia: Fulminating pneumococcal septicemia is common with asplenia. These individuals have greatly increased risk of infection with encapsulated bacteria, e.g. Klebsiella or *E. coli* in infants, Pneumococci or *H. influenzae* in older children. In view of prevalence of pneumococcal and *H. influenzae* sepsis in patients of congenital asplenia continuous antibiotic prophylaxis is recommended.

KARTAGENER SYNDROME

Triad of

1. Situs inversus totalis,

2. Paranasal sinusitis,

3. Bronchiectasis.

Described in 1933 by Kartagener.

This syndrome typically occurs in children with mirror image dextrocardia and functionally normal heart.

Bronchiectasis occurs in 25% cases with situs inversus. Cause of bronchiectasis in this syndrome is congenital anatomic and hence functional defect of mucocilliary epithelium. Cilia do not move or beat in normal fashion. Lack of dynein arms in cilia of respiratory epithelium leads to immotile respiratory cilia thereby setting stage for development of bronchiectasis.

Infertility may occur due to lack of dynein arms in tails of spermatozoa leading to immotile spermatozoa.

Situs inversus totalis is due to single recessive autosomal gene. Layton's hypothesis is that situs inversus and situs ambiguous both are randomly occurring results of absence of dominant gene for situs solitus.

Clinical Features and Diagnosis

1. *Dextrocardia with normal type of heart*: Chest X-ray shows right sided liver shadow and left sided stomach bubble.

   ECG shows spatial AP being oriented anteriorly, inferiorly and leftward. RS complexes from V8R to V2 suggest presence of large right sided right ventricle. QRS complexes from V3 to V5 suggest that left ventricle is left sided.

   Angiocardiography confirms right sided right ventricle and left sided left ventricle.

   Associated malformation: Hemivertebrae can be seen through stomach bubble. This suggests possibility that dextrocardia is secondary to aplasia or hypoplasia of right lung. Right pulmonary artery may be hypoplastic. There may be anomalous systemic arterial supply, anomalous right pulmonary venous drainage to superior *vena cava* and inferior *vena cava*.

   Due to severe hypoplasia of right lung normal heart is right sided and posterior. Normal left aortic arch as it passes from right to left side compresses trachea anteriorly. Severe tracheal compression and respiratory distress thus occurs without vascular ring.

2. *Dextrocardia with corrected transposition*: Situs solitus is indicated by liver shadow and stomach bubble in X-ray chest, P-wave in ECG and catheter location of inferior *vena cava*.
   ECG: QRS complex in V6 suggests left sided left ventricle. Angiocardiographically L TGA is present.

   Associated malformation: subpulmonary VSD, permitting large left to right shunt may cause CHF.

3. *Dextrocardia with corrected TGA in situs inversus*: X-ray chest shows right sided stomach bubble and left sided liver shadow. ECG P-wave and catheter in left sided inferior *vena cava*.

   Angiocardiography confirms left sided and anterior left ventricle and right sided and posterior right ventricle. Bilateral conus is present.

   TGA is rule with discordant ventricular loop (when ventricles do not correspond to atria).

Associated malformation: Pulmonary stenosis, VSD of AV canal type, hypoplastic right ventricle, overriding tricuspid valve, right sided aortic arch.

Conclusion

Approach to diagnosis of right sided heart should be like that of left sided heart using segmental and morphological approach. ECG, X-ray chest and angiocardiogram should not be "corrected" for dextrocardia except for mirror image dextrocardia with inversion of both atria and ventricles, then "correction" of ECG by reversal of arm and precordial leads may assist interpretation. Dextrocardia in an infant with tracheoesophageal fistula may be secondary to aspiration and atelectasis of right lung. Isolated levocardia means heart is left sided.

There is situs inversus or ambiguous which is associated with visceral heterotaxy and splenic dysgenesis.

47

Rheumatic Fever

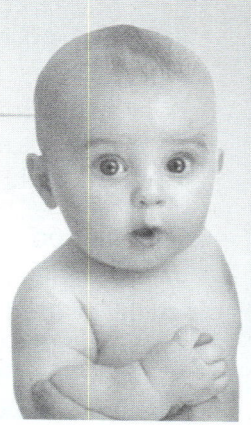

Rheumatic fever is a clinical syndrome chief manifestations of which are arthritis, heart disease, subcutaneous nodules, erythema marginatum and chorea.

- Either gender may be involved.
- Maximum incidence between 5 and 15 years age.

Etiology

1. *Infection*: Group A hemolytic streptococcus. First attacks of rheumatic fever are precipitated by streptococcal infection at an interval of few days to five weeks. During this interval there may be an immune response to hemolytic streptococcus which is considered a manifestation of hypersensitivity to streptococcus. Appearance of rheumatic fever is not dependent upon antibody rise but more likely is related to persistence of organism in throat or other focus of infection in body. Special type of reaction in collagen tissues of body occurs in response to streptococcal disease. A protein enzyme has been suggested as intermediary factor. In recurrence of rheumatic fever and initial attack some evidence of current streptococcal infection can be found, e.g. antistreptolysin O antibody in significant dilution in 80% cases. When this is not found one should also test for antihyaluronidase, antiDPNase, antistreptokinase or antiDNAse.

In rheumatic arthritis antibody response is at or close to its peak. In chorea antibody rise has fallen to a lower level. Laboratory tests may be negative when chorea appears.

2. *Individual susceptibility*: Hemolytic streptococcal infection produces recurrence in 50% children. There may be an inherited susceptibility. If one child in a family has rheumatic fever approximately 10% of other children will develop it, an incidence which is 50–100 times higher than in general population.

Incidence of rheumatic heart disease 5 years after primary attack of rheumatic fever depends to a greater extent on individual susceptibility and response to disease as revealed initially.

3. *Streptococcal antigens*: There is lymphocytic sensitization to streptococcal antigens in rheumatic fever or in patients who have had rheumatic heart disease. This type of hyperreactivity to streptococcal membrane antigen is noted in patients during acute rheumatic fever and in follow-up period 1–5 years after initial attack. It is also seen in chronic valvular disease or previous history of rheumatic fever. Study of HLA antigens show that parents of children with rheumatic fever have increased incidence of shared antigens as compared with parents of disease free individuals. This explains why rheumatic fever tends to occur in families which may result from predisposition to an abnormal type of reactivity to streptococcal membrane antigens leading to rheumatic fever response.

MAJOR MANIFESTATIONS

Revised Jones Criteria

Five major manifestations are arthritis, heart disease, subcutaneous nodules, erythema marginatum, chorea.

Diagnosis of rheumatic fever is made when two major manifestations exist or one major two minor.

Typical picture of rheumatic fever is characterized by onset of symptoms a few days to five weeks after streptococcal throat infection. Heart disease, erythema marginatum or sub-cutaneous nodules may accompany arthritis or follow it in a matter of few days to few weeks. Chorea occurs a few weeks to few months later.

Arthritis

Occurs in 75% of first attacks of rheumatic fever and 50 to 75% of recurrences. Joints may appear swollen, tender and red. Several joints are commonly involved, sometimes together sometimes one after another. Typically large joints, such as knee, wrist, ankle and elbow. There is migratory type of arthritis moving from joint to joint in acute illness. Occasionally involvement may be a single joint. Fever is usually present at outset and ESR is elevated. As a rule there is prompt improvement when salicylates are administered but whether salicylates are given or not it is rare for signs and symptoms to persist for more than a week. Rheumatoid arthritis persists longer than a week and shows less response to salicylates.

Arthralgia consists of aches and pains in joints described more as a discomfort than as direct tenderness on motion. It is more commonly associated with carditis than more blatant joint involvement of classic arthritis.

Growing pains are nonrheumatic and benign leg pains after the child has gone to bed. It usually occurs a number of times over several weeks often months before mother seeks medical attention. Pain is commonly in thigh, calf or behind knee and not directly in joint. It is gone the next morning and child runs about and plays normally. Heat rubbing and analgesic is all that is required for therapy. ESR is found to be normal.

Heart Disease

In rheumatic fever it embodies endocarditis, myocarditis and pericarditis.

Pericarditis

There may be no audible or visible signs of pericarditis and it may appear as an incidental finding at autopsy. Pericarditis is most commonly recognized clinically by hearing the characteristic friction rub of fibrinous type. This is a superficial scratchy noise heard over precordium especially near sternum and has a to and fro character in systole and diastole. It is accompanied by fever and leukocytosis and sometimes an abnormal ST segment in ECG with flattening or inversion of T-waves in left precordial leads. In rheumatic fever the rub lasts a few days to a week or two. In pyemic infection it is gone in 2 or 3 days.

Pain over precordium is a characteristic feature in adults. Rare in children.

When effusion forms it produces an area of enlarged cardiac dullness and somewhat distinct heart sounds. A rapid enlargement of cardiac shadow clinically and by X-ray is usually due to pericardial effusion. Gross enlargement due to carditis takes 3 to 4 months to occur whereas pericardial effusion occurs rapidly and subsides in 3 to 4 weeks.

MITRAL INSUFFICIENCY

Apical systolic murmur occurs in 70% of cases of acute rheumatic fever. It is prolonged, filling most of systole, best heard at apex, well transmitted to axilla and does not change significantly with position and respiration. An organic apical systolic murmur is blowing in quality but it may become more high pitched until it is described as 'seagull murmur'. Mitral insufficiency is not always accompanied by its characteristic murmur.

First Heart Sound

Reduced in intensity in 50% children with acute rheumatic fever during an attack due to increased conduction time which facilitates early closure of mitral valve and thus diminishes valvular component of first heart sound.

Pulmonary Second Sound

Pulmonary second heart sound may appear slightly accentuated but this is usually due to relative diminution of first heart sound.

Third Heart Sound

Found in 30% cases of acute rheumatic fever with mitral insufficiency during acute stage of disease. It should not be confused with opening snap of mitral valve which occurs more promptly after second sound and is indicative of mitral stenosis.

Mitral Diastolic Murmur

Short diastolic murmur may be heard in children with mitral insufficiency. It usually occurs with audible third heart sound. It is short early or mid diastolic always associated with apical systolic murmur. It occurs in approximately one-third to half of patients with mitral insufficiency during acute attack and in one-third of these cases disappears during ensuing year. A loud mid diastolic murmur may occur in children with large hearts due to relative stenosis of mitral ring in presence of dilated left ventricle cavity.

Cardiac Impulse

Apical thrust due to left ventricle hypertrophy in mitral regurgitation occurs in older children who have had mitral regurgitation for long time. Electrocardiographically LVH is present in only 15% cases.

Heart Size

Heart may vary in size from normal to grossly enlarged organ nearly filling chest. Largest hearts seen in childhood are usually associated with mitral regurgitation rather than with mitral stenosis. Mitral ring is dilated rather than narrowed and whole heart is enlarged. There is usually a relationship between degree of mitral insufficiency and heart size. Under fluoroscope one may see an enlarged left atrium with mitral regurgitation which is similar in size and shape to that found in mitral stenosis. There may be systolic expansion of left atrium in region of esophagus best visualized by barium swallow. Such pulsations when they are associated with marked degree of insufficiency and considerable enlargement of heart are due to mitral regurgitation. Slight pulsations are commonly visible and are more likely transmitted by ventricles. They do not reflect a diagnosis of mitral insufficiency.

ECG

Normal tracing in majority of children with mitral insufficiency. LVH occurs in 15% cases. Common in older children and those children where insufficiency has been present for quite sometime. In mitral stenosis right ventricle hypertrophy is commonly found. RVH in MS appears to be parallel to pulmonary vascular resistance. Cardiac catheterization reveals an elevated pressure in right ventricle and pulmonary artery as well as wedge pressure but this is usually of moderate severity and not sufficient to produce right ventricle dominance in mitral insufficiency.

Differential Diagnosis

There are other murmurs that simulate rheumatic mitral insufficiency. Most common is functional murmur when it is heard between apex and sternum, has a 'twanging string' quality, may cause diagnostic difficulty in children between 2 and 7 years. It is short and coarse and not as loud as rheumatic heart disease. Heart is not enlarged and child is perfectly well. Other functional murmurs in aortic or pulmonary areas or down LSE are less likely to be confused with rheumatic heart murmur.

Faint transient murmurs heard during acute illness of any origin are usually associated with tachycardia and tend to disappear when fever subsides.

Short systolic apical murmur of anemia should be ruled out. There are a number of nonrheumatic pathological conditions that produce apical systolic murmur:

1. Abnormal insertion of chordae tendineae producing insufficiency of posterior cusp of mitral valve.
2. Congenital defect of mitral valve with splitting and insufficiency.
3. Endocardial fibroelastosis in child who has reached the age of rheumatic group, producing insufficiency due to either enlarged heart or actual enlargement of mitral valve.
4. Infective endocarditis which may ulcerate mitral valve near its margin and produce mitral insufficiency.

5. Congenital heart defects that produce dilatation of ventricles and insufficiency of mitral valve, e.g. coarctation of aorta, VSD, ASD, Eisenmenger complex.
6. Anemia causing dilatation of mitral valve ring.
7. Isolated myocarditis.
8. Cardiorespiratory murmur.
9. Tricuspid insufficiency.

MITRAL STENOSIS

It is possible to have MS without MR. MV may be thickened well back from free margins to the extent that these thickened areas meet with systole and prevent regurgitation. Such cases may have a diastolic murmur only and no systolic murmur. An apical systolic murmur may occur due to thickening and damage of anterior cusp of MV at outflow tract to LV thus producing a murmur that simulates mitral insufficiency.

Diagnosis is based on several characteristic features: Presystolic murmur

• Accentuated first heart sound
• Accentuated pulmonary second heart sound
• Opening snap of mitral valve
• RV heave on precordium
• Some degree of cardiomegaly
• Presence of RVH in ECG.

Mitral diastolic murmur: Long in duration leading up to accentuated first heart sound.

There is no interval between murmur and first heart sound.

First Heart Sound

Almost always accentuated. When MR is associated with MS it may be soft. Accentuated first heart sound is due to sudden reversal in direction of MV in systole. Previously the valve was kept pointing to LV by high LA pressure. Combination of presystolic murmur with loud first heart sound is good evidence of MS but is not indicative of degree of stenosis.

Pulmonary Second Sound

Accentuated when pressure is raised in pulmonary circuit. It may be accentuated in presence of normal or slightly raised pulmonary resistance with result that clinical value of this sign is limited.

Opening Snap

If mitral insufficiency is also present this sound is not heard. Third sound is frequently heard in mitral insufficiency. Although timing of this sound is slightly later than that of opening snap it may at times be difficult to tell the two apart. Third heart sound is rarely heard in MS unless MR is also present.

Cardiac Impulse

Presence of mitral stenosis leads to an elevated pressure in LA, pulmonary vascular bed, pulmonary artery and RV. Over a period of time RVH occurs and results in heave over precordial area covering RV. This heave is useful point in making diagnosis of MS and can be readily distinguished from apical thrust of mitral insufficiency.

Heart Size

Radiologically heart appears slightly or moderately enlarged with some enlargement of RA and RV. In AP view LA may show on right and left borders and in RAO view its dilatation may be demonstrated by barium swallow. Wood in 1953 concludes from his studies that mitral insufficiency is more likely to produce enlargement of LA than is MS. This is particularly true in children where marked mitral insufficiency is common but advanced mitral stenosis rare.

ECG

In MS P-wave is broad and bifid. Less frequently in mitral insufficiency. Precordial leads show RVH if PVR is elevated sufficiently to raise pressure in RV. LVH is rare in pure MS but is commonly present in combined MS and MR.

Diagnosis

This is based on presystolic murmur leading up to loud first heart sound. Precordial impulse near sternum points to mitral stenosis. Apical thrust to mitral or aortic insufficiency. Opening snap is associated with MS whereas MR is associated with third heart sound. MS has RVH whereas MR has LVH. A short MDM with 3rd HS is common accompaniment of MR but this combination is not unusual in pure MS.

AORTIC INSUFFICIENCY

Diastolic murmur of aortic insufficiency is characteristically heard over down the LSE, sometimes out to apex and above. High pulse pressure is due to carotid sinus reflex and is vascular in origin. It occurs in last half of systole before regurgitation has taken place. Same phenomenon occurs in hyperthyroidism. Occasionally in early phase of disease aortic diastolic murmur will disappear but commonly once it has been established for a few months it will remain indefinitely.

Diagnosis

Nephritis, toxic myocarditis, coarctation of aorta and syphilis may produce aortic insufficiency. Pulmonary insufficiency may occur in certain types of congenital heart disease but this is commonly associated with RVH, accentuated pulmonary second sound and often pulsating hilar shadows.

Congestive Heart Failure

Occurs in 7% of children with rheumatic fever. There are two types: chronic and acute. Former occurs in children with well established RHD with marked valvular involvement and insufficiency rather than stenosis. These children have distended neck veins, edema, weight gain, enlarged liver, dyspnea, rales in chest, an ESR depressed to normal range, little or no fever, no leukocytosis but considerably enlarged hearts. Such children respond well to digitalis.

Acute failure is characterized by overwhelming infection with fever, leukocytosis, high ESR, dyspnea, tachycardia, enlarged liver but little or no edema, moderate heart enlargement and poor response to digitalis.

In acute rheumatic fever with heart failure ESR is usually high. Failure itself may lower the rate in patients who prior to failure had elevated level. ESR is lowered to a minor degree. When child is in chronic failure or when failure is precipitated by increased physical activity ESR may be normal or increased slightly. Thus with above listed minor reservations ESR continues to be a most useful guide to presence or absence of rheumatic activity. There are three symptoms in congestive heart failure that are frequently noted in children but are uncommon in adults. These include nausea, cough and right upper quadrant discomfort in abdomen. This is due to hepatic tenderness. RHD in its most severe form in childhood is usually associated with marked degree of mitral regurgitation and failure. In past this was treated with supportive therapy, digitalis, antibiotics. Surgery was rarely attempted. Yuan and coworkers in 1964 pointed out that surgery could be most useful. Marked improvement in CCF can occur with mitral annuloplasty. Since pericarditis may have a markedly enlarged cardiac shadow coupled with some dyspnea it may be difficult to identify from heart failure. A friction rub indicates pericarditis. But one may have heart failure with pericarditis.

SUBCUTANEOUS NODULES

They are found on skin over back of hands, knuckles, elbows, knees, ankles, back of head, vertebrae and spinal areas. Approximately 75% of patients have nodules have them on elbows. Such nodules are characteristic of rheumatic infection and when they are present there is invariably an associated heart lesion. They disappear at end of 6 weeks in 75% cases and 100% four months after onset of illness.

Erythema Marginatum

It is characterized by circinate or annular rash occurring on arms, trunk and legs. It is usually faint with no elevation and has dull purplish hue. Rash changes gradually from hour to hour. Similar rash occurs in allergic conditions particularly in children below usual rheumatic fever age. Here the circles of rash may be larger, margins raised and hive like and rash redder and more palpable.

Chorea

A neurologic manifestation that is closely related to rheumatic fever. It is characterized by abnormal movements of voluntary muscles the origin of which appears to be in basal ganglia. Onset is relatively rapid. Usually a week or two in developing and then one sees multiple purposeless movements of arms, legs, feet, facial muscles and respiratory muscles. The original movement may be purposeful as in reaching for an object but the hand and arm undergo many accessory writhing movements before reaching that object. When chorea is moderate or severe the child is upset emotionally by this unusual movement over which he has no adequate control. An attack can begin unilaterally involving face, arm and leg on one side. This is referred to as hemichorea. Eating, writing and speech may be interfered with. Muscles are hypotonic and in severe cases arms and legs may be thrown about in a flail like fashion. An occasional rare case may appear almost paralyzed by choreiform involvement of muscle control.

Only 10% of rheumatic fever have chorea. 50% cases of chorea develop heart disease but this is of a milder degree and thus prognosis is better than in other manifestations of rheumatic fever. Some cases may develop rheumatic valvular disease insidiously over years, about 25% over 20 year period, mostly mitral stenosis.

Chorea is to be Differentiated from Habit Spasm

1. In more than two-third cases of chorea there is at sometime a history of other rheumatic stigmata, such as heart disease, joint pains, nose bleeds and erythema marginatum. In habit spasm these are lacking. The history is of high strung child who is susceptible to emotional strain.
2. Onset of chorea is relatively rapid. One to two weeks and parents can give an approximate date of beginning. In habit

spasm the onset is insidious gradually becoming more exaggerated and parents cannot give an approximate time of onset.

3. In chorea the whole body usually becomes involved. Face, arms, legs and respiratory movements. These may be limited to one side of body as in hemichorea. In habit spasms movements are limited to one particular area of body, such as eye, mouth and neck and rarely do they become generalized.

4. In chorea the movements are writhing and purposeless. A child with chorea may reach for an object and that movement is purposeful but many accessory writhing movements are made before main movement is completed. In habit spasm the movements are spasmodic, short and quick and are originally purposeful, such as adjusting the collar or hair but become exaggerated and are made frequently without necessity. In chorea the eyebrows movements are usually upwards whereas in habit spasm the eyes may blink and eyebrows are compressed. In chorea writhing movements may interfere with eating, writing and speech. These faculties are not interfered with in habit spasm.

5. Muscles tend to be hypotonic in chorea whereas they are either normal or hypertonic in habit spasm.

6. Chorea usually subsides in about 2 months. Habit spasm may last for many months. Although if newly acquired it may disappear rapidly.

MINOR MANIFESTATIONS

FEVER: Approximately 50% children have some fever when first seen by doctor, usually between 100–103°F and after few days tend to subside to normal. Fever is adequately controlled by administration of salicylates.

Two problems may arise with regard to fever. Firstly the child may recover completely and yet may have a fever between 99 and 100°F. ESR and TLC may become normal. In management of such children it should be remembered that some children usually have a normal temperature between 99 and 100°F and if other signs of disease have subsided it is not adequate reason for keeping the child in bed.

Second problem in diagnosis arises when a child has fever and a functional heart murmur and no other rheumatic manifestations. This may be diagnosed as acute rheumatic fever and child kept in bed. Other causes for fever should be searched for. A careful examination of heart and an evaluation of history and physical signs should be made before a decision is reached to keep child in bed for any significant period of time.

Abdominal Pain

An occasional accompaniment with little or no heart involvement. Two causes are pericarditis and hepatic enlargement but the usual type of abdominal pain is not associated with either of these. Pain is similar to that found in acute respiratory infection and is usually vague and not too acute. It will disappear in a day or two. However at times it may be more severe and present a diagnostic problem when it simulates appendicitis. In such cases presence of other rheumatic stigmata is useful in differential diagnosis.

Precordial Pain

It rarely occurs under age of 15 years in children with rheumatic fever and RHD. Even those with pericarditis do not have this symptom. In older children it may occur with enlargement of heart, pericarditis, aortic insufficiency or aortic stenosis. It is more characteristic of AS than any other form of RHD.

Epistaxis

Nontraumatic nose bleeds are common in rheumatic fever. They appear to be less severe and less frequent nowadays.

Pulmonary changes: Increased bronchial markings to complete consolidation are described. Children with mitral insufficiency tend to have congested lung fields and hilar areas. Increased pulmonary markings are a feature of mitral stenosis. When an acute overwhelming infection occurs the child may die with signs in chest and with CCF and at autopsy one may find rubbery red lung with some interstitial hyperplasia and an outpouring of some epithelial cells and fluids.

X-ray may show an increased bronchial markings of varying degree and consolidation of lung fields. This is referred to as rheumatic pneumonia.

Clinically a known rheumatic may have a primary atypical pneumonia which may be mistaken for rheumatic pneumonia especially when it occurs in a patient who has several other rheumatic stigmata. An attack of primary atypical pneumonia is occasionally accompanied by joint symptoms in early stage of disease.

Elevated ESR

The ESR and leukocyte count remain abnormally high for longer than other signs mentioned above and therefore are most useful deciding how long a patient should be kept in bed. Degree of alteration from normal is greater in ESR than leukocyte count. TLC is often a little bit above the normal upper limit. When ESR returns to normal it is taken as an evidence that rheumatic process has subsided. It is a nonspecific test. It may be elevated by any infection or by a tonsillectomy. In heart failure ESR may be normal inspite of the fact that active rheumatic disease is present.

ECG

Sinus tachycardia is commonly found in acute attack of illness especially with fever. With administration of aspirin temperature and pulse rate fall and by the end of second or third week less than 10% show tachycardia as demonstrated by sleeping pulse (tachycardia being defined as sleeping pulse rate of 100/minute or more). Bradycardia of sleeping pulse less than 60 occurs in a number of cases between second and fourth week. This is more likely to occur in those with no heart disease or a mild degree than severe heart involvement. Such bradycardia is apparent considerably before TLC, ESR and other signs of rheumatic activity subside completely.

PR interval is frequently increased in children with rheumatic fever. Upper limit of normal in a child is taken as 0.2 second. But if a child's previous PR interval is 0.12 second and it increases to 0.16 second, this is a significant increase.

Clarke and Keith in 1972 have devised a PR index that is a simplified method for demonstrating these changes. They showed that in 84% of patients with acute rheumatic fever abnormalities of conduction occured. Simple streptococcal infection or glomerulonephritis per se were not associated with similar abnormalities of conduction. Slight or moderate lengthening of conduction time may occur with certain CHD, e.g. in 57% cases of L TGV, 50% of ebstein anomaly, 43% of ASD, 12% of coarctation of aorta, 8% of TAPVD, 6% of VSD, 3.4% of PDA, 3% in PS, 3% in TOF. It rarely occurs in otherwise normal children. It appears therefore that lengthening of PR interval when above CHD are ruled out is relatively specific for rheumatic fever either with or without carditis particularly when conduction lengthening is reversible. It is suggested therefore that a significantly reversible PR interval prolongation could well be used as a measure criterion among the Jones criteria in diagnosis of rheumatic fever. In chronic rheumatic heart disease conduction time is characteristically lengthened than average for child's age usually between 0.18 and 0.21 second and does not change much during acute stage, although occasionally a child with grossly enlarged heart in third or fourth attack will show marked prolongation of PR interval. This lengthening of conduction time is rare in diseases other than rheumatic fever and therefore has some diagnostic significance when other findings are in doubt. Varying degrees of lengthening conduction time up to complete heart block are apparent. Complete heart block is uncommon. Flat or inverted T-waves over left precordium are characteristic findings in acute rheumatic pericarditis. Such findings revert to normal when pericarditis subsides.

Corrected QT interval or rate lengthening is evidence of active rheumatic heart disease. Drugs, CCF, electrolytes, ventricular hypertrophy and ventricular dilatation affect QT interval. Normal values may occur in presence of gross carditis. Thus, it is of doubtful value.

Premature beats may occur with acute rheumatic heart disease particularly in aortic valvular disease, pericarditis and mitral valvular disease. They may occur in normal child.

Atrial fibrillation is likely to occur when mitral stenosis is present. There will be ECG changes of MS and MR. LAD and LVH may be seen in mitral insufficiency. Presence of RAD is of little help in diagnosis of MS.

IMMUNOLOGICAL EVIDENCE

An increased titre to any of the several antistreptococcal antibody: ASO, antihyaluronidase, antistreptokinase, antiDPnase. 80% children show increased titre of ASO. In other 20% tests for other antibodies will be required. After a hemolytic streptococcal infection these antibodies show a sharp and sudden increase for first 4 weeks and then a gradual drop extending over several months. Thus when rheumatic fever follows a streptococcal infection the ASO titre usually reach its peak until about 2 to 4 weeks after onset of rheumatic symptoms. Several estimations of this antibody showing a progressive rise or fall may be of diagnostic value.

C reactive protein in serum of patients with rheumatic fever, even a small amount, is suggestive of rheumatic activity. C reactive protein is completely absent from normal blood. However a positive reaction may be obtained in diseases other than rheumatic fever. These include malignant tumor, acute nephritis and rheumatoid arthritis.

Treatment

Rest in bed. Child should be kept in bed until ESR is normal. If heart damage has been considerable it may be wise to keep the child in bed for 2 to 4 weeks after ESR has returned to normal. One can increase activity by 10 minutes each day by allowing the child up to 10 minutes first day after ESR is normal, 20 minutes second day, 30 minutes third day and so on. When no heart disease is present the time up may be increased 15 to 20 minutes a day. Activity may gradually be increased over next 2 to 3 months depending upon severity of heart damage. Five categories are suggested:

1. No restriction.
2. *Slight restriction*: Abstinence from strenuous games like hockey, football, races.

3. *Moderate restriction*: Cycling on level ground is permitted. Lead a quiet average life.
4. *Fairly marked restriction*: Can take part in short walks only.
5. *Semi invalidism*: Where a good part of day would be spent on a couch with a minimum of physical activity.

Occupational Therapy

"Have fun get well". To keep up the morale of rheumatic patients. Many things to interest and teach children in way of games, sewing, leather works, etc.

Schooling

Visiting teacher for children who are convalescent but well enough to accept some teaching. This helps the child to keep abreast of work going on in class and occupying some of his hours during the day.

Drug Therapy

Salicylates: Their efficacy is judged by the effect on following manifestations of the disease during past few decades—fever, arthritis, sedimentation rate, murmurs, heart size, erythema marginatum, chorea, nodules, heart failure and conduction time in ECG. Heart disease is not prevented or diminished by salicylates. A blood level of 20 to 25 mg/100 ml is safe and effective. Aspirin contains no sodium and can be used in failure. Toxic signs are nausea, deafness and tinnitus, acidosis and tachypnea. In event of toxicity the dosage should be reduced.

Steroids

Temperature is equally controlled by ACTH and aspirin. ESR decrease is more with steroids than in those treated with aspirin. There is greater proportion for bradycardia during treatment in aspirin group than in those treated with steroids. Arthritis responds equally in both groups. Nodules take longer to disappear in cases treated with aspirin. No difference in response to treatment of chorea. Neither the appearance nor disappearance of erythema marginatum is related to therapy. During first 3 to 4 weeks of treatment a larger proportion of those treated with steroids show an increase in heart size than those treated with aspirin. Steroids are useful in early stages in making the patient feel better, improving appetite and speeding up disappearance of murmurs. Salicylates are useful in suppressing rheumatic activity at all stages but particularly when steroids are stopped and rebound phenomenon needs prevention.

Salicylates permit ESR to be used as a guide to activity in later stages of disease.

Summary

1. Start with salicylates when there is no evidence of cardiac involvement.
2. In seriously ill patients with cardiac involvement start salicylates with steroids for two weeks.

FAMILIAL INCIDENCE

Although appearance of more than one case of rheumatic fever in same family is reported from time to time role of genetics as etiological factor remains to be clarified. There is interplay of an inherent susceptibility and an infective agent.

Possible modes of inherited susceptibility:

1. Single autosomal dominant gene with complete penetrance (Beers 1948)
2. Autosomal recessive gene with reduced penetrance (Wilson 1937)
3. No definite Mendelian mechanism (Stevenson 1953)
4. Susceptibility to rheumatic infection is inherent in host (Quinn 1967)

Twin studies: Low concordance rates in monozygotic twins indicate that enviornmental factors are important. An inherent susceptibility is present in host but it is less important.

Association with blood group:

(Glynn 1956) these patients carry the nonsecretor gene (secretor gene allows ABO antigens to be secreted in saliva but this gene is not linked with ABO gene).

Prevention

To prevent streptococcal infection 1.2 mega units of benzathene penicillin is given initially and then once a week for 3 weeks. 50% of known cases of rheumatic fever will develop rheumatic recurrence if they have a rheumatogenic streptococcal recurrence infection. To prevent recurrence 1.2 mega units of benzathene penicillin intramuscular is given every 3 weeks for at least 10 years and ideally for life.

Prognosis

1. *Pericarditis*: This is considered as a serious form of heart involvement in rheumatic fever.

2. *Arthritis*: Not the most severe manifestation of disease. Incidence of carditis increases with decreasing severity of joint symptoms. Severity of carditis is related inversely to severity of arthritis. Most severe form of heart disease occur in patients who have no evidence of arthritis.

3. *Heart size*: Cardiomegaly increases mortality.

4. *Valvular lesions*: Mitral regurgitation predominates. Mitral stenosis cases develop atrial fibrillation and congestive cardiac failure. Aortic regurgitation group provide a site for bacterial endocarditis.

5. *Chronic rheumatic carditis*: Term reserved for those patients who following an attack of rheumatic fever continue to show evidence of active infection and active carditis for more than 6 months and at times extending over years. This term does not include cases whose only sign of activity is an elevated ESR, nor the prolonged cases of chorea. These children have progressive signs of carditis as well as raised ESR. Usually they have had 3 or 4 previous attacks of rheumatic fever but the continuing activity is not accompanied by immunological evidence of fresh streptococcal infection. The mortality is high in this group and they need constant antirheumatic treatment, preferably salicylates because of long administration required. Fresh valvular disease is identified frequently.

6. *Functional ability*: 95% of children who have recovered from initial attack of rheumatic fever are able to lead an essentially normal life. 5% live a somewhat restricted life but majority are able to go to school and take part in regular activities. Those with significant aortic or mitral valvular disease are kept out of strenuous and competitive sports. Improvement in prognosis is caused by many factors: reduced severity of hemolytic streptococcal infection in community, improvement in socio economic conditions and prophylaxis in known rheumatic cases with penicillin.

48

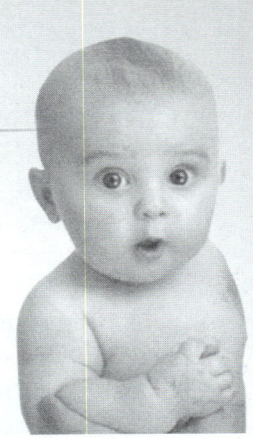

Pericarditis

ETIOLOGY

1. Rheumatic: 55% cases.
2. Purulent or septic 28% cases.
3. Idiopathic: acute, benign.
4. Rheumatoid arthritis.
5. Coxsackievirus.
6. Constrictive pericarditis.
7. Tuberculosis.
8. Traumatic.
9. Miscellaneous:
   - Uremia.
   - Polyarteritis nodosa.
   - Disseminated lupus.
   - Postoperative pericardial tamponade.
   - Thrombocytopenic purpura.
   - Congenital hypoplastic anemia.
   - Cooley's anemia.
   - Glycogen storage disease.
   - Friedreich ataxia.
   - Ulcerative colitis.
   - Chronic nonspecific pericarditis.
   - Rupture of aorta in pericardium.
   - Meningococcal sepsis.
   - Gaucher disease.

Clinical Features

Precordial pain in childhood is not as frequently a feature of pericarditis as it is in adults. When it does occur it is not a marked feature of illness and lasts only a day or two.

Visceral and parietal pericardium inner surfaces are not sensitive to pain. Pain is produced by involvement of pleura either mediastinal, diaphragmatic or costal. Most children with pericarditis develop moderate effusion which itself is not sufficient to cause symptoms. If effusion is marked there may be interference with diastolic filling of heart and resulting congestion of great veins, with distension of neck vessels and enlargement of liver. Thus, it may be difficult to differentiate features from cardiac failure.

Characteristic feature of pericarditis is friction rub usually heard best along left sternal edge but may be audible over entire precordium. Friction rub must be distinguished from pleuro-pericardial rub and also from mediastinal emphysema, such as may occur in pneumonia in childhood. At times a bulging pulmonary artery of cor pulmonale may produce a rubbing sound against pericardium that simulates pericarditis.

Heart sounds are difficult to hear in presence of friction rub whether or not effusion is present.

With developing pericardial effusion lung is pushed back posteriorly and laterally and in many instances bronchial breathing becomes audible at left base posteriorly (Ewart sign). When this is a marked feature there will also be dullness on percussion in same area.

With marked effusion pulse becomes weak especially during inspiration, producing the paradoxic pulse.

Tachycardia is common.

Radiologic Examination

As effusion increases the cardiac borders fill out and produce a pear shaped shadow. Cardiophrenic angles become less acute. Angiocardiogram will reveal size and position of chambers of heart and demonstrate distended pericardial sac.

Same information can be obtained by cardiac catheterization. Under fluoroscope the shape and size of cardiac shadow with absence of usual pulsations of borders will permit suspicion in absence of pericardial rub.

In rheumatic fever when no friction rub is heard and cardiac outline is suggestive diagnosis can be made when marked change of shadow size takes place in a month or less. Change in heart size due to myocarditis is a more gradual process and usually takes several months to accomplish.

ECG

In early acute stage of disease ST segment is elevated usually in leads over left precordium. This is best recognized over serial ECG's. ST segment may be concave. T-waves become flat and finally invert. These changes last for 2 to 3 weeks but may persist for months or occasionally years in tuberculous pericarditis. Amplitude of QRS and T-waves are diminished when effusion is present.

Alterations in ECG are considered to be due to involvement of myocardium immediately under pericardium causing ST and T-wave changes and pericardial effusion causing a diminution of voltage.

DIAGNOSIS

Most reliable signs of pericarditis are:
- Friction rub.
- Rapid and significant change in heart size occurring over a period of 1 to 4 weeks.
- Detection of fluid by pericardial tap or echocardiography.
- ECG changes.
- Faint heart sounds.
- Bronchial breathing.

Normally both visceral and parietal layers of pericardium are slightly separated (1 to 2 mm) at peak of anterior motion of posterior ventricular wall on echocardiography. As fluid accumulates the parietal pericardium flattens and separates from visceral pericardium. These changes are usually best seen at level of posterior wall of left ventricle. Anterior fluid may be seen as echo free space just posterior to anterior chest wall.

Sweep up left ventricle will show progressive decrease in amount of fluid with apposition of layers of pericardium as one approaches the left atrium. Differentiation from normally occurring echo free space just posterior to pericardium is required from an effusion.

A pleural friction rub occurring in general area of pericardium needs differentiation from pericardial friction rub. Such a rub may be altered by force of heart beat and thus may resemble pericarditis. Pleural rub disappears when patient holds his breath. ECG shows a raised ST segment, inverted T-wave over left precordium and diminished QRS and T voltage. Similar patterns are seen in myocarditis.

When pericarditis occurs in rheumatic fever it has to be differentiated from acute or chronic heart failure.

1. Edema and weight gain are seen in chronic heart failure but they are rare in acute heart failure and do not occur in acute pericarditis.

2. Dyspnea is present in all three conditions.

3. Friction rub is characteristic of pericarditis and not of heart failure.

4. Although heart shadow may appear enlarged in all three conditions there is a rapid increase or decrease in heart size when effusion is present. Such is not the case with acute or chronic heart failure.

5. Hilar shadows may be congested in all three but are more likely to be so with heart failure.

6. With chronic heart failure there is a long history of previous rheumatic fever activity. Such is usually not the case with pericarditis.

7. In chronic heart failure there is usually evidence of marked valvular involvement. This may or may not be present in acute heart failure but is often not present with pericarditis.

8. patients with acute heart failure are usually acutely and seriously ill. Those with pericarditis are less so.

9. ESR may be elevated or normal in chronic failure. It is usually high in acute failure and pericarditis.

10. Neck veins are distended with acute or chronic heart failure. They may be distended with pericarditis but often are normal.

11. Rales in chest are common when failure is present but are absent in pericarditis.

12. Response to digitalis is good when chronic failure is present. There may be a slight response with acute failure and no response with pericarditis.

13. Pericarditis and failure may occur together.

DIFFERENTIAL DIAGNOSIS

If there are signs of pericarditis in a child under 2 years it is not rheumatic in origin but is most probably septic. If the child is 3 to 5 years of age it is more likely rheumatoid in origin. Rheumatic is possibility over 5 years of age.

Pyogenic pericarditis occurs secondary to pneumonia, osteomyelitis or any other purulent infection. This is most commonly seen in first 2 years of life. A friction rub may be present but more commonly the diagnosis is suggested by cardiac shadow.

Rheumatoid pericarditis occurs in first five years of life, usually between 2 and 5 years. There is usually high fever uncontrolled by salicylates, pericardial friction rub and transient arthritis, eventually followed by typical joint swellings.

Uremic pericarditis is diagnosed by underlying nephritis.

Periarteritis nodosa has run quite a prolonged course before pericarditis appears.

Diagnosis of acute idiopathic benign pericarditis is made by exclusion. A friction rub is noted in a child who is over 5 years of age, is not desperately ill any has no evidence of rheumatic fever or pyogenic infection. No stigmata of rheumatic fever or rheumatoid arthritis develop. Cause is variable but usually benign.

Chronic constrictive pericarditis is a different diagnostic problem. There is no friction rub, heart usually is not enlarged to a significant degree. Traumatic pericardial effusion and tamponade may occur from a swallowed safety pin.

Treatment

The underlying disease must be treated primarily, e.g. rheumatic fever, pyogenic infection, tuberculosis, etc. *Staphyllococcus aureus* is the commonest causative agent. *Streptococcus pneumoni* and *hemolytic streptococci* are second and third most commonly found. Thus if purulent pericarditis is suspected and etiology has not been determined therapy should be aimed primarily to cover these three organisms.

Pericardial paracentesis needs to be performed if there is a large effusion that is producing a high degree of temponade. This may be judged by tachycardia, hepatomegaly and engorgement of vessels.

Surgical intervention and introduction of a drainage tube into pericardium may be necessary.

Aspiration is performed in 4 th or 5th LICS, 1 cm inside the border of the pericardial margin. This can be established from X-ray or fluoroscopic examination.

Percardial paracentesis is rarely needed in rheumatic pericarditis because the prime difficulty is in myocardium rather than pericardium and the pericardial effusion is rarely sufficient to interfere seriously with cardiac function. Pericardial paracentesis is of more value in pyogenic pericarditis in both diagnosis and relief of cardiac tamponade when such is present.

In benign idiopathic pericarditis mortality is nil and such patients have no apparent residual defects although it is possible that some of them eventually develop constrictive pericarditis. Constrictive pericarditis has a poor prognosis without surgery. There is an 18% mortality.

RHEUMATIC PERICARDITIS

Incidence and mortality has been decreasing. Rheumatic pericarditis is associated with irregular accumulation of fibrin over pericardium that becomes adherent primarily to one surface but not uncommonly develops on both surfaces and this often leads to complete obliteration of pericardial sac. At autopsy the pericadium presents a shaggy rough appearance.

Normally 10 to 15 ml of fluid is present in pericardial cavity. With effusion there may be hundreds of ml.

Rheumatic fever patient with pericarditis appears acutely ill at onset and presents other stigmata of rheumatic fever. There is an audible rub and rapid change in heart size.

ECG changes are similar to other forms of pericarditis but the pattern may be altered by underlying myocarditis of rheumatic infection. Elevation of ST segment followed by inversion of T-wave is common.

Those children who have pericarditis are likely to have more underlying disease and therefore a poorer prognosis. There is no evidence that rheumatic pericarditis leads to constrictive pericarditis in later years. Steroids are rarely needed.

Purulent Pericarditis

This forms an exudate of varying consistency. Thick or thin. Fibrin mass coated with purulent material is seen at autopsy.

Causative Organisms

- *Staphyllococcus aureus.*
- *Streptococcus pneumoni.*
- *Hemolytic streptococci.*
- *Haemophilus influenzae.*
- *E coli.*
- *Pseudomonas aeruginosa.*
- *Streptococcus anaerobius.*

Most cases are associated with pneumonia, empyema or osteomyelitis. Only 15% cases develop a friction rub. There may be a large or enlarging cardiac shadow shown by X-ray. ECG shows ST and T-wave changes which can appear early before pericardial effusion is enough to produce a tamponade. Prognosis is usually grave. Pericardial aspiration is important for determination of organisms and initiation of appropriate antibiotic therapy. Open drainage may be required at times if response is not satisfactory.

Meningococcal Pericarditis

Pericarditis complicating meningococcal meningitis is rare in children. In patients known to have meningococcal meningitis one should look for friction rub, chest pain, ECG changes or progressive pericardial compression. Removal of pericardial effusion may show an immediate improvement in patient. Recovery is slow but complete in few months. Heart function and size return to normal and ultimate prognosis is good. Large doses of crystalline penicillin will control the disease adequately. Constrictive pericarditis may occur occasionally.

Rheumatoid Pericarditis

Age group 4 years and less. Illness always begins with high spiking fever of unknown origin which persists. This is soon accompanied by joint pain. Friction rub is heard at this stage 1 month after onset of fever and joint pain. Typical periarticular swellings of rheumatoid arthritis appear later usually 6 to 8 weeks after appearance of illness and one month after hearing friction rub.

Diagnostic Points

1. Maculopapular rash suggestive of rheumatoid arthritis.
2. Joint pain suggestive of rheumatic infection.
3. Fever that does not respond to aspirin suggest rheumatoid arthritis. Fever shows response to steroids.
4. High leukocytosis.
5. Age between 3 and 5 years.

X-ray may show pericardial effusion. ECG has typical changes.

Most cases of rheumatoid pericarditis recover and show no residual cardiac signs. Many of those who survive develop an adherent pericardium.

IDIOPATHIC PERICARDITIS

Age group 3 to 11 years. Chest pain is not a marked feature. Pain may be referred to abdomen. Onset of pain is insidious.

Tachypnea is common. Fever is usual in acute stage. Friction rub is heard. ECG changes persist for 1 to 3 months. X-ray findings are similar to those in other forms of pericarditis.

On pericardial paracentesis the fluid is sero sanguineous. Leukocytosis may reach 25000/cu mm. ESR is high.

All cases survive. Recurrence rate is 15%.

Diagnosis is by exclusion of other forms of pericarditis. It is difficult to exclude rheumatic fever entirely because it is well known that rheumatic fever may show no signs of arthritis and still have heart disease and it is possible that signs of heart disease are limited to pericardium only.

Purulent pericarditis must be ruled out. This usually occurs in younger age group children who are desperately ill. Response to antibiotic is satisfactory. On paracentesis purulent exudate is obtained. On occasions the organism is cultured.

Tuberculous pericarditis is usually painless and friction rub may last for long-time, from several weeks to several months. There should be evidence of tuberculosis in lungs.

Symptomatic treatment with rest in bed until the illness is subsided is usual therapy. Shortening of course occurs with ACTH and cortisone.

Tuberculous Pericarditis

More common after 10 years age. Primary invasion of pericardium by tuberculosis bacillus is an uncommon event. The lesion is always due to a direct extension from lungs. It may spread from an infected hilar gland or directly from caseous lung tissue. Tubercles may be scattered over visceral or parietal pericardium but usually there is a diffuse pericardial reaction with considerable fibrosis. Eventually there is obliteration of pericardial sac. The early acute stage proceeds to one characterized by effusion but if the patient survives the fluid is absorbed and fibrotic reaction remains. Pericardial fluid is watery. Leukocytes in pericardial fluid vary from 500 to 1000/cu mm. Lymphocytes predominate. In few cases mycobacterium may be demonstrated in fluid.

Clinically all have evidence of pulmonary tuberculosis. Some have miliary tuberculosis and some tubercular meningitis. Duration of illness before onset of pericarditis varies from 2 weeks to 7 months. Onset is slow and insidious. Pyrexia and tachycardia occur. There may be friction rub. Heart sounds are muffled and occasionally a gallop rhythm is present. Cardiac failure may occur. ESR is high. Leukocytosis is 15 to 21 thousand/cu mm. Diagnosis is based on pericardial friction rub that lasts for weeks. In other forms of pericarditis it rarely lasts longer than 10 days to 2 weeks. Appearance of pericardial effusion in a known case of tuberculosis is suggestive. Presence of a significant tachycardia occurring in a tuberculosis patient without obvious explanation is suspicious. Appearance of heart failure in tuberculosis patient is indicative of pericarditis. ECG may show elevation of ST segment and T-wave inversion. In some cases diagnosis is at autopsy. Constrictive pericarditis is fatal complication

Treatment is with full course of antituberculosis therapy.

CHRONIC CONSTRICTIVE PERICARDITIS

Very rare in children. Most cases have an insidious onset. Some develop following acute respiratory infection. Others after tuberculosis infection, suppurative lesion or nonspecific pericarditis.

Pyogenic infections that cause pericarditis are meningococcal and tularemia.

10% cases are due to coxsackievirus infection.

Other causes are trauma and tumor.

Pathology

There is fibrous thickening of visceral and parietal pericardium. Pericardial sac is obliterated. Constriction may occur from visceral pericarditis alone. Fibrosed pericardium is 1 to 5 mm thick, covers the whole of pericardium and may involve great veins as well. Calcification is not seen in children. Myocardial involvement may at times contribute to clinical picture. When the heart has been compressed by constrictive pericardium for considerable period of time the myocardium is reduced in power. When tuberculosis is etiological factor there may be evidence of direct infection from hilar glands or from a caseous pulmonary infection close to pericardium.

Clinical Features

Dyspnea with effort, ascitis, edema and orthropnea develop insidiously over a period of time. Heart murmurs are absent. Diastolic murmur may be produced by calcium penetrating the heart producing valve narrowing or by constricting bands around the edges of ventricular grooves. Third heart sound is present due to rapid inflow filling at beginning of diastole due to high venous pressure. Venous pressure is always elevated and varies between 150 and 400 mm of water. Neck veins are distended and superior *vena cava* is seen enlarged under fluroscope. Blood pressure is low and decreases with inspiration producing paradoxic pulse. Patient may appear well. Cyanosis does not occur. Heart rate is more than 100/minute. There is no precordial thrust and heart sounds are distant. Ascitis is more common than pitting edema. Serum proteins are reduced and A:G ratio is reversed. Vital capacity is reduced. Stroke volume is reduced slightly.

ECG

P-waves are broad and notched. Inverted T-waves over left precordium and diminished QRS voltage, atrial fibrillation, flutter and extrasystole are seen. These changes disappear with pericardiectomy.

Radiological Features

Heart may be triangular, globular or boot shaped. There is absence or diminution of cardiac pulsations. Cardiac shadow remains fixed during inspiration and expiration. In 50% there may be cardiomegaly. Superior *vena cava* may appear widened due to engorged great veins and normal outline of aorta and pulmonary artery are obscured. Vascular markings of lungs may be increased due to passive congestion. Calcification is an unusual finding in childhood but is reported.

Diagnosis

Differentiation from heart failure, cirrhosis of liver and idiopathic benign pericarditis is required. In childhood heart failure is due to congenital heart disease which can be easily differentiated from constrictive pericarditis. Presence of ascitis, normal size heart, lack of activity of heart under fluoroscope, ECG, distended neck veins and raised venous pressure. Cardiac catheterization reveals high right atrial pressure, precipitous fall in right ventricle pressure at end of systole proceeding to a sharp dip in diastole and rising to an elevated diastolic pressure which correspond to pressure in right atrium.

Acutely developing constrictive pericarditis may occur in 21 days due to purulent origin, e.g. meningococcal and coxsackie virus infection. Signs are those of early tamponade without significant pericardial effusion. Occasional case begins with subacute effusion and ends up with constrictive pericarditis.

Treatment

Bedrest may be necessary depending upon the severity of constriction of pericardium. Diuretics and low sodium diet is indicated when there is ascitis and edema. Paracentesis should be done when ascitis does not respond to therapy. Digitalis is of help when myocardium is weak.

Pericardiectomy is treatment of choice. Ventricular fibrillation and cardiac standstill can occur during surgery. Preoperative use of digitalis may reduce cardiac arrhythmia and reduce the possibility of failure. Postoperative hemorrhage may occur.

COXSACKIEVIRUS PERICARDITIS

Epidemics of Bornholm disease are associated with pericarditis. Coxsackievirus type B5 and B3 are most frequently reported. There are multiplicity of signs and symptoms relating to coxsackievirus. These include fever, malaise, headache, tachycardia, pleurodynia, lymphadenopathy, splenomegaly, meningeal signs, cardiac enlargement, congestive cardiac failure and pericardial friction rub. Myocarditis is common in neonate. It can precipitate cardiac failure. This is indicated by gallop rhythm, cardiac enlargement (apart from pericardial effusion) congestive cardiac failure with enlargement of liver and visible JVP. Friction rub may persist for a few hours or few days. It is rarely accompanied by precordial pain. Occasionally coxsackievirus infection leads to constrictive pericarditis. Strict bedrest is most important factor in treatment of these cases. Steroids have not been found to alter course of disease significantly. Salicylates are helpful in relieving symptoms and reducing fever in acute stage of disease. Prognosis is good in vast majority of cases. Recovery is rule. Even when myocarditis is present recovery is rule. Prognosis is poor when there is accompanying meningoencephalitis and disease occurs with myocarditis in first few weeks of life. Surgery is occasionally needed if constrictive pericarditis occurs as a sequelae to this condition.

Postpericardiotomy Syndrome

Syndrome occurs as sequelae to cardiac surgery and appears to be a delayed response to opening of pericardium. It is characterized by fever, chest pain and signs of pleural or pericadial reaction with or without a friction rub. Chest pain is likely to be minimal or absent in children. Onset is 2 to 3 weeks following cardiac surgery. X-ray reveals abnormalities of heart and lungs. Cardiac shadow may show enlargement or lack definition. Pleural involvement may be evident with effusion, thickening of pleural layer and tenting of diaphragm. Both pericardium and pleura are involved more on left side of chest than right. ECG may show ST and T-wave changes. Presence of conduction defect, RBBB, digitalis effect make it difficult to defend this approach to diagnosis. Early ambulation is responsible for causing or prolonging symptoms. Steroids are used. Occasionally they prolong course of disease. A short course with moderate doses is indicated.

Congenital Absence of Pericardium

Columbus in 1559 was first to recognize. Most cases have no symptoms. Most common symptom is a vague chest pain.

Dizziness has been recorded occasionally. Systolic ejection murmurs are noted in most patients usually along LSE. Apex beat is shifted to left. Apical precordial activity may be obvious. In complete absence of left pericardium heart is shifted to left with trachea in midline. There is prominence of pulmonary artery and right heart border may not be visible, may be indistinct and hidden by spine. Lung tissue may be seen between left hemi diaphragm and inferior border of heart. A tongue of lung projects between aorta and main pulmonary artery in left anterior oblique view. In partial pericardial defect heart is in normal position. There is prominence of pulmonary artery or left atrial appendage, right axis deviation, right bundle branch block. Angiogram will show herniation of left atrial appendage through partial defect in pericardium ECG shows RAD, partial RBBB and leftward displacement of transitional zone in precordial leads. Some children have sinus bradycardia.

Prognosis

Absence of left pericardium does not interfere with normal life unless other cardiac anomalies are present. In smaller or partial defects of pericardium which permit herniation of left atrial appendage with consequent strangulation of the portion of heart sudden death may occur.

No treatment is indicated for complete absence of pericardium. In presence of symptoms or possibility of sudden death in partial defect surgical procedures include left atrial appendectomy, division of adhesions, pericardioplasty or extension of defect to prevent herniation. Very small defect that is unlikely to cause herniation do not require surgery.

49

Transient Pulmonary Vasoconstriction in Newborn

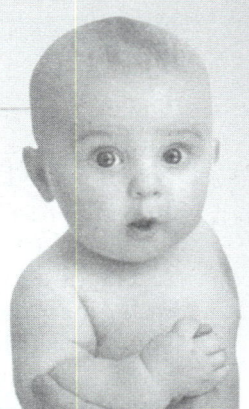

SYNONYMS

- Persistent fetal circulation.
- Persistent pulmonary vascular obstruction in newborn.
- Persistent transitional circulation.
- Progressive pulmonary hypertension.
- Early respiratory distress syndrome.
- Transient myocardial ischemia.

So many names suggest that pathogenesis of this disorder is still uncertain and full clinical spectrum of disease is not appreciated widely.

Most common form of disorder is reflected in disturbed right heart hemodynamics. A striking disturbance of pulmonary circulation that could occur in term infants that cause distressed breathing, hypoxia and fetal direction of ductal flow which later follow the trend toward normal transitional hemodynamics in pulmonary circulation, e.g. lowering of pulmonary artery pressure to mature limits. Left to right shunt through ductus and eventual closure of both duct and foramen ovale. Data from cardiac catheterization confirm high pulmonary vascular tone and suggest hypoxia as trigger mechanism. Atrioventricular valvular regurgitation and right ventricular failure are known associations. There is evidence of left ventricular failure in addition to right heart stress. ECG evidence of myocardial ischemia or infarction occurs during recovery phase.

It is postulated that intense pulmonary vascular constriction impose a major load on right ventricular work with resultant ischemia of right ventricle as well as that of posterior wall of left ventricle, an area frequently supplied by branches of right coronary artery.

A third category of disease exists in which selective and less extensive subendocardial ischemia of posterior wall of left ventricle occurs without striking right sided manifestations.

Clinical Features

Affected infant is born at term. There is history of perinatal stress. Tachypnea and cyanosis are present within 24 hours of delivery. Development of respiratory distress and appearance of chest X-ray is not characteristic of respiratory distress syndrome of prematurity. Respiration is suggestive of severe cardiac disease. There is right ventricle lift parasternally. Second heart sound is accentuated always and usually is split. In more severe form there will be gallop rhythm and tricuspid regurgitation murmur at lower left sternal edge. Liver is often enlarged. Frank cardiac failure is present. There is cardiomegaly in X-ray. Overdistended lungs may be seen. Hypoglycemia and hypocalcemia are present. Arterial blood gas analysis shows hypoxemia and varying values of PCO_2. Hyperoxic test shows an increase in PaO_2 values but in very severe cases response to very high ambient oxygen may be limited.

ECG shows right ventricle dominance or right ventricle hypertrophy. Occasionally shows T-wave changes suggestive of myocardial damage. QRS voltage is normal but may exceed normal values.

Differential Diagnosis

Extracardiac causes of hypoxia, e.g. birth asphyxia, tracheoesophageal fistula, aspiration pneumonia, diaphragmatic hernia. Echocardiography is useful in demonstrating normal cardiac anatomy. In cases of doubt cardiac catheterization and angiocardiography may be required. Catheterization data show systemic or close to systemic levels of pressure in right ventricle and pulmonary artery, right to left shunt at both ductus and foramen ovale and normal left atrial pressure.

Angiocardiogram following right ventricular injection frequently show tricuspid regurgitation. A wide open duct with pulmonary artery to aorta contrast shunting and normal pulmonary venous return to left atrium.

When there is left ventricular failure in addition to gross congestive cardiac failure pulses weaken and clinical picture simulates abrupt vascular collapse. Symptoms are similar to hypoplastic left heart syndrome with aortic outflow obstruction or interruption of aortic arch. Chest X-ray shows cardiomegaly and pulmonary venous congestion. ECG shows severe right ventricle hypertrophy with subendocardial ischemia often present during recovery phase.

Echocardiogram demonstrate reduced left ventricle wall movements and other indices of left ventricular function. Serial studies indicate improvement of ventricular performance. There is sluggish contraction of left ventricle in left sided angiocardiograms.

Treatment

In usual form of disease oxygen is most important form of therapy. Blood glucose, calcium and pH should be normalized. In congestive heart failure digitalis and diuretics are employed. Vasodilator drugs are used in severe form of disease to reduce pulmonary vascular resistance. Such drugs should best be administered directly into a major pulmonary artery division since right to left shunting at pulmonary artery level might otherwise produce hypotensive changes on systemic side. In practice intravenous use is effective. Progressive improvement in condition occurs over a period of several days. In case of patients with severe form involving left ventricle failure response is dramatic. Development of loud mitral regurgitation murmur and continuing left ventricular failure are ominous.

Confirmation of an ischemic basis for clinical picture has recently been obtained through myocardial imaging techniques. Patients with left ventricular failure may have ventricle dysfunction at later age, particularly of left side.

50

Primary Pulmonary Hypertension

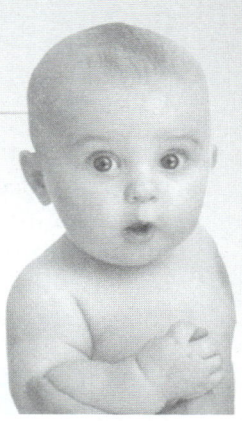

This term should be used specifically for the distinctive syndrome that is associated with intrinsic, idiopathic, obstructive disease in small terminal arterioles and arteries of pulmonary vascular bed.

Etiology

There is no sex preponderance in infancy or childhood. It has been suggested that disease may represent persistence off fetal type of pulmonary vasculature with secondary intimal proliferative changes. In immediate postnatal period elastic fibers in pulmonary artery are arranged in parallel manner similar to those in aorta. After birth with a fall in pulmonary artery pressure this arrangement of elastic fibers normally gets distorted but if pulmonary hypertension persists postnatally then fetal type of histologic pattern in pulmonary trunk is retained.

Histologic pattern in pulmonary trunk varies.

An autoimmune basis is suggested and familial occurrence is reported.

Changes in lung vessels are identical to those seen in congenital heart disease complicated by pulmonary hypertension as in large VSD. On basis of these studies it is speculated that alterations in primary pulmonary hypertension are initiated by vasoconstriction produced by variety of stimuli.

433

Pathology

At autopsy right atrium and right ventricle are dilated and hypertrophied. Foramen ovale may be open or closed. In small vessels of lungs there is usually medial hypertrophy, laminar intimal fibrosis, fibrinoid necrosis, arteritis and plexiform lesions. In some cases thrombosis and thromboembolism complicate picture. Occasionally necrotizing arteritis is present.

Clinical Features

Principal symptoms are dyspnea, fatigue and syncope and these may be related to exertion. Syncope may mimic a convulsive disorder. In infancy dyspnea may interfere with feeding and weight gain may be poor. Chest pain may occur in infants as well as in older children. Most fatal cases in childhood develop symptoms before 5 years of age.

Cyanosis when present is due to associated intracardiac shunting usually via a patent foramen ovale or from intra-pulmonary shunting.

Clubbing rarely occurs unless there is significant right to left shunt.

Prominent 'a'-wave is visible in neck.

There is right ventricle lift and increased pulmonary component of second heart sound.

There is usually a loud pulmonary ejection click.

Murmurs are absent. Some patients have a soft mid systolic murmur at left sternal edge. With progress in severity of pulmonary hypertension a loud pulmonary regurgitation early diastolic murmur may develop and as right ventricular decompensation occurs murmur of tricuspid regurgitation appears.

Congestive cardiac failure is a terminal feature.

Arrhythmias usually herald decline of patient.

ECG

QRS axis is deviated right ward usually in excess of + 100°. Marked right ventricular hypertrophy is present in precordial leads with a tall R-wave in V1 and or a QR complex in V1 and deep T-wave inversion in right precordial leads. P-waves are tall and peaked but may be normal. PR interval is usually normal. Serial tracings may be valuable in following progression of disease. Appearance of T inversion in lead 2, 3, and avf is a late sign.

Radiology

Chest X-ray shows prominence of main pulmonary artery and some degree of cardiac enlargement with normal peripheral pulmonary vascularity. Vascular markings at hilum are occasionally normal. Right atrial enlargement is slight but may be prominent when heart failure or tricuspid regurgitation occurs. Barium swallow is normal and lung parenchyma is always normal.

Pulmonary Function Tests

A decrease in PaO_2 is found if there is a right to left shunt at intra cardiac or pulmonary level. $PaCO_2$, PaO_2, pH are normal unless altered by dyspnea, hyperventilation or heart failure.

Echocardiography

Useful in assessing cardiac chamber dimensions and particularly assist in exclusion of left atrium and mitral obstructive lesions. Patients with high pulmonary vascular resistance and congenital heart defects, such as in Eisenmenger complex should be clarified by sweep from ventricular septum to aorta, to search for overriding of that vessel. Ratio of right ventricle projection period/right ventricle ejection time as obtained from right heart and pulmonary valve echocardiogram to determine the presence of pulmonary hypertension has been used. Whenever, pulmonary artery diastolic pressure or pulmonary vascular resistance is increased this ratio rises above normal value of 0.25.

Cardiac Catheterization

This demonstrates right ventricle and pulmonary artery pressure. Calculated levels of pulmonary vascular resistance are extremely high. Pulmonary artery wedge pressure is normal but may be difficult to obtain. Cardiac output is low in contrast to a low normal or even slightly increased output when pulmonary hypertension is due to disorder of pulmonary function or parenchymal lung disease. If right ventricular failure is present right ventricle end diastolic pressure and right atrial pressure are elevated.

Angiocardiography

Reveals dilated pulmonary vessels with pruned appearance and slow passage of contrast through lung. There is risk of sudden death associated with right side injection of contrast in these circumstances.

DIFFERENTIAL DIAGNOSIS

A wide variety of diseases are associated with an elevated pulmonary vascular resistance. Patients with severe pulmonary hypertension and Eisenmenger syndrome with intracardiac or intervascular communications are usually cyanosed. Lesions associated with pulmonary venous hypertension, such as pulmonary venous stenosis and malformations affecting left side of heart may give rise to an elevated pulmonary vascular resistance. The radiological findings of interstitial or alveolar edema may be helpful. Slightly enlarged left atrium indicate congenital mitral stenosis. An elevated pulmonary artery wedge pressure is helpful in confirming presence of pulmonary vein stenosis or left heart obstructive lesion.

Echocardiography clarifies anatomic type of obstruction whether it is cor triatriatum, supravalvular stenosing ring, mitral valve stenosis, mitral atresia, diseases of left ventricle myocardium or aortic outflow tract obstruction.

Evaluation of clinical picture and X-ray help to rule out diseases of pulmonary parenchyma.

Pulmonary artery elevation seen pulmonary parenchymal disease is not as marked as that in primary pulmonary hypertension.

Evidence of a thromboembolic disease or an associated systemic disease process should also be sought for carefully.

Prognosis and Treatment

The condition is progressive. Average duration of life after onset of symptoms in childhood is 1 year. Survival longer than 7 years is not reported. In older children severe and frequent syncopal episodes usually precede sudden death. It may also follow right ventricle failure which is progressive. No effective treatment is available though steroids, anticoagulants, digitalis and diuretics have been tried without success since fixed pulmonary vascular changes are unlikely to be influenced enough to change the natural course of the disease.

Miscellaneous Pulmonary Vascular Diseases

1. *Sickle cell anemia*: This is associated with occlusive pulmonary vascular disease. Pulmonary infarction and vascular changes occurring secondary to aggregation of abnormal red blood cells.
2. Connective tissue disorders: SLE causes arteritis of small pulmonary arteries.
3. *Nephrotic syndrome*: Primary thrombosis of pulmonary artery occurs when patients are on steroids and in diuretic phase of disease.
4. Anorexigenic drugs.
5. *Portal hypertension*: Substances released from platelets enter pulmonary circuit in portal hypertension and produce pulmonary vasoconstriction.
6. High altitude hypoxia elevates pulmonary artery pressure which returns to normal on descent to sea level.

Thromboembolic Pulmonary Vascular Diseases

1. *Acute thromboembolism*: Pulmonary embolization may follow prolonged immobilization or some diagnostic or therapeutic intervention. One-third of cases die dramatically. Others have an abrupt onset of severe respiratory symptoms. Many remain undiagnosed or believed clinically to have pneumonia. Primary causes of emboli are sepsis of lower abdomen, cachexia and Spitz Holter valve inserted for hydrocephalus management.

Hemodynamic changes: Decreased cardiac output, systemic hypotension, increased pulmonary artery pressure, increased pulmonary arterial resistance. Probably both mechanical and vasoconstrictive factors are responsible for pulmonary hypertension. In massive pulmonary embolism the clinical picture is dramatic. There is sudden collapse with hypotension, cyanosis, dyspnea, tachypnea, distended neck veins, prominent 3rd or 4th heart sounds, gallop and accentuation of pulmonary component of second heart sound. Death may occur immediately due to ventricular fibrillation. In some cases marked slowing of heart rate together with low stroke volume produces poor tissue perfusion with acidosis and cardiac standstill. ECG shows sinus tachycardia, right bundle branch block and nonspecific T-wave changes. ECG may be normal. X-ray chest may show vascular branching and prominence of main pulmonary artery but lobar atelectasis, consolidation and elevation of diaphragm are more frequent.

Pulmonary angiograms provide more reliable evidence of embolism than do pulmonary perfusion scans.

Management is conservative. External cardiac massage may be necessary when cardiac arrest occurs. Ionotropic and vasoconstrictive agents are useful. Removal of a massive embolus under cardiopulmonary bypass may be carried out. Lung scanning is used increasingly in diagnosis of pulmonary embolism with a high degree of sensitivity but not the specificity of pulmonary angiography.

In phlebothrombosis heparin should be started. Urokinase and streptokinase are thrombolytic agents. Massive pulmonary emboli lyse more rapidly with these than with heparin alone.

2. *Chronic thromboembolism*: Recurrent embolism with progressive pulmonary hypertension can complicate rheumatic fever, endocarditis and schistosomiasis.

Pulmonary hypertension also occurs as a complication of ventriculovenous shunts for treatment of hydrocephalus. Causes are infective emboli from superior *vena cava* and right atrium, spontaneous thrombosis and an autoimmune reaction of pulmonary vessels to cerebrospinal fluid. Clinical features of chronic thromboembolism are identical to primary pulmonary hypertension. Therapy consists of prevention of further embolism and regression of vascular changes secondary to previous emboli.

Air Embolism

A rare cause of acute cor pulmonale in childhood may complicate a variety of medical and surgical procedures including changing intravenous packs. Lethal dose varies with age, condition and position of patient and rapidity with which air enters the circulation. It may be as little as 5 ml/kg. Death results from an air lock within right ventricle or from embolism to lungs with secondary reflex pulmonary vasoconstriction. The infant becomes suddenly cyanosed and stops breathing. A loud continuous murmur or noise may be heard over precordium from air and blood trapped in right ventricle. Treatment consists of turning the patient onto left side with head in dependent position and administration of 100% oxygen. Aspiration of air through needle or catheter inserted into right ventricle may be helpful.

Fat Embolism

Very rare in children may occur in advanced systemic connective tissue diseases. In these even minimal trauma may cause rapid fulminating clinical course characterized by sudden onset dyspnea, tachypnea, cyanosis and tachycardia. Assisted ventilation may be necessary with steroids in massive doses.

51

Congestive Cardiac Failure

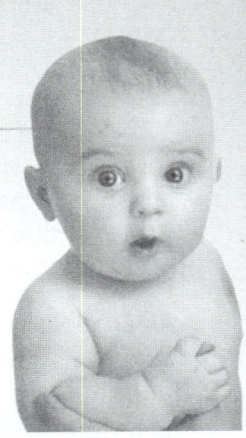

An inability of heart to increase its output adequately to meet normal demands of body tissues at rest and with exercise. Heart provides oxygenated blood to various organs of body by its pumping action. When it fails to do so it is evident initially only with exercise but if the process is progressive the signs are recognized with individual inactive. In first year of life clinical signs are usually not identified until they are evident at rest. Infection rather than activity is more likely to precipitate failure in infancy.

Causes of Cardiac Failure

1. Aortic and ductal defects:
   - Aortic regurgitation. Congenital or acquired.
   - Aortic valvular stenosis.
   - Congenital subaortic stenosis.
   - Subaortic stenosis with infundibular obstruction of right ventricular outflow.
   - Supra-aortic stenosis.
   - Absent aortic valve.
   - Aortic atresia.
   - Patent ductus arteriosus.
   - Isolated aorticopulmonary septal defect.
   - Persistent truncus arteriosus.
   - Preductal coarctation of aorta.

- Coarctation of aorta with patent ductus arteriosus, isolated coarctation, coarctation with patent ductus arteriosus and atrial septal defect, coarctation with PDA, ASD, VSD.
- Coarctation with TGV, PDA, VSD.
- Coarctation with TGV and PDA.
- Coarctation with ASD. With VSD.

2. Arrhythmias:
   - Complete heart block.
   - Complete heart block with endocardial fibroelastosis. Paroxysmal atrial tachycardia.
   - Paroxysmal ventricular tachycardia.
   - Persistent paroxysmal tachycardia.
   - Atrial flutter.
   - Atrial fibrillation.
   - Ventricular fibrillation.

3. Atrial septal defects:
   - Atrioventricularis communis.
   - Complete absence of atrial septum.
   - Persistent ostium primum.
   - Persistent ostium secundum.
   - Left ventriculo right atrial defect.
   - Lutembacher's syndrome (atrial septal defect with mitral stenosis).

4. Fistulae:
   - Arteriovenous fistulae.
   - Aneurysms.
     (systemic, congenital, acquired).

5. Common ventricle:
   - CV with completed transposition.
   - CV with normal great vessels.
   - CV with corrected L transposition of great vessels.
   - CV with aplasia of right ventricle sinus (single ventricle with rudimentary outlet chamber).
   - CV with aplasia or hypoplasia of left ventricle sinus.

- CV with absent or rudimentary ventricular septum.
- CV with absent right or left ventricular sinuses and ventricular septum.
- CV with common atrioventricular valve (with pulmonary atresia).

6. Mitral valve disease:
   - Mitral atresia.
   - Congenital mitral stenosis.
   - Congenital mitral regurgitation.

7. Pericarditis:
   - Constrictive.
   - Idiopathic.
   - Rheumatic.
   - Tubercular.
   - Viral.
   - Uremic.
   - Postpericardiotomy syndrome.

8. Pulmonary vein anomalies:
   - Anomalous pulmonary veins total cardiac (APVTC) into coronary sinus.
   - APVTC into right atrium.
   - APVT infracardiac into portal vein.
   - APVTI into ductus venosus.
   - APVT mixed.
   - APVT supracardiac into left superior *vena cava*.
   - APVTS into superior *vena cava*.

9. Pulmonary artery and valve anomalies:
   - Coarctation or stenosis of pulmonary artery branches.
   - Pulmonary atresia with normal aortic root.
   - Acute cor pulmonale.
   - Chronic cor pulmonale with emphysema.
   - CCP with pulmonary hypertension.
   - Fibrocystic disease.
   - Primary pulmonary hypertension.
   - Absent pulmonary valve.

10. Rheumatic fever:
    - Acute rheumatic fever.
    - Rheumatic aortic regurgitation.
    - Rheumatic aortic stenosis.
    - Rheumatic mitral regurgitation.
    - Rheumatic mitral stenosis.
11. Tetralogy of Fallot:
    - Atypical TOF (acyanotic).
    - cTOF with tricuspid regurgitation.
12. Transposition of great vessels:
    - Taussig Bing malformation (TGV with overriding pulmonary artery).
    - D and L TGV with cardiac shunts.
13. Tricuspid valve anomalies:
    - Tricuspid atresia.
    - Congenital.
    - TA with VSD.
    - TA with dextrocardia.
    - TA with D TGV.
    - TA with L TGV.
    - Congenital tricuspid stenosis.
    - Tricuspid regurgitation.
14. Ventricular septal defect:
    - Isolated primary simple VSD.
    - VSD with anomalous aortic cusps.
    - VSD with TR.
    - VSD with tricuspid valve perforation.
    - Ventriculoatrial defect.
    - Left ventricle to right atrium shunt.
15. Miscellaneous causes:
    - Bacterial endocarditis.
    - Systemic lupus erythematosus.
    - Polyarteritis nodosa.
    - Dextrocardia.
    - Levocardia

- Mesocardia with various types of cardiac shunts.
- Ebstein disease.
- Primary endocardial fibroelastosis with valvular involvement.
- Primary endocardial fibroelastosis without valvular involvement.
- Secondary endocardial fibroelastosis with or without valvular involvement.
- Glycogen storage disease of heart.
- Systemic hypertension.
- Hyperthyroidism.
- Hypothyroidism.
- Marfan's syndrome with cardiac involvement.
- Muscular dystrophies.
- Friedreich ataxia.
- Myocarditis idiopathic, viral, toxic.
- Cardiac tumors.

AGE OF ONSET OF CARDIAC FAILURE: NEWBORN

First two months of life.

1. Volume overloading from tricuspid regurgitation and pulmonary regurgitation.
2. Arteriovenous fistula.
3. Hypoplasia of left heart chamber with pulmonary venous congestion and closed foramen ovale.
4. Asphyxia at birth.
5. Endocardial fibroelastosis.
6. Massive placental transfusion—twin to twin.
7. Paroxysmal tachycardia in first few hours of life.

Birth to One Week

Aortic atresia or hypoplastic left heart syndrome. This is accompanied by patent ductus so that the only way blood can get to coronary arteries is from right heart via ductus in reverse direction down a small thread like ascending aorta. Blood reaching coronaries is not fully saturated. Patent ductus may itself constrict thus threatening entire circulation. Perfusion of lungs is at systemic pressure and blood returning from lungs enters small left atrium from which it may or may not be able to escape adequately through foramen ovale. If foramen ovale is closed this leads to pulmonary edema and death. Many of these cases develop hypoglycemia during first few days of life. Transposition of great vessels and coarctation of aorta also cause cardiac failure in first week of life.

First Month of Life

1. Coarctation of aorta with PDA.
2. VSD.
3. Atrioventricularis communis.
4. Paroxysmal atrial tachycardia.
5. Total anomalous pulmonary venous drainage.
6. Tricuspid atresia.
7. Common ventricle.
8. Persistent truncus arteriosus.
9. Bizarre lesions associated with dextrocardia.

Second Month of Life

Transposition of great vessels is the commonest cause.

Second to Third Month

1. VSD with large opening between ventricles and low pulmonary vascular resistance. In severe cardiac failure ASD and PDA are associated.
2. Endocardial fibroelastosis.

Three to Six Months

1. VSD isolated or associated with other anomalies.
2. Anomalous left coronary artery origin from pulmonary artery.
3. Truncus arteriosus with large left to right shunt.

Six to Twelve Months

1. Endocardial fibroelastosis.
2. Atrioventricularis communis.
3. Total anomalous pulmonary venous drainage.
4. Ventricular septal defect.

HEMODYNAMICS

First response to increased load on heart is hypertrophy of ventricle concerned. This occurs usually before there is an increase in venous pressure but eventually pressure rise appears. This may be kept within physiological bounds by increased strength of contraction of cardiac muscle and also by an increased heart rate. In time however these mechanisms of increased rate and strength become inadequate. Now the compensation is by means of increased venous pressure.

1. *Venous pressure*: First rise in venous pressure is physiological and does not lead to signs of cardiac failure. When burden is excessive and cardiac muscle is fatigued signs of cardiac failure begin to appear. This state of cardiac muscle fatigued is referred to as hypodynamic. Hypodynamic hearts are the ones most likely to respond to digitalis therapy. Starlings law states that contractile power of heart muscle is a function of initial length of muscle fibers. More the heart is filled in diastole greater is the force of following cardiac contraction. Starlings mechanism is augment by neural and hormonal influences. In a healthy baby ventricle can increase its output without any change in filling pressure because of these additional mechanisms. Initially a slight increase in heart rate, respiration or myocardial contractility will be adequate to supply baby's physiological needs in heart failure. Eventually arterial pressure will rise.

Mechanisms of rise in systemic venous pressure:

a. Decreased effectiveness of cardiac muscle leading to damming back of blood and raised arterial pressure.

b. Reflex increase in sympathetic vasomotor tone throughout body increasing rate of flow through veins to right atrium.

c. Retention of fluid by kidneys causing an augmentation of both interstitial fluid volume and blood volume.

2. *Right atrial pressure*: In children rise is slight because failure is not accompanied by much fluid retention and it is of acute onset. Thus not enough duration of high capillary pressure to develop edema. Disturbed renal function due to hypoxia, myocardial metabolites, vasoconstriction, neural or hormonal factors will cause progressive retention of fluid.

3. *Redistribution of blood flow*: Local vasodilatation may occur in certain muscles of body and in other areas flow may be restricted. Reduced flow occurs in skin, liver and kidneys. In this way aortic pressure is maintained for selective flow to vital organs of body.

4. *Right and left heart failure in various defects*: Primary right heart failure occurs in pulmonary stenosis, ASD osteum secundum, osteum primum, atrioventricularis communis, total anomalous pulmonary venous drainage and aortic atresia.

Primary left heart failure occurs in aortic stenosis, PDA, coarctation of aorta, endocardial fibroelastosis, myocarditis, paroxysmal atrial tachycardia, tricuspid atresia, mitral insufficiency.

60% of both right and left heart failure are due to TGV and 10% are due to VSD.

VSD is primarily a burden on left heart as long as resistance and pressure in pulmonary circuit is less than in aorta. When pressure in pulmonary artery is same as in systemic work of both ventricles is similar. Failure under such circumstances is biventricular.

TGV is associated with VSD in 50% cases. Failure in this combination occurs early in life once pulmonary vascular resistance is fallen sufficiently to greatly increase pulmonary flow and increase left ventricular pressure to systemic level. As a result part of left ventricle blood is expelled into systemic circulation. Thus a considerable systolic and diastolic overload is established for both ventricles.

In children with intracardiac or vascular shunts pulmonary circulation may get congested without failure being present. Digitalis differentiates between these two conditions.

5. *Volume load, pressure load*: Myocardial efficiency is greater with an increased diastolic load at moderate or low pressure than in presence of significantly increased pressure load.

Increased diastolic overloading is common in congenital heart disease in childhood.

Right ventricle can sustain systemic pressure readily. Eisenmenger complex is rare. Shunt may reverse itself with ASD, VSD or PDA. Right ventricle failure may occur now with diastolic overload.

In infancy a combination of high pressure and large flow leads to failure in VSD.

High pressure defects, such as AS, PS, coarctation do not cause failure in isolated form but when they are associated with diastolic load CHF may occur.

Tricuspid regurgitation is commonly the result of insufficiency of right ventricle than the cause of it. In right ventricle dilatation anterior and posterior cusps of tricuspid valve are inadequately approximated to prevent reflux of blood into right atrium. Pulmonary valve regurgitation is common in pulmonary hypertension owing to dilatation of pulmonary artery. Incompetence is minimal. If pressure is high in pulmonary artery and right ventricle insufficiency of pulmonary valve is likely to precipitate failure or augment it if other causes are operating already. Failure of left ventricle causes a rise in left ventricle end diastolic pressure and left atrial, pulmonary venous and pulmonary capillary pressure. Lungs become congested and less compliant. Rhonchi are frequently heard in children but crepitations of full blown pulmonary edema are uncommon.

6. *Pulmonary vascular bed*: Hypoxia in slight degree increases pulmonary vascular resistance and lowers degree and prevalence of heart failure in children.

7. *Ventilatory capacity*: There is great increase in resistance to air flow. Transudate in alveolar wall, alveoli and air passage

may cause sufficient interference with oxygen transfer to reduce arterial oxygen concentration to produce visible cyanosis. Nocturnal dyspnea is less common in children. With restlessness, irritability and crying the activity during waking hours may raise blood pressure and systemic resistance and tend to increase load in pulmonary circulation during day.

CHF when occurs in AS is likely to occur in first year of life than later. AR rarely causes CHF unless associated with VSD. MR is regular accompaniment of osteum primum ASD and atrioventricular communis. It augments left to right shunt and precipitates CHF.

8. *Systemic resistance in coarctation of aorta*: There is increased resistance in upper part of body. On exercise or crying pressure may rise above 200 mm Hg and add to left ventricle load. When it is accompanied by an intracardiac shunt, such as VSD or PDA signs of CHF are likely to appear in neonatal period.

9. *Chemical to mechanical energy*: Membrane pumps continually use energy to preserve the gradient of sodium, potassium and calcium ions. Substrates, such as carbohydrates, fats, proteins are taken up from coronary blood stream leading to production of ATP, stores of which provide energy for cellular activity. In failing myocardium there is a decrease in maximum intrinsic velocity of shortening (V max) and decrease in rate of pressure rise (DP/dt). Frank Starling mechanism plus increased sympathetic stimulation helps to maintain overall compensation of circulation in early stages of failure. Increased stress beyond capacity to respond adequately leads to further failure of deepening degree. Specific biochemical limitations of cardiac function appear to be responsible. Uptake of substrates and oxygen is not a primary problem and energy utilization is not significantly decreased. There is defect in excitation—contraction coupling. This involves release and uptake of calcium ions from sarcoplasmic reticulum. Ability of digitalis to improve contractile state of myocardium is related to cellular action of drug to potentiate excitation—contraction coupling by

enhancing concentration of calcium ions in endoplasm enveloping myofibrils at moment of cardiac contraction. Toxic manifestations of digitalis are due to loss of intracellular potassium ions.

CLINICAL FEATURES

1. *Dyspnea*: Children with large heart may have dyspnea on effort without CCF. Dyspnea at rest is present in heart failure in infancy. Tachypnea (respiratory rate more than 50/minute) is abnormal in a baby. Dyspnea may be precipitated by feeding. Sucking and swallowing lead to exhaustion and breathlessness.

2. *Venous pressure*: External jugular vein in babies in first year of life can be seen clearly. Struggling, crying or respiratory distress will raise venous pressure. In small children when back of hand is not chubby venous pressure may be assessed by prominence of veins in that area by raising and lowering the hand above position of right atrium one may notice the point at which emptying may occur in vein. These veins should empty if hand is held at or just above sternal angle with child at an approximate angle of 45°. In older children external jugular vein may be seen and the top of its distended pulsating column may be recognized easily. Position of emptying of veins at back of hand can be assessed more accurately. Top of venous column should not exceed 3 cm above sternal angle.

3. *Liver size*: Enlargement means 3 to 4 cm down the costal margin. It is accompanied by pain or tenderness of organ. Liver pulsations are usually due to impulse transmitted from heart movement. Occasionally it is due to an atrial pressure wave during ventricular systole especially in presence of tricuspid regurgitation.

4. *Pulmonary rales*: In infants a considerable degree dyspnea is present before basal rales are heard. A respiratory infection may complicate pulmonary plethora due to CCF. Infection may also precipitate failure and at times rales can be due to infection or failure or both.

5. *Vital capacity*: There is reduced vital capacity in rheumatic fever even before failure appears. With onset of failure there is greater reduction due to congestion of lung fields.

6. *Radiological signs*: Pulmonary congestion in X-ray chest. There is widespread increase in density of lung fields specially in hilar area. In acute pulmonary edema a diffuse mottling appears that is apparent right out to periphery of lung fields.

7. *Circulation time*: Normal is 6 to 12 seconds. In CCF it may be prolonged to 30–50 seconds. This delay is in part to engorgement of systemic veins and vascular bed of lungs.

8. *Gallop rhythm*: Presence of gallop rhythm in congenital heart disease, myocarditis and nephritis denotes CCF. In rheumatic heart disease presence of gallop is of more benign yet significant import. Sounds that simulate gallop rhythm are third heart sound, atrial or presystolic sound, systolic click and opening snap of mitral stenosis. Most commonly heard gallop in children is a protodiastolic sound coming 0.10 second after second heart sound. It is due to sudden distension of ventricles in rapid filling stage of diastole. Same mechanism produces physiological third heart sound. In normal infants and in older children this is not heard or is so faint as to be insignificant. Presence of a well heard third heart sound is considered to be pathological.

9. *Cyanosis*: Three groups of causes of cyanosis in children are:

   a. *Congenital heart disease*: Cyanosis results from a shunt of cyanotic blood into systemic circulation. In presence of failure shunt may be augmented. TGV, aortic atresia and single ventricle are good examples.

   b. *Central cyanosis*: This is due to pulmonary congestion or disease with inadequate oxygenation in lungs. In this failure is not accompanied by shunt, e.g. coarctation of aorta, isolated myocarditis, endocardial fibroelastosis.

   c. *Vasomotor*: Effect in small vessels and capillaries leading to a slowing of bloodstream and desaturation of hemoglobin. This may occur in heart failure and is accompanied by cold extremities. Oxygen saturation of arterial blood is normal indicating its peripheral origin, e.g. pulmonary stenosis without a shunt, endocardial fibroelastosis, isolated myocarditis and coarctation of aorta.

A baby with large VSD and pulmonary congestion may be cyanotic because of inadequate oxygenation of blood in lung fields or because of a partial shunt between right to left ventricle and aorta.

10. *ESR*: An elevated ESR in rheumatic fever drops to normal level when failure supervenes. This effect is related to edema and gain in body weight in more chronic type of failure with rheumatic heart disease. In acute rheumatic fever with an overwhelming infection and heart failure the ESR remains high. In chronic failure with edema when edema decreases the ESR returns to previous high levels until the infection subsides.

11. *Blood pressure*: In slight cardiac decompensation blood pressure is usually in normal range. In severe failure a low systolic blood pressure is common (normal systolic blood pressure is between 75 and 95 mm Hg).

12. *Heart rate*: Heart rate is usually increased to levels over 100–150/minute in children over 1–2 years in CHF. This is due to Bainbridge reflex which occurs with a rise of pressure in right atrium and by which vagal effect is diminished and heart rate increased.

Right Heart Failure

This occurs in aortic atresia, TGV, TAPVD, ASD, VSD, atrioventricularis communis, preductal coarctation. Signs are increased venous pressure, dyspnea, edema and enlargement of liver.

Left Heart Failure

Dyspnea, rales in chest, gallop rhythm, radiological evidence of congested lung fields.

Commonly both ventricles fail together.

DIFFERENTIAL DIAGNOSIS

In first 24 hours of life there are a number of conditions that either simulate CHF or produce it:

1. *Aortic or mitral atresia with closed foramen ovale*: The blood returning to heart has no opportunity to escape and pulmonary edema with cyanosis and failure occur in few hours usually associated with large heart and no murmur. Angiography confirms.

2. *Anomalous pulmonary vein below diaphragm*: This produces excessive pulmonary congestion and pulmonary edema. An injection contrast medium in pulmonary vein will show anomalous vein.

3. *Infant of diabetic mother*: They have cardiomegaly. There is no CHF in most cases. If there is associated PDA or severe hypoglycemia CHF may occur.

4. *Placental transfusion*: At birth it increases blood volume and causes cardiomegaly with plethoric baby. This produces extra load on myocardium. This condition can be recognized by finding maternal red cells in fetal blood and may require an exchange transfusion.

5. *Twin to twin transfusion*: One baby must be anemic while other plethoric.

6. *Idiopathic polycythemia*: Cardiomegaly occurs with a high hematocrit over 65% and may occasionally be associated with convulsions.

7. *Respiratory distress syndrome*: With patent ductus may be difficult to differentiate from CHF. RDS is more responsive to oxygen and raised carbon dioxide is present in this condition.

In children with left to right shunt CCF is expected to occur at sometime but may not have occurred as yet. These infants have enlarged heart, tachycardia and tachypnea. If liver is not enlarged, right atrial pressure not elevated and there is no edema and activity is good, failure is not considered to be present.

Many infants with heart defect develop respiratory infection involving lungs, especially those with left to right shunt. Such children may have tachypnea without failure.

Finally babies with right to left shunt who are cyanotic and have reduced flow to lungs may at times have dyspnea. These infants are rarely in failure unless they have accompanying tricuspid regurgitation. Their dyspnea does not require digitalis.

Treatment

It is preferable to keep patient at an angle of 45°. Baby should be turned from side to side to minimize pulmonary stasis.

1. *Digitalis*: Slowing of heart rate is due to restored compensation of failing organ. Digitalis appears to have an effect on rate in certain arrhythmias of which atrial fibrillation is prime example. Therapeutic doses of digitalis do not produce much slowing of normal heart but do so in presence of failure. Slowing of heart with a conventional dose is usually not a sign of toxicity but simply an improvement in child's cardiac function or moderate effect of digitalis mediated through vagus nerve.

   In heart failure chief effect of digitalis is on myocardium itself. It causes an increased force of systolic contraction with more adequate emptying of heart. One minor effect of digitalis is diuretic action which is independent of its effect on heart. Digoxin has rapid action, duration of effect is shorter and its toxic effects are short lived. Therapeutic effect is reached before toxic level is approached.

   Dose: Digoxin absorption averages 80% of orally administered dose. Peak levels are reached in serum in 30 to 60 minutes. A plateu curve is achieved in 4 to 6 hours. Digitalizing dose of digoxin is 0.04 to 0.08 mg/kg body weight given in 4 divided doses over 24 hours. Maintenance dose is one fifth to one fourth of digitalizing dose. In urgently needed cases rapid digitalization can be achieved by intravenous route.

   Toxicity: Anorexia, nausea, vomiting are early signs followed by visual symptoms, dizziness, headache, ectopic beat, first degree heart block, bundle branch block, intraventricular conduction impairment, shortening of QT interval, ventricular tachycardia, sinoatrial block, intra-atrial block.

These are rare in children. Characteristic abnormality on ECG are scooping of ST segment with inversion of first portion of T-wave. Digitalis poisoning can occur in absence of ECG changes. Atrial fibrillation may be produced with an overdose of digitalis.

2. *Oxygen*: When there is desaturation of arterial blood oxygen administration increases saturation by 10 to 20%. A concentration of 50% is maintained by flow rate 5 liter/minute. High concentration irritates nasal mucosa and favor atelectasis by washing away pulmonary alveolar nitrogen. In cor pulmonale, chronic hypoxia and carbon di oxide retention may be present. Respiratory center is acclimatized to high CO_2 and ceases to respond, respirations being stimulated largely by hypoxia. Administration of oxygen abolishes this hypoxic drive and patient goes into carbon dioxide narcosis.

3. *Diuretics*: Fluid retention is almost always present in CHF. Frusemide can be given orally. One daily dose is sufficient. Intravenous dose is 1 mg/kg body weight. Orally 2–3 mg/kg body weight. Serum potassium level should be monitored and potassium chloride should be given orally when serum level falls.

Treatment of Associated Pathological Features

1. *Electrolyte imbalances*: Mercurial diuretics cause more chloride loss than sodium loss. Hypochloremic alkalosis may occur.

2. Hyponatremia:

   a. *Dilutional hyponatremia*: In edema serum sodium concentration may be lowered because of retention of greater quantities of water. This is best treated by restricting fluid intake to 500 ml per day.

   b. Acute sodium depletion may occur in early stage when diuretic is used with salt restriction. Symptoms include lethargy and sleepiness.

   c. Chronic sodium depletion may occur in a strict dietary regime of low sodium plus prolonged use of diuretic.

Signs are muscle weakness and cramps and poor tissue turgor. Gradual increases of salt in diet will correct.

3. *Acidosis*: In TGV where failure is associated with cyanosis severe acidosis may occur requiring prompt therapy with sodium bicarbonate 2–5 meq per kg intravenously. Amount of bicarbonate required may be arrived at by formula. The desired HCO_3 (23 mEq/litre)–existing HCO_3 concentration × 0.6/kg body weight = HCO_3 in mEq.

4. *Respiratory acidosis*: In reduced pulmonary ventilation CO_2 retention occurs. Acidosis may develop in cor pulmonale. Treatment is of underlying lung disease.

5. *Potassium depletion*: This may occur with excessive diuresis or prolonged administration of cortisone. Potassium ion exerts an antagonistic effect on digitalis activity. Orally potassium chloride should be given 1 gm per day.

6. *Edema*: Low sodium diet helps to clear edema. Normal diet contains 5–12 gm of salt per day. A reduction to 0.5 to 1 gm per day will prevent fluid retention in body.

Pulmonary edema occurs in aortic atresia, primary endocardial fibroelastosis, VSD, TAPVD below diaphragm. Wheezing in CHF is characteristic of pulmonary edema. Causes are increased capillary permeability, reduced plasma oncotic pressure (more likely to occur in premature) and increased capillary pressure in pulmonary vascular bed. Treatment is with upright posture, morphine 1 mg per year of age, oxygen 50% concentration 5 liter per minute flow.

7. Treatment of associated respiratory infection by appropriate antibiotic.

DIGITALIS INTOXICATION

There are two types:
1. Therapeutic toxic levels.
2. Digitalis poisoning.

Therapeutic Toxic Levels

One or more of the following ECG signs may be present:
1. Supraventricular tachycardia (atrial or atrioventricular junctional) with atrioventricular block.

2. Frequent or multifocal ventricular premature beats, ventricular bigemini or ventricular tachycardia.
3. Atrial fibrillation with high grade atrioventricular block (ventricular response less than 50 beats per minute) and ventricular premature beats.
4. Sinus rhythm with second or third degree atrioventricular block. Digitalis toxicity is less common in pediatric age group, occurring in less than 2% of infants and children receiving a digitalis maintenance dose for chronic failure.

    Serum levels of 2 nanogram per ml or above are associated with signs of toxicity.

    There are a number of factors which influence an individual's sensitivity to digitalis. These include serum potassium, sodium, calcium, magnesium, hypoxia, pH, autonomic tone, thyroid status, associated cardioactive drug.

    Radioimmuno assay of digoxin should be done.

    Bradycardia in children is rarely a sign of digitalis toxicity in children. The drug may be continued unless the bradycardia is associated with Arrhythmias or heart rate falls below 60/ minute. Improvement associated with digitalis therapy in CCF is accompanied by diminution of sympathetic activity and this may be the factor that reduces rate rather than action of digitalis on vagus nerve or sinus pacemaker.

Treatment

1. Dilantin is particularly useful in treating tachycardia of digoxin toxicity since it depresses the enhanced ventricular automaticity without affecting intraventricular conduction. It also reverses the digitalis induced prolongation of PR interval. Dilantin is particularly useful in supraventricular arrhythmia due to digoxin.
2. Lidocain is effective in digoxin induced ventricular tachycardia. It does not affect conduction velocity of AV node and ventricular myocardium.
3. Propranolol is useful in tachyarrhythmias and ventricular premature beats. Its disadvantage is that in addition to its depressing effect on cardiac contractility and heart rate it has a beta blocking action that diminishes sympathetic support for failing heart.

4. Electric overdrive by either atrial or ventricular pacing may be used for suppression of ventricular arrhythmias induced by digitalis. The electrical stimulus is delivered at a more rapid rate than frequency of idiopathic ventricular focus thus suppressing the later.
5. Countershock: Shock energy should be kept at lower than average levels since this diminishes the possibility of shock induced Arrhythmias.
6. Atropine and electrical pacing in the event of complete heart block (potassium is contraindicated in complete heart block).

Digitalis Poisoning

Majority of children are between 18 months and 4 years old. Signs are nausea, vomiting, diarrhea, drowsiness, headache, confusion, convulsions, color vision, blurred vision and other personal idiosyncracy to the drug. Effect on heart are development of cardiac failure, arrhythmia or heart block.

Guide to management of digitalis poisoning:

1. Determine time, amount, type of ingestion.
2. Empty the stomach.
3. Monitor ECG and vital signs.
4. Determine serum electrolytes potassium, sodium, chloride, magnesium.
5. Treat cardiac arrhythmias with dilantin, lidocain or propranolol.
6. Sodium Ethylene Diamine Tetra Acetic acid (EDTA) is of value. It has rapid onset of action but its effects are transient and it occasionally produces hypotension.
7. Give intravenous potassium chloride when patient is voiding and serum potassium is low. Potassium is contraindicated in heart block or with heart rate less than 50/minute.
8. Use an external electrical pacemaker for cardiac arrest or extreme bradycardia.
9. Dialysis.
10. Digitalis antibodies.

52

The Distressed Newborn

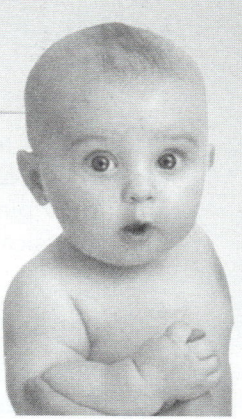

Cardiac malformations as well as other disturbances in newborn with architecturally normal heart can produce cardiorespiratory distress in neonatal period.

Among the newborn with congenital heart disease infants in distress in first week of life are at greatest risk. Diagnosis after cardiac catheterization gives the most useful indication of the frequency with which specific cardiac disorders present:

1. TGV: 17.4%
2. VSD: 11.2%
3. Coarctation complex: 13.6%
4. Fallot's tetralogy: 7.1%
5. Hypoplastic left heart: 6.9%
6. Patent ductus arteriosus: 5.3%
7. Single ventricle: 5.2%
8. Transitional circulation: 5.3%
9. Hypoplastic right heart: 7.6%
10. Truncus arteriosus: 1.7%
11. AV canal defect: 3%
12. Tricuspid atresia: 2.1%

Clinical Features

Physical signs of cardiovascular system normally change after birth during transition of circulation from fetal to postnatal life. Physical signs of both normal and abnormal newborn infants, such as right ventricular dominance, behavior of second

459

heart sound and color of mucous membranes are governed largely by level of pulmonary artery pressure, rate of constriction of ductus arteriosus, metabolic status of infant and amount of placental transfusion. These variables can add to or mask physical signs in infants with CHD.

Most severe CHD in early infancy are not associated with loud murmurs and many malformations that eventually are associated with loud murmurs most often do not show them immediately after birth. Heart sounds in severe CHD are abnormal and loud. These sounds together with a rapid rate may constitute the first signs of serious illness. A gallop rhythm is an extremely helpful sign that indicates presence of CHF. Presence of a single heart sound after 12 hours of birth is always abnormal and should stimulate search for other signs of cardiopulmonary disease. An ejection click is normally noted during only first few hours of life when it may accompany normal hypertension that characterizes transitional pulmonary circulation. Thereafter presence of loud click may signify a large aorta, such as in pulmonary atresia, a large pulmonary artery, such as in hypoplastic left heart syndrome or a large single vessel as in truncus arteriosus.

In newborn period there is considerable propensity for peripheral cyanosis, blood arterial oxygen tensions are significantly lower shortly after birth. Cardiac malformations that are usually associated with severe arterial oxygen desaturation later in neonatal period may present in first few days of life in a relatively acyanotic form, owing to good mixing of oxygenated and unoxygenated blood that can result temporarily from continued patency of ductus arteriosus or foramen ovale.

Reduced amplitude of arterial pulses is an important sign in this age group and implies reduced cardiac output into aorta. This may result from anatomical malformations, such as hypoplastic left heart, severe aortic stenosis and coarctation of aorta or from acute left ventricular failure due to other causes, such as ischemia. Bounding pulses usually imply a large aortic run off, e.g. in large PDA or truncus arteriosus.

Tachypnea is a useful sign of cardiopulmonary difficulty. Respiratory rate of more than 50/minute is indicative of a cardiorespiratory disorder. Tachypnea without much respiratory effort is characteristic of congenital heart disease of congestive type. In severe pulmonary disease obvious labored breathing is a striking feature.

Large liver is associated with other signs of CHF.

X-RAY CHEST

In frankly cyanotic infants cardiomegaly or a strikingly unusual cardiac contour is often present. Presence of considerable cyanosis in association with normal appearing lung vascular marking favors transposition complex. Presence of severe cyanosis in association with extreme pulmonary stenosis is associated with oligemic lung fields.

In early newborn period chest film may appear normal and change later, e.g. in transposition complex or may have an abnormal configuration in absence of cardiac malformation. Diagnostic nihilism with respect to X-ray film can be avoided by detailed consideration of cardiac contour, lung vascular pattern, abdominal and cardiac situs and the appearance of thoracic cage.

ECG

In first few days of life abnormal right ventricular hypertrophy is difficult to interpret. Subtle changes are abnormal frontal plane QRS axis, Q-waves in V3R and V1 or abnormally peaked P-waves. After 72 hours an upright T in V1 is a useful sign of moderate RVH. Presence of LVH can be easily recognized in infant's ECG.

Blood Measurement

Arterial blood gases and pH. Arterial oxygen desaturation can be quantified. Response to high oxygen breathing evaluated and acidosis combated. Samples from right radial or brachial artery or temporal vessels better indicate oxygen tension of blood leaving left heart. Umbilical cord artery samples may be affected by a fetal direction of flow through ductus arteriosus.

Hyperoxic studies are useful in distinguishing transitional disturbances from true major cardiac malformations of cyanotic type when a low PaO_2 is discovered. Values of PaO_2 during hyperoxia in excess of 100 mm Hg exclude TGV. Blood sugar calcium, magnesium estimation are useful in treatment.

Echocardiography

Useful in hypolastic left heart syndrome and right heart syndrome, TOF, TGV and truncus arteriosus. Serial study of left to right shunt particularly PDA of premature infants is also of great help.

Cardiac Catheterization and Angiocardiography

This technique is still the gold standard by which others may be judged. Detailed anatomic information is obtained preoperatively. In addition to separating severe cardiac malformations from distressed newborn with no cardiac malformation in first week of life there is also difficulty in deciding whether an infant with evidence of CHD has a mild or severe defect or whether early absence of symptoms will soon be replaced by more important events, such as CHF. Physical signs are often subtle and may be misleading.

NONSTRUCTURAL HEART DISEASE

1. *Respiratory distress syndrome*: Incidence 14 to 33% of premature live births. 0.2% in term infants. Deficiency of lung surfactant as a result of immaturity and intranatal stress leads to alveolar atelectasis. Hypoxia resulting from perfusion of poorly ventilated areas of lungs leads to pulmonary arteriolar vasoconstriction. Right to left shunting occurs at foramen ovale, ductus arteriosus and in lungs early in disease because of increase in pulmonary vascular resistance. With collapse of alveoli shunting becomes mainly intrapulmonary. On way to recovery a variable left to right shunt may occur and persist for a time.

   Tachypnea is apparent from birth or shortly thereafter with progression subcostal and intercostal drawing, edema, sternal recession will appear. Central cyanosis occurs in few hours. Signs of CCF do not appear unless a large ductal left to right shunt occurs in recovery phase.

Chest X-ray confirms diagnosis in 85% cases. A granular pattern on inspiration or a uniform opacity on expiration along with an air bronchogram is a typical sign.

ECG changes are nonspecific to aid in diagnosis.

Treatment is with oxygen, relief of acidosis and assisted ventilation. Drug therapy for pulmonary vasoconstriction has not altered course. Surgery for PDA complicating RDS is controversial. Maximum mortality occurs on second day.

2. Polycythemia: Hyperviscosity syndrome is characterized by cyanosis, plethora, neurological signs, RDS, CHF and tachycardia. Heart is enlarged. Hyperbilirubinemia and hypoglycemia occurs. Partial exchange transfusion will improve viscosity. Polycythemia is due to placental twin to twin or maternal to fetal transfusion. Intrauterine hypoxia stimulating excess erythropoietin production and small size for gestational age are contributing factors.

3. *Infants of diabetic mother*: Pregnancy is hazardous in diabetic female and perinatal mortality is higher in diabetic because of increased incidence of complications during pregnancy, cesareen section and premature births.

The typical infant of diabetic mother is large for gestational age. Increased cell size and nuclear size is noted in liver, thymus, adrenals, lungs and heart.

Heart is larger than expected week of gestation. CHF due to hypertrophic cardiomyopathy is reported. Cardiac and spinal congenital anomalies are most frequent. VSD and TGV are common defects.

Special metabolic problems occur in infants of diabetic mother that influence cardiac function:

a. *Hypoglycemia*: 50% newborns have blood glucose concentration less than 30 mg % in first 6 hours of life. Symptoms are jitteriness, tremors, convulsions, sweating, cyanosis or limpness. Hypoglycemia may accompany CHF and produce cardiac enlargement clinically and in X-ray chest.

b. *Hypocalcemia*: Tetany may occur in 23% of newborn.

4. *Transient myocardial ischemia of newborn*: Cardiovascular changes induced by hypoxia in term newborn are noted. Persistent high pulmonary vascular resistance leads to maintenance of fetal type of circulation in severe cases. Cyanosis RDS and CHF suggest possibility of CHD. There is evidence that ischemic changes in right ventricle create tricuspid regurgitation in distressed term infants. Ischemia basis has been obtained from myocardial perfusion scanning.

Echocardiography and isotope angiocardiography may exclude anatomical cardiac abnormalities and cardiac catheterization most certainly does. On the cine angiocardiogram a striking feature is poor contractility of left ventricle. Therapy with oxygen, digoxin and diuretic will support sick neonate until effects of hypoxia subside in days to a week.

ECG and X-ray chest revert to normal in 3 months.

HEART MALFORMATIONS

A. Frank Cyanosis in First Week of Life

1. *Transposition of great arteries*: Physiologically systemic and pulmonary circulations run in parallel instead of running in series. Necessary connections between two circuits is dependent on patent foramen ovale and ductus arteriosus. Hypoxia develops when these fetal connections become inadequate or close within a few days of birth. In few cases natural connections may remain adequate for 1 to 4 weeks. Additional defects, such as VSD will allow greater obligatory mixing in two circuits. Most patients are males of good size at birth. Associated extra cardiac anomalies are rare. Cyanosis due to mixing of blood in two circuits appears at birth. In those with an intact septum and without pulmonary stenosis murmurs are absent or trivial. CHF may appear at this time. Classically chest X-ray after first week shows an egg shaped tilted heart with a narrow supracardiac segment or pedicle and increased vascularity. In first few days heart is nearly normal in size, shape and vascular markings. ECG in majority without

additional lesions will present with right axis deviation
and right ventricle hypertrophy. A small number may
have left axis deviation. Arterial oxygen tension, a crucial
investigation will show values of 15 to 30 mm Hg with
little effect on breathing 80 to 100% oxygen. Two
dimensional echocardiography is useful in diagnosis.
Sudden deterioration in neonate's condition may occur
due to hypoxia and acidosis. These patients constitute a
major medical emergency and require prompt diagnostic
confirmation and balloon atrial septostomy.

2. *Hypoplastic right ventricle syndrome*: Right ventricle is of
small size associated with pulmonary stenosis. There may
be accompanying hypoplasia of tricuspid valve and ring.
The smaller the right ventricle the smaller the ring and
valve. In 20% cases there is atresia of main pulmonary
artery without detectable pulmonary valve atresia.
Although in majority the right ventricle is small a minority
has normal or nearly normal chamber size. Enlarged right
atrium has an exit route through foramen ovale or through
an ASD.

Most patients are cyanotic soon after birth. Degree of
cyanosis varies with patency and flow across ductus
arteriosus. Prominent 'a' waves may be visible in jugular
vein. Liver may be enlarged as CHF develops in time.
Second heart sound single and aortic. Ejection clicks are
common. There may be no murmurs, a variable mid and
late systolic murmur of tricuspid regurgitation or a faint
continuous murmur of flow through PDA. In chest X-ray
majority of patients show cardiomegaly and prominent
right atrium and oligemic lung fields. ECG estimation of
chamber size is possible. Normal ventricular or right
ventricular hypertrophy pattern suggest a reasonable size
ventricular cavity. Left ventricular hypertrophy suggests
small right ventricle and small tricuspid valve. At cardiac
catheterization giant 'a' waves may be present at right
atrium and mean right atrial pressure will exceed mean
left atrial pressure. Right ventricle pressure is elevated
over left ventricle or aortic pressure. Angiographic

evidence from right and left ventricular injections is most useful.

3. *Ebstein anomaly*: Cardiomegaly, clear lung fields and right atrial hypertrophy are useful in diagnosis. CCF is rare.

4. Total anomalous pulmonary venous drainage entering systemic veins below diaphragm. Chest X-ray shows pulmonary venous congestion and slight cardiomegaly. ECG shows right ventricle dominance or hypertrophy.

5. *Tricuspid valve atresia*: ECG is most characteristic showing left axis deviation and left ventricular hypertrophy.

B. Frank Cyanosis in 1 to 4 Weeks of Life

In this category are placed complex lesions with pulmonary stenosis that develop cyanosis with increasing time and obstruction. Example is Fallot tetralogy. Cyanosis on crying may be first sign, progressing to cyanotic spells. Heart is quiet and second sound is single or widely split with soft pulmonary closure sound. Ejection systolic murmur varying with severity of cyanosis is heard at left sternal border. ECG shows right ventricle hypertrophy and in half of cases transitional zone over right precordial leads.

C. Congestive Cardiac Failure in First Week of Life

Two main groups of cardiac defects without significant cyanosis but which cause CCF occur in immediate newborn period.

1. *Hypoplastic left heart syndrome*: In this syndrome with small left ventricle, mitral valve and ring and ascending aorta the commonest group has congenital aortic valve atresia. A tiny cavity with a thick wall or only a potential cavity may constitute left ventricle.

   Endocardial fibroelastosis is observed in 50% of cases and also only in presence of patent mitral valve.

   Mitral atresia occurs in 25% cases or mitral valve if patent is small.

   Only 10% of the hearts show VSD.

In 85% cases atrial septum is patent but in 15% atrial septum is intact.

With aortic valve atresia onset of CCF is early and death occurs in 4 to 5 days. At birth condition and weight of baby appear normal. Within first two days varying degree of cyanosis appears and cyanosis becomes progressive with increasing age. Tachypnea is present from shortly after birth but right ventricle failure may not be apparent for 2 to 3 days. Along with CCF peripheral pulses are poor. Precordium is hyperactive. Second sound is loud and single in pulmonary area and pulmonary ejection click may be present. Soft pulmonary ejection systolic murmur may be heard at left sternal border. X-ray chest shows marked cardiomegaly, increased vascular markings and pulmonary congestion by the time CCF is recognized. Barium swallow shows normal left atrial size and normal descending aorta, despite an associated coarctation of aorta. ECG shows right axis deviation, right atrial enlargement, right ventricle hypertrophy and QR pattern in right precordial leads. 10% cases show left axis deviation and left ventricle hypertrophy which is due to thick left ventricle wall. Echocardiography demonstrates small left sided structures nicely. Treatment of cardiac failure with digitalis, diuretic and oxygen will not improve condition substantially. In some transient improvement may occur when atrial connection is enlarged by creating an ASD. Physiologically pulmonary blood flow must be controlled and adequate systemic perfusion must be provided with banding of pulmonary artery branches for the former and creation of a central shunt for the latter. Ascending aorta must be adequate to receive shunt.

2. *Coarctation of aorta syndrome*: In newborn period coarctation of aorta as an isolated lesion producing CCF is rare. However, when there are associated intracardiac defects serious difficulties may develop early. Anatomic setting for coarctation is produced in fetus by infolding of aortic wall opposite to entrance of ductus arteriosus when there is abnormal flow through the ductus. In order of frequency

the cardiac defects associated with coarctation of aorta are PDA, VSD, complete TGV, bicuspid aortic valve, mitral valve disease and aortic stenosis.

Onset of CCF in newborn is on seventh day. Main sign is absent or faint pulses in legs as compared to arms. Small pressure difference between legs and arms indicate that either a large VSD or PDA is present. Large pressure difference with hypertension in arms indicates an intact ventricular septum. In presence of PDA femoral pulse may change in quality from hour to hour depending upon degree of patency of ductus arteriosus. On auscultation gallop rhythm may be present. There may be no murmur or there may be systolic murmur of VSD or atrioventricular valvular regurgitation. In chest X-ray there is cardiomegaly, pulmonary congestion and increased flow in presence of left to right shunt. An enlarged left atrium is common. In cases of associated defects ECG always shows right ventricle hypertrophy. Echocardiogram shows enlarged right ventricle and left atrium. Cardiac catheterization is important to determine associated malformations. Resection of coarctation of aorta, ligation of ductus and banding of pulmonary artery for control of VSD are necessary when the three defects are present. For patients with aortic stenosis preliminary resection of coarctation will be needed.

D. Congestive Cardiac Failure in one to four Weeks of Life

There are two major malformations:

1. *VSD*: In first month of life in those with isolated VSD, CCF occurs on average at 15 days of life. As pulmonary vascular resistance is still elevated due to increased pulmonary blood flow, physical signs are modified. Systolic murmur is short of pansystolic and pulmonary second sound is accentuated. Mid diastolic murmur is not present usually. In ECG only right ventricle hypertrophy may be present. Cardiac catheterization is essential. If on angiocardiographic measurement of a clearly delineated defect the diameter is greater than 3/4 of diameter of aortic root, most cases will require surgical treatment early.

2. *PDA*: Ransient continuous murmur can be detected in 15% of term newborn infants up to the age of 12 hours. Spontaneous closure of PDA may occur in term infant up to 3rd month of life. Surgery will be required thereafter. Onset of CCF averaged 20 days in term infants and 29 days in those with respiratory distress syndrome.

Typically the patient with PDA has continuous murmur or an abbreviated murmur of left to right shunt. A minority have atypical murmur which may be indication of very large or very small PDA. An associated bounding pulse in all limbs is an important sign. Chest X-ray shows an enlarged heart, plethoric lung fields and left atrium and left ventricle enlargement. Biventricular and left atrial hypertrophy will be present in patient with CCF. Echocardiographic assessment of left atrial size in these patients has been a reliable guide to size of shunt across the PDA. Medical treatment of heart failure is indicated initially. In term infant late spontaneous closure may occur but after 3 months surgery is indicated if substantial flow remains. Closure of PDA with prostaglandin antagonists, indomethacin, brufen or aspirin holds promise.

Aortic Valve Stenosis

Infants with less severe obstruction appear normal at birth. Typical precordial thrill of aortic stenosis is uncommon in newborn. Right ventricle thrust is usual sign rather than left ventricle impulse. Weak pulses are present in severely obstructed patients. Ejection systolic murmur best heard in second right intercostal space may in low output states is soft or absent or located in left sternal edge. Second heart sound is closely split though the aortic element may be absent. Chest X-ray in CCF will show cardiomegaly and venous congestion with enlargement of left atrium. In severely affected neonate ECG will show right ventricle hypertrophy. ST segment and T-wave abnormalities are common. After initial treatment of CCF diagnostic catheterization and angiocardiography should be carried out. Attempts at surgical correction should be made provided contracted endocardial fibroelastosis can be ruled out.

Truncus Arteriosus

Often there may be no cyanosis. Bounding pulses, ejection click, single second heart sound and early diastolic murmur are characteristic. Very early presentation can occur with gross truncal valve regurgitation or when interrupted arch is associated. A typical feature on chest X-ray apart from cardiomegaly and plethora is the anterior shelf seen in lateral projection because of absence of bulge of main pulmonary artery. Right aortic arch is common. Cardiac catheterization and cineangiography will determine anatomy and type of pulmonary artery branching. Surgical treatment of choice is palliative pulmonary artery banding until the age till reconstruction of outflow tract of right ventricle can be done.

ARRHYTHMIAS

In normal newborn autonomic nervous control may not be fully developed. Holter (constant multi hour rhythm monitoring) ECG recordings have demonstrated that rapid changes in heart rate may occur changing from sinus tachycardia to bradycardia. This varying heart rate with physiological mechanisms is exaggerated and occurs in a large percentage of cases in premature infants.

1. *Congenital supraventricular tachycardia*: Varying presentations, such as cyanosis, CCF, ascitis or edema and hypoglycemia. congenital atrial tachycardia may occur in association with heart defect, such as ASD, ebstein anomaly, TGV, coarctation of aorta, endocardial fibroelastosis. Some show WPW syndrome in ECG. Digoxin is drug of choice adding early cardioversion if there is not a prompt response. Fetal ECG may be more useful in diagnosing cases in future.

2. *Congenital heart block*: Uncommon in newborn. Some cases are familial. Most are due to prenatal disturbances, such as infection. Some congenital malformations are associated with slow heart rate. CCF occurs when heart rate is less than 30–50 per minute. Adam Stokes attack may occur. Even without a heart defect an aortic ejection systolic murmur or apical mid diastolic murmur may be heard. Diagnosis is by ECG.

No treatment is indicated for asymptomatic newborn. Isoproterenol is used when symptomatic pending intravenous temporary pacemaker insertion. Permanent pacing may be necessary.

Myocarditis

Coxsackie B virus and rubella syndrome. Pathologically necrosis and destruction of muscle fibers is present with round cell infiltration. Clinically infant refuses feeds and becomes irritable. Associated fever, cyanosis, gallop rhythm and hepatomegaly appear. Heart enlarges with increasing severity. ECG shows low QRS complexes with flat or inverted T-waves and depressed ST segment. Diagnosis is by recovery of virus from blood, urine, stool, throat with demonstration of rising neutralizing antibodies titre against virus. Treatment is digitalis, diuretics and oxygen. Prognosis is guarded.

Anemia

CCF with volume overload *in utero* can occur with severe anemia of hemolytic disease.

Tumors

Rare. Rhabdomyoma and mesenchymal tumors of apex are detected in neonatal period. Diagnosis is by echocardiography and nuclide study.

Management

A. Cyanotic heart disease:
  1. *TGV*: In absence of heart murmur exclusion of other causes of cyanosis in neonate particularly pulmonary and neurological causes is essential. Hyperoxic test is most useful. Since sudden deterioration may occur with hypoxia leading to acidosis early and urgent diagnosis by non invasive methods as well as by cardiac catheterization is essential. Ballon septostomy is the safest initial technique to create an adequate communication between two circulation. When response to ballon septostomy is poor other palliative surgical procedures

should be done. When these fail serious consideration to placement of an atrial baffle should be given.

2. *Pulmonary valve atresia and tricuspid valve atresia with pulmonary stenosis*: Neonate with normal or near normal right ventricle chamber size will require a valvotomy only. A combination of procedures including ballon atrial septostomy, ligation of PDA, systemic to pulmonary shunt (usually Potts) increases survival rate. In those patients with closing PDA which is main source of natural systemic artery to pulmonary artery shunt, use of prostaglandins to promote dilatation of this channel while awaiting surgery has met with success. With tricuspid valve atresia and pulmonary stenosis initial palliative surgical treatment of choice has been aortopulmonary artery shunt.

B. Congestive heart failure:
   1. *Digitalis*: Digitalizing digoxin dose:
      • Premature infant: 0.03 mg.
      • Newborn to 2 years: 0.05 mg.
      • Maintenance dose:
      • Premature: 0.003 mg.
      • Newborn to 2 years: 0.005 mg.
      Total digitalizing dose is divided into three parts:
      • First is given stat.
      • Second after 6 hours.
      • Third after 8 hours of second dose.
      • Maintenance dose is started 12 hours later.
      • ECG monitoring should be done to watch for toxicity.
   2. *Diuretics*: In neonate saluretics are drug of choice. Furosemide has less ototoxicity. Adverse effects are hypovolemia, hypokalemia and hyponatremia. Aldecton may be used in conjunction with lasix. Sodium restriction is not employed.
   3. *Treatment of cause of CCF*: Many congenital malformations require surgery whether palliative or curative, e.g. ligation of large PDA, AV fistula, resection of coarctation

of aorta, relieving aortic or pulmonary valve stenosis, creation of ASD in D TGV with intact ventricular septum.

Prognosis

That stage of the course of serious congenital heart malformation when it is appreciated that baby is abnormal is obviously a very important element in future outlook for that individual. Early detection is thus pre-eminent consideration of those concerned with reducing infant mortality from congenital heart disease. Although the data that come do not guarantee successful end result it surely gives best chance for such outcome by allowing measured assessment and opportunity for precise diagnosis before patient's condition deteriorates.

53

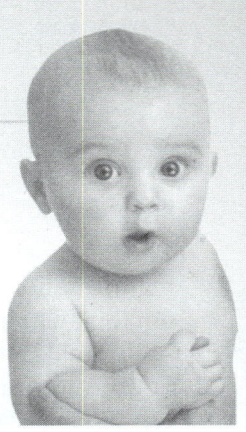

Sudden Infant Death Syndrome

Incidence of sudden infant death syndrome (SIDS) varies from 1.4 to 3/1000 live births.

General Causes

In newborn period weak immature babies may die suddenly owing to their prematurity alone. Death may result from aspiration of vomitus, congenital defects of diaphragm, lungs, gastrointestinal tract, heart and central nervous system. Hyperadrenalism or hypoadrenalism is rare cause.

Syndrome of SIDS has peak age incidence at 2–3 months. Preponderance in males, low birth weight babies and lower socioeconomic group of families. Nearly all infants die during sleep in silent fashion during early morning. Infection plays a vital role but several factors are involved:

1. Magnesium deprivation in rapidly growing infant may occur particularly in a mother who has diet poor in magnesium.
2. Infant who is found dead lying face down may have had a vasovagal effect on raising head particularly one who is recovering from infection.

Cardiac Causes

- Acute myocarditis.
- Endocardial fibroelastosis.
- Congenital pulmonary stenosis.
- Congenital aortic stenosis.

- Paroxysmal tachycardia.
- Congenital heart block.
- Stokes-Adams attack.
- Bacterial endocarditis.
- Cerebral embolism.
- Ventricular fibrillation.
- Pulmonary embolism.
  Drugs: digoxin. Potassium.

In congenital pulmonary stenosis minor events, such as breath holding, vomiting or minor infection in first year of life may precipitate SIDS.

In hypoxia myocardium is more sensitive to digoxin.

Fibrillation may occur in hypokalemia.

Potassium chloride administration may cause heart block.

Four Main Groups of SIDS

1. *Left ventricular outflow tract obstruction*: Aortic valve stenosis or discrete subvalvular stenosis. 1% of cases.
   ECG shows left ventricular hypertrophy or strain.
   Idiopathic hypertrophic muscular obstruction. 17% of cases.
2. *Pulmonary valve disease*: Primary pulmonary hypertension, increased pulmonary vascular resistance in association with VSD.
3. *Heart block*: During surgical repair of VSD, procedure may damage left anterior fascicle of left bundle branch giving rise to left anterior hemiblock that has characteristic pattern with swing of axis from positive to negative usually – 60°. Failure of pacemaker can cause sudden death.
4. *TGA*: After Mustard procedure.
5. *Anomalous coronary artery*: Left artery arising from right sinus of Valsalva in association with right coronary artery. From this origin it passes anteriorly between aorta and main pulmonary artery before dividing into two branches. The vessels can get narrowed at a point where it passes between two great arteries.

Anomalous coronary artery arising from pulmonary artery causes ECG features of myocardial infarction.

Prevention

In case of aortic stenosis it is important to know degree of narrowing. Patients should be restricted in activity.

In Eisenmenger syndrome identify the cause that may lead to pulmonary vascular disease in early life and correct them surgically before the damage has been done to pulmonary branches.

Pacemaker will prevent Stokes-adams attack in congenital heart block.

Conditions amenable to surgery are Ebstein anomay, aortic valve deformity in Marfan's syndrome and accessory conduction tissue of WPW and related syndrome.

Mitral valve replacement in relief of refractory ventricular arrhythmia associated with mitral valve prolapse should be considered.

54

Physical Growth in Children with Congenital Heart Disease

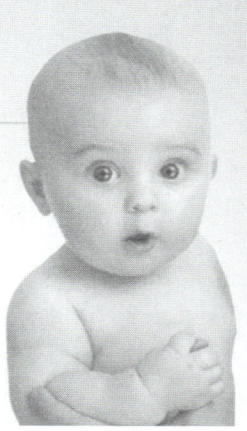

Children with severe congenital heart disease have inadequate growth of height or weight or both. When such children are operated upon successfully they are likely to have an increase in weight and height. Greatest acceleration is seen in children who had their operation early in life. Growth retardation is more marked in boys than girls. There is a greater lag in weight than in height.

Problem of nutrition in CHD is a specialized one particularly in infants who are deeply cyanosed and those with large shunts with or without heart failure.

Growth retardation of some degree is commonly noted these children.

Altered growth pattern may be due to chronic hypoxia, repeated respiratory infection, inadequate calories, etc. such infants may be in a hypermetabolic state.

If infant has a large shunt or is cyanotic feeding becomes complicated. Some babies with large shunt appear to loose fluid through skin excessively and need replacement of such loss. Diet should contain high calorie density with adequate fluid intake.

In small babies frequent small feeds may add to total daily intake in calories and thus nourish infant. Occasionally tube feeding may be resorted to. If baby is anemia iron therapy is indicted.

In care of babies with severe cyanosis or those with large intracardiac shunts a number of parameters should be monitored. Daily weight, weekly length, daily urine output, osmolality, blood urea and skin turgor. If diuretics are being given serum sodium and potassium should be determined three times a week.

A feeding problem often evaporates after successful correction of cardiac lesion by surgery.

55

Cerebral Complications in Congenital Heart Disease

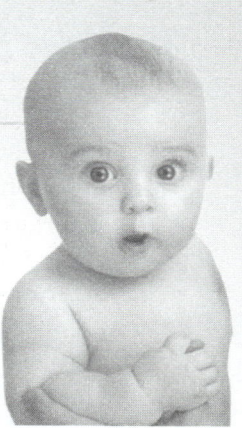

Many pathological changes may be found in children with congenital heart disease. These include venous congestion, petechial hemorrhages, inflammatory reactions, focal necrosis and encephalomalacia, patchy demyelination, vascular occlusions and cerebral abscess.

Clinical Classification

1. Hypoxic episodes with or without loss of consciousness or convulsions. Brief blue spells or apneic episodes with or without evident loss of consciousness or convulsions may be seen in child with congenital cyanotic heart disease related to low arterial oxygen content and precipitated by febrile illness or by other more obscure factors. Most such spells occur under 2-year age group. Severe or repeated hypoxic damage will cause convulsions and hence need for anticonvulsant medication. Hypoxic attacks are treated with oxygen, correction of anemia and where possible cardiac surgery.

2. *Cerebrovascular accidents*: Incidence is 3.8% of congenital heart disease. Majority of children are under 2-year. 70% children below 4-year. Accidents are associated with anemia and hypoxia but in older children association is with polycythemia and hypoxemia. Tetralogy of Fallot and transposition of great vessels account for 90% of all patients.

   Pathologically there are areas of infarction related to arterial or venous occlusion.

Prognosis is better with older children but sequaele are common and include hemiplegia, convulsions and mental retardation.

Diagnosis lies in exclusion of cerebral abscess and bacterial endocarditis and the age range (younger patients) is useful in this respect. Investigations, such as CT scan, radionuclide brain scan, EEG, blood culture and progression of clinical picture are useful.

Treatment is symptomatic. Preventive measures include early correction of relative anemia and early corrective surgery.

3. *Cerebral abscess*: When brain abscess is considered from all causes about 10% have an associated congenital heart lesion. In childhood years cyanotic congenital heart disease remains single common correlate with brain abscess formation.

Brain abscess with congenital heart disease is rare under age of 2 years. Half the cases occur between age 3 and 10 years. Brain abscess is rarely associated with bacterial endocarditis. Development of abscess may be preceded by recognized infection, such as otitis, pharyngitis, dental infection.

Onset is insidious. Headache, vomiting and convulsions with focal neurological signs are present while signs of infection, such as leukocytosis, increased ESR, fever may be minimal or absent. Signs of increased intracranial tension as papilledema, split sutures on X-ray skull, bradycardia are late features and indicate abscess of considerable size and duration. In presence of cyanotic congenital heart disease in child over 2 years age any cerebral symptoms or signs should be considered to indicate an abscess until proved otherwise.

Noninvasive investigations, e.g. CT scan, radionuclide scan, EEG are useful. Information may be supplemented by cerebral angiography. In suspected cases lumbar puncture should not be performed.

Very rare posterior fossa or brainstem abscess is difficult to diagnose clinically.

With rare excepts cerebral abscess is found in cyanotic congenital heart disease with right to left shunt. TOF and TGV providing most of patients. 2.8% of TOF and DORV, 1.9% of complete AV canal, 1.3% of tricuspid atresia and 1% of dextro transposition.

Abscess may occur in any part of brain but very rarely in posterior fossa or brainstem.

Culture of organisms involved in abscess formation show great variety of bacteria both aerobic and anaerobic.

Two conditions are prerequisite for abscess formation:

1. Intermittent bacteriemia.
2. Focal encephalomalacia.

Because of presence of right to left shunt there is an absence of normal phagocytic filtering action of pulmonary vascular bed so that transient bacteriemia may result in infection reaching brain. Focal encephalomalacia is increased by hypoxia and decreased cerebral blood flow.

Infection may also reach brain by direct extension from ears and sinuses.

Mortality and morbidity in brain abscess are inversely related to oxygen saturation levels. High blood viscosity may also play a part by decreasing blood flow and predisposing to arterial and venous occlusion.

Treatment: It is an axiom that any child with cyanotic congenital heart disease with cerebral symptoms has brain abscess until proven otherwise especially if child is over two year age. Once diagnosis is made treatment is neurosurgical and generally repeated aspirations will be satisfactory. Use of antibiotic is routine but value is uncertain once abscess formation is begun. Prognosis is better with early diagnosis depending upon cardiac condition but 50% of survivors have some neurological sequelae.

Prevention: In view of etiological factors involved—age, right to left shunt, hypoxia, decreased cerebral blood flow it might be expected that corrective surgery in first two years of life will reduce incidence of brain abscess in future life.

56

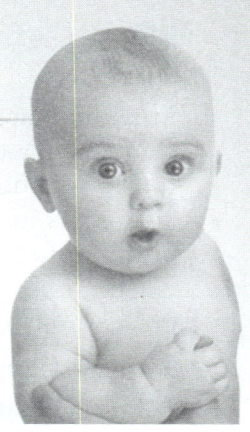

Infective Endocarditis

IN INFANTS UNDER 2 YEARS AGE

- Acute infection superimposed on one or more heart valves.
  - Incidence 0.8%.
- Mitral valve is more frequently involved and pulmonary valve least.
  - Organisms are streptococcus, *staphyllococcus, pneumococcus, gonococcus* and mycobacteria.
  - Incidence in congenital heart disease is 8%.
  - Large proportion is in first week or month of life.

Clinical picture is of acute infection and progressively severe illness. In large proportion there is evidence of sepsis elsewhere in body, e.g. skin, pneumonia, enteritis, empyema, osteomyelitis, tuberculosis. Spleen is palpable in few cases and embolic phenomenon rare. Tachycardia is usually out of proportion to fever. In few there is precordial murmur which appears as disease progresses.

In children Over two Years Age

Organisms: *Streptococcus viridans, nonhemolytic streptococci including enterococcus, staphyllococcus pyogenes, staphyllococcus albus, hemolytic streptococci, diplococcus pneumoni, E coli, pseudomonas, haemophillus influenzae, klebsiella.*

There is preceding history of congenital or rheumatic heart disease. Infection of teeth, tonsils and glands are predisposing factors.

Disease spectrum has altered since introduction of cardiac surgery and hemodynamics, hemodialysis and intravenous narcotics.

Clinical Features

Staphyllococcal disease is suspected when there is high septic type of fever rising to 104°F in early stage of illness. High leukocyte count of 15–20 thousand is also suggestive. Duration of illness varies from 3 days to 3 weeks.

Signs of infection are less serious in streptococcus viridans. Fever is not high. Insidious onset with loss of appetite and pallor are common. Anemia is not marked. Clubbing and splenomegaly may be present. Petechae may be seen and obvious embolism uncommon. Osler nodes are tiny red raised nodules seen at tip of finger and toes.

Hematuria should be looked for as possible embolic phenomenon. Mouth should be examined for infected gums or alveolar abscess. Sinus X-ray film may be indicated. Echocardiography identifies vegetations on cardiac valves.

Diagnosis

Recognition of infective endocarditis is most important factor influencing survival. Diagnosis is based on presence of an underlying heart lesion accompanied by fever lasting for few days to few weeks with evidence of embolic phenomenon, palpable spleen and positive blood culture.

Predisposing events may lead to diagnosis, such as recent tooth extraction, paronychia and impetigo. Exposure to rats may cause spirillum or streptobacillus moniliformis and cat bite to pasturella infection. An operation involving intestinal tract may cause *E coli* or streptofecalis infection. Association with recent heart surgery is more common. When diagnosis of infective endocarditis is suspected a series of blood cultures is taken at beginning of fever, 15–30 minutes apart, can be repeated in 24 hours. Routine broth media are ordinarily used. Special media permit growth of fastidious organisms. Blood culture may be taken from bone marrow, urine and arterial blood.

Echocardiogram demonstrates shaggy or fuzzy echoes resulting from vegetations that have a distinct appearance.

PROPHYLAXIS

A significant number of cases follow a tooth extraction in an individual who has congenital or rheumatic heart disease. Removal of tonsils and adenoids, antepartum and postpartum manipulations, diagnostic procedures, such as cardiac catheterization have been implicated.

Incidence of positive blood culture after dental extraction varies between 16 and 17%.

Risk of bacterial endocarditis following a tooth extraction in a patient with congenital heart disease or rheumatic heart disease is 1 in 533.

These children should be given prophylaxis before tooth extraction as follows:

1. *Prophylaxis for dental procedures, tonsillectomy, adenoidectomy, bronchoscopy*: Penicillin intramuscular one hour prior to procedure and once daily for two days following the procedure.

   For patients allergic to penicillin or resistant to penicillin erythromycin 20 mg/kg two hours prior to procedure followed by 10 mg/kg/6 hours for remainder of the day and for two days following the procedure.

2. *Prophylaxis for genitourinary and gastrointestinal tract surgery over infected tissues*: Penicillin intramuscular one hour prior to procedure and once daily for two days following procedure and amikacin one hour prior to procedure and then once daily for two days following the procedure.

   For patients with penicillin allergy vancomycin intravenously every 6 hourly for that day and next two days.

   Lincomycin 250 mg orally can be used four times a day for older children and 40 mg/kg/day in three divided doses for younger children. It may be given on day of procedure and the following day.

3. *Prophylaxis in relation to catheterization of heart and heart surgery:*
Predisposing factors are underlying heart lesion, cardiac
surgery open or closed, cardiac catheterization, use of
polyvenyle or polyethylene intravenous catheters, drug
administration or addiction, debilitating disease, prolonged
steroid administration and bone marrow depression.

Prophylactic vancomycin and third generation
cehalosporins are used.